Attention Deficit Hyperactivity Disorder

Attention Deficit Hyperactivity Disorder

Adult Outcome and Its Predictors

EDITED BY LILY HECHTMAN, MD, FRCP, ABPN

PROFESSOR OF PSYCHIATRY AND PEDIATRICS
DIRECTOR OF RESEARCH
DIVISION OF CHILD PSYCHIATRY
MCGILL UNIVERSITY HEALTH CENTRE
MONTREAL CHILDREN'S HOSPITAL

OXFORD
UNIVERSITY PRESS

OXFORD
UNIVERSITY PRESS

Oxford University Press is a department of the University of Oxford. It furthers the University's objective of excellence in research, scholarship, and education by publishing worldwide. Oxford is a registered trade mark of Oxford University Press in the UK and certain other countries.

Published in the United States of America by Oxford University Press
198 Madison Avenue, New York, NY 10016, United States of America.

Library of Congress Cataloging-in-Publication Data
Names: Hechtman, Lily Trokenberg, editor.
Title: Attention deficit hyperactivity disorder : adult outcome and its predictors / edited by Lily Hechtman.
Other titles: Attention deficit hyperactivity disorder (Hechtman)
Description: Oxford ; New York : Oxford University Press, [2017] |
Includes bibliographical references.
Identifiers: LCCN 2016014436 | ISBN 9780190213589 (pbk.)
Subjects: | MESH: Attention Deficit Disorder with Hyperactivity | Adult |
Treatment Outcome | Longitudinal Studies | Case Reports
Classification: LCC RC394.A85 | NLM WM 165 | DDC 616.85/89—dc23
LC record available at http://lccn.loc.gov/2016014436

I would like to dedicate this book to my inspiring mentor Dr. Gabrielle Weiss who started me on this exciting journey, my wonderful supportive colleagues who contributed chapters and with whom it is a pleasure to work, and our patients who share their courageous struggles and teach us so much.

Finally, this book and much of my career would not be possible without the encouragement, humour, and support of my husband Peter, who usually sees the glass as half-full.

CONTENTS

CONTRIBUTORS

Russell A. Barkley, PhD
Clinical Professor of Psychiatry
Medical University
of South Carolina
Charleston, South Carolina

Joseph Biederman, MD
Chief, Clinical and Research
Programs in Pediatric
Psychopharmacology and
Adult ADHD
Director, Bressler Program for
Autism Spectrum Disorders
Massachusetts General Hospital
Professor of Psychiatry
Harvard Medical School
Boston, Massachusetts

Mariya V. Cherkasova, PhD
University of British Columbia
Vancouver, British
Columbia, Canada

Mariellen Fischer, PhD
Associated Mental Health
Consultants
Milwaukee, Wisconsin

Lily Hechtman, MD, FRCP, ABPN
Professor of Psychiatry and
Pediatrics
Director of Research
Division of Child Psychiatry
Montreal Children's Hospital
McGill University Health Centre
Montréal, Québec, Canada

Stephen P. Hinshaw, PhD
Professor of Psychology, University
of California, Berkeley
Berkeley, California
Professor of Psychiatry, University
of California, San Francisco
San Francisco, California

Sylviane Houssais, MA
McGill University Health Centre
Montréal, Québec, Canada

Rachel G. Klein, PhD
New York University School of Medicine
New York, New York

Brooke S. G. Molina, PhD
Professor of Psychiatry and Psychology
University of Pittsburgh
Pittsburgh, Pennsylvania

Elizabeth B. Owens, PhD
Institute of Human Development
University of California, Berkeley
Berkeley, California

Sarah L. Pedersen, PhD
Department of Psychiatry
University of Pittsburgh
Pittsburgh, Pennsylvania

William E. Pelham, Jr., PhD
Department of Psychology
Center for Children and Families
Florida International University
Miami, Florida

Arunima Roy, MBBS
McGill University Health Centre
Montréal, Québec, Canada

Margaret H. Sibley, PhD
Florida International University
Department of Psychiatry and Behavioral Health
Center for Children and Families
Miami, Florida

Mai Uchida, MD
Psychiatry Department
Massachusetts General Hospital
Harvard Medical School
Boston, Massachusetts

Gabrielle Weiss, MD
Former Professor of Psychiatry (Retired)
McGill University
Montréal, Québec, Canada
University of British Columbia
Vancouver, British Columbia, Canada

Christine A. Zalecki, PhD
University of California, San Francisco
Children's Center at Langley Porter
San Francisco, California
University of California, Berkeley
Institute of Human Development
Berkeley, California

1

Introduction

LILY HECHTMAN

A good deal of interest and controversy currently exist regarding the high rate of diagnosis of Attention Deficit Hyperactivity Disorder (ADHD). Some reports by specialists in the field and in the media have suggested that ADHD is overdiagnosed and thus overtreated. This sentiment is particularly true for ADHD in adulthood. In fact, there is some skepticism regarding the existence of ADHD in adults, given that early on it was believed that children outgrew this condition as the hyperactivity and impulsivity tended to decrease with age.

However, well-controlled prospective follow-up studies (which will be reviewed in this book) first showed that symptoms of ADHD, particularly symptoms of inattention, continued into adulthood and caused significant functional and clinical impairment, thus laying the groundwork for the diagnosis of ADHD in adulthood. These prospective follow-up studies have appeared in the literature intermittently over the last 20 to 30 years and, therefore, did not have the impact they deserved in helping establish the validity of the diagnosis in adulthood. No other publication to date brings together in one place these various well-controlled prospective follow-up studies, which show that more than half of the children with ADHD continue to have significant symptoms and impairment in adulthood.

This book thus addresses an important controversy—namely the validity of an ADHD diagnosis in adults, which is of great interest currently. The fifth edition of the *Diagnostic and Statistical Manual of Mental Disorders* (DSM-5) has contributed to the support of this diagnosis, not only by providing an Adult ADHD diagnostic category but also recognizing that the symptom criteria requiring six out of nine symptoms in either the Inattentive or Hyperactive–Impulsive symptom category was not appropriate for adults because it required adults to score above the 99th percentile whereas most conditions require scores above the 93rd percentile. DSM-5 thus lowered the symptom criteria to five out of nine symptoms for anyone over the age of 17 years. This modification in symptom criteria for adults clearly recognized the presence of ADHD in adulthood and does much to validate the diagnosis in this age group.

These studies also show, however, that not all children with ADHD go on to have the symptoms and impairment in adulthood. Professionals; researchers; pediatricians; child, adolescent, and adult psychiatrists; family physicians; psychologists; social workers; and teachers frequently are asked about the prognosis of this condition. Will the child always be impaired? Will he grow up to be a delinquent or addict? Will he be able to complete school? Go on to university? These studies provide a comprehensive view of the prognosis of this condition—a view that professionals cannot obtain elsewhere.

Finally, what factors may influence long-term outcome and prognosis? Identifying such prognostic factors is critical because this has current treatment implications if more positive outcomes are sought. Again, professionals (outlined above) will be able to access these relevant factors in one place and use them in their treatment planning.

At this point in time no other book brings all these diverse studies together and provides a sound basis for the diagnosis of ADHD in adulthood. These chapters offer a clear view of possible outcomes and prognosis, which professionals require to address patient concerns adequately, along with evidence of factors that may influence prognosis and outcome, all of which professionals can use in treatment planning.

The book reviews current data from a number of prospective controlled follow-up studies that have traced the outcomes of children diagnosed with ADHD into adolescence and adulthood. Outcomes explored include continuation of ADHD symptoms and diagnosis; comorbidities (e.g., anxiety, depression, and substance abuse); and social, academic, and emotional functioning. These outcomes are compared with matched control groups.

In addition, potential predictors of outcomes are explored. These predictors may be related to the characteristics of the child (e.g., IQ, severity of initial ADHD symptoms, initial comorbidity), characteristics of the family (e.g., socioeconomic status [SES], single parenthood, parental pathology, family functioning), and/or treatment (e.g., medication and psychosocial treatments).

These factors and their interactions are explored with regard to their impact on long-term adult outcome. Potential interventions that may affect these predictive factors and thus result in more positive long-term outcomes also are explored. The book provides professionals, parents, and the general public with a view of the possible long-term outcomes of ADHD, what factors influence these outcomes, and potential interventions that may positively impact these factors and thus result in better long-term functioning.

This edited book consists of chapters by the leading researchers in the field of ADHD and describes well-controlled prospective follow-up studies of children with ADHD into adolescence and adulthood. These studies and authors include:

- The Montreal Study (mean age at follow-up, 26 years), conducted by Dr. Gabrielle Weiss and Dr. Lily Hechtman (authors: Dr. Mariya Cherkasova, Dr. Gabrielle Weiss, and Dr. Lily Hechtman)
- The New York Study (mean age at follow-up, 41 years), conducted by Dr. Rachel Klein and Dr. Salvatore Mannuzza (authors: Sylviane Houssais, MA, Dr. Lily Hechtman, and Dr. Rachel G. Klein)

- The Milwaukee Study (mean age at follow-up, 27 years), conducted by Dr. Russell A. Barkley, Dr. Kevin R. Murphy, and Dr. Mariellen Fischer (authors: Dr. Russell A. Barkley and Dr. Mariellen Fischer)
- The Pittsburgh Study (mean age at follow-up, 22 years), conducted by Dr. William E. Pelham, Jr. and Dr. Brooke S. G. Molina (authors: Dr. Brooke S. G. Molina, Dr. Margaret H. Sibley, Dr. Sarah L. Pedersen, and Dr. William E Pelham, Jr.)
- The Massachusetts General Hospital Study (mean age at follow-up, 21 years), conducted by Dr. Joseph Biederman (authors: Dr. Mai Uchida and Dr. Joseph Biederman)
- The Berkeley Girls Study (mean age at follow-up, 20 years), conducted by Dr. Stephen P. Hinshaw and Dr. Elizabeth Owens (authors: Dr. Elizabeth Owens, Dr. Christine Zalecki, and Dr. Stephen P. Hinshaw)
- The Multisite Multimodal Treatment of ADHD Study (MTA) (mean age at follow-up, 24 years), conducted by the MTA Cooperative Group at seven sites (authors: Dr. Arunima Roy and Dr. Lily Hechtman).

2

Adolescent and Adult Outcomes of Childhood Attention Deficit Hyperactivity Disorder

The Montreal Study

MARIYA V. CHERKASOVA, GABRIELLE WEISS, AND LILY HECHTMAN

INTRODUCTION

Attention deficit hyperactivity disorder (ADHD) has been historically conceptualized as a disorder of childhood. Several decades ago, clinicians believed that children outgrew this condition as they entered adolescence (Bakwin & Bakwin, 1966). The developmental course of ADHD was thought to resemble that of disorders such as specific language impairment, where a child's command of language is developmentally inadequate early in life, but typically reaches normative levels later on. Long-term prospective follow-up studies of children with ADHD have challenged that assumption, however, and clearly demonstrated that many, though not all of these children continue to have significant symptoms and impaired functioning as adolescents and adults. Currently, adult ADHD is a well-accepted diagnosis, with epidemiological studies suggesting prevalence estimates of about 4% (Faraone, Sergeant, Gillberg, & Biederman, 2003; Kessler et al., 2006)—approximately half the prevalence of ADHD in childhood. Besides demonstrating persistence of ADHD beyond the childhood years, prospective follow-up studies have provided a wealth of information on the evolution of ADHD across the life span in terms of both presentation and associated impairments. These studies also have highlighted the individual developmental variability in ADHD: As we will see, some children do indeed appear to outgrow ADHD and attain essentially unimpaired functioning, while others continue to have impairing symptoms and function poorly in a number of life domains. Although questions still remain regarding the determinants of such developmental variability, data from prospective follow-up studies have helped identify some predictors of developmental course and outcome.

The first prospective follow-up studies of children with ADHD, which challenged the notion of ADHD being a childhood-only disorder, were conducted by a group of researchers at the Montreal Children's Hospital.

METHODOLOGY

The Montreal group studied 104 hyperactive children, ages 6 to 13 years, referred to the psychiatric outpatient clinic of the Montreal Children's Hospital. The children were initially enrolled between 1961 and 1965. They were followed and evaluated in 5-year intervals over the subsequent 15 years (5-year, 10-year, and 15-year follow-up; see Figure 2.1). In order to be eligible, sustained hyperactivity reported by both parents and teachers needed to be the primary complaint. Other eligibility criteria included normal intelligence (IQ > 85), absence of neurological disease (e.g., epilepsy, cerebral palsy) and psychosis, and living arrangement at home with

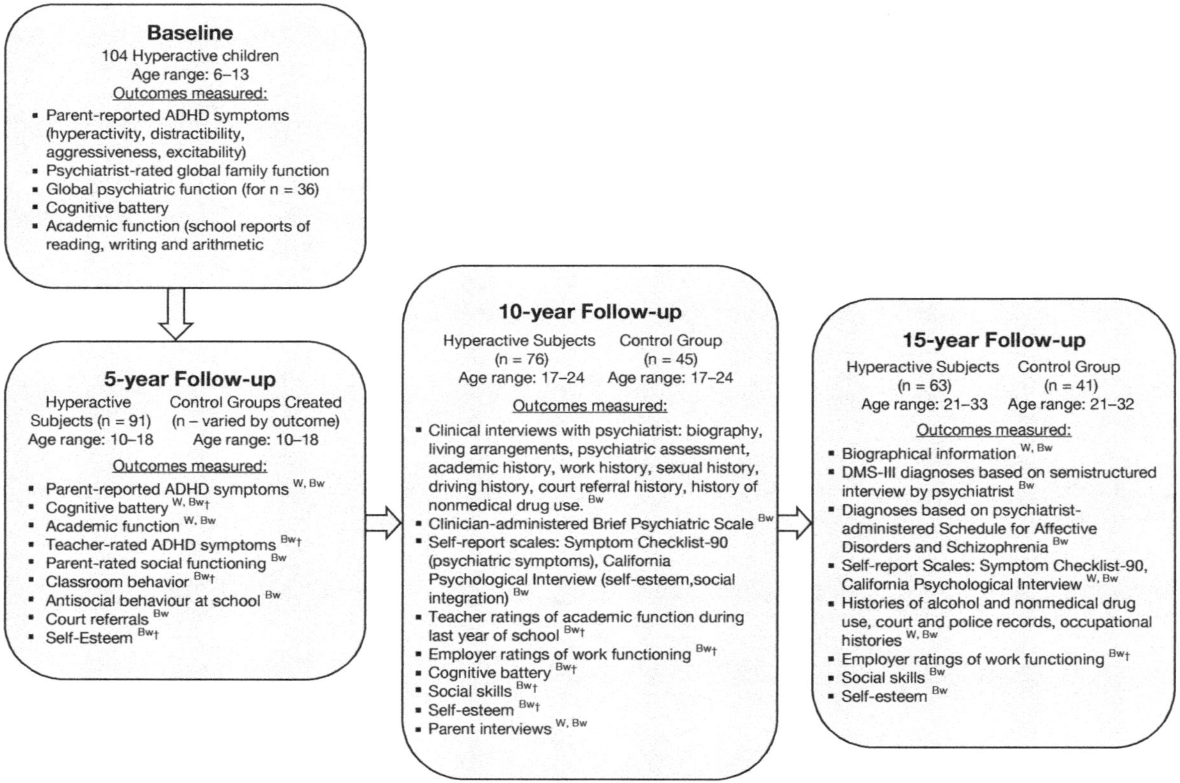

Figure 2.1 Flow of hyperactive probands and controls through the 15-year follow-up and outcomes evaluated at each point. W = an outcome was compared to baseline functioning or an earlier assessment point for the same subjects (within-group longitudinal analysis). Bw = probands' outcome was compared to that in a group of matched controls (between group cross-sectional analysis). † = outcome evaluated in a smaller subsample.

at least one parent. These children participated in acute drug studies of chlorpromazine and dextroamphetamine at the onset of follow-up but subsequently received no sustained pharmacological treatment. Some children, however, were intermittently medicated at various points. The initial baseline evaluations included measures of:

1) Parent-reported ADHD-like symptoms: hyperactivity, distractibility, aggressiveness, and excitability, assessed via the Werry-Weiss-Peters scale locally designed by the study group (Werry, 1968).
2) Global psychiatric function via the Peterson-Quay Checklist (Peterson & Quay, 1967), for a subsample of 36 of the subjects, starting in 1964.
3) Psychiatrist-rated global family functioning, including parental marital relationship, child-rearing practices, maternal deprivation, mother-child relationship, mental health of the family members, socioeconomic status, with each facet scored on a scale, and scores summed up of a global rating.
4) Neurological status (including electroencephalogram [EEG], neurological exam, and medical history).
5) Battery of cognitive and motor tests: Wechsler Intelligence Scale for Children (1949); Bender Visual-Motor Gestalt Test (Bender, 1938); Good-Enough Draw-a-Man Test (Harris, 1963); Lincoln-Oseretsky Motor Development Scale (Sloan, 1955).
6) School reports of reading, writing, and arithmetic.

Note that the *Diagnostic and Statistical Manual of Mental Disorders–III* (DSM-III) was not in use at the time, and the only formal diagnostic criteria for the syndrome were the DSM-II criteria for Hyperkinetic Reaction of Childhood, which were rather nonspecific; hence, the reliance on the locally custom-designed scale to assess the relevant symptoms. Based on the impression of the authors, however, who have worked clinically with children with ADHD over a number of decades with evolving diagnostic criteria, the subjects would have met the current criteria for ADHD combined subtype, with many also having associated conduct problems.

At the 5-year follow-up 91 probands were re-evaluated; subjects lost to follow-up did not significantly differ from those retained on any of the baseline characteristics. Probands' ages at the 5-year point were 11 to 18 years (mean age 13.4 years), and 89% of the sample were boys. An initial follow-up evaluation of the majority of this sample (n = 64; 92% boys; age range 11–18, M = 13.34) focused on the above and several additional outcomes: teacher-rated hyperactivity, distractibility, aggressiveness, and antisocial behavior at school, court referrals, and parent-rated social functioning (Weiss, Minde, Werry, Douglas, & Nemeth, 1971). In addition, self-esteem was examined in a subsample of 15 probands using Davidson and Lang (Davidson & Lang, 1960) and a modified Ziller Self-Other (Ziller, Hagey, Smith, & Long, 1969) tests. Because there was no healthy nonhyperactive control group at baseline and not all 5-year outcomes had been evaluated at baseline, matched healthy control groups were created at the time of the 5-year follow-up by recruiting the probands' classmates. Control subjects were required to have IQs > 85 and no significant problems academically or behaviorally at school. The control subjects were matched to probands for comparison on specific outcomes, so the size of the control groups varied as a function of outcomes evaluated.

At 10-year follow-up, 76 hyperactive probands from the initial cohort were re-evaluated. One proband was dropped from analysis due to suspected brain damage from glue sniffing, so the findings were based on 75 probands. There were no significant differences between the probands lost to follow-up and those retained on any of the baseline measures except a trend for those lost to have higher baseline parent-rated aggressiveness. The probands were compared with 45 healthy controls. This control sample included 35 subjects from the 5-year cohort plus additional 10 subjects, generally referred to the study by existing controls and meeting the same inclusion criteria. The age range was 17 to 24 years for both groups (hyperactive probands: mean = 19.5; controls: mean = 19). The two groups did not differ in terms of age, sex ratio (probands: 91% males; controls: 89% males), and socioeconomic status, but there was a trend for the probands to have lower IQ on the Wechsler Adult Intelligence Scale (WAIS) (probands: 105 vs. controls: 108). The evaluation differed from that at baseline and 5-year follow-up in that it relied less on parent reports and more on the adolescents' self-reports. Subjects underwent in-depth interviews with one of the study's two psychiatrists (psychiatrists were blind to group membership). In addition to a global psychiatric assessment, these interviews collected information on biography, living arrangements, academic and work history, sexual history, driving history (e.g., car accidents), court referral history, and history of nonmedical drug use. The clinician-rated Brief Psychiatric Rating Scale also was administered (Overall & Gorman, 1962). Subjects also completed the Symptom Checklist–90 (SCL–90) (Derogatis, Lipman, & Covi, 1973) and the California Psychological Interview (CPI) (Gough, 1975) self-report scales. The former scale assesses a broad range of psychiatric symptoms, and the latter is designed to measure self-esteem and social integration. In addition, self-esteem and social skills were examined in more depth in a subsample 18 probands and 18 controls (matched to the probands on age, sex, IQ, and socioeconomic status). The self-esteem scales were the same as used in the 5-year substudy; social skills were assessed via the Situational Social Skills Inventory (Clark, 1974), which evaluates a subject's responses to a set of hypothetical social situations, and the Means-Ends Problem Solving Procedure (Platt, Spivack, & Bloom, 1971), which evaluates a subject's understanding of social scripts. Though impressions of ADHD and other symptoms were primarily based on the clinical interviews and not on reports from parents or teachers, parents of 65 probands and 43 controls were interviewed regarding aspects of family and their child's functioning. Finally, locally designed rating scales were mailed to subjects' school teachers and employers to assess school functioning (for the last grade completed) and work functioning.

At 15-year follow-up, 63 probands and 41controls from the 10-year cohort were re-evaluated. Six of the probands could only be interviewed by telephone, and the information provided by two of these six subjects was deemed unreliable and excluded from analysis. Hence, the analyses focused on 61 hyperactive probands (90% males, age range 21 to 33 years, mean age: 25.1 years) and 41 controls (90% males, age range 21 to 32 years, mean age: 25.2 years). Again, the two groups were not different with respect to age, sex ratio, and socioeconomic status, but there was a trend for the controls to have a higher IQ on the WAIS (probands: 105 vs. controls: 108). As at the 10-year point, probands lost to follow-up did not differ significantly on baseline characteristics from the ones retained, except for a trend for higher aggressiveness in the probands lost to follow-up. The evaluation included:

(1) A semistructured interview by one of two study psychiatrists (not blind to group membership), from which the DSM-III diagnoses were made jointly by the psychiatrists.
(2) The Schedule for Affective Disorders and Schizophrenia (SADS-L) (Endicott & Spitzer, 1978) modified to focus on the past five years, except for the category of Antisocial Personality Disorder, and administered by another trained psychiatrist blind to group membership.
(3) Self-report scales—the SCL-90 and the CPI—were again completed by the subjects.
(4) Histories of alcohol and nonmedical drug use and abuse, court and police records, and occupational histories collected by research assistants.
(5) Tests of social skills and self-esteem, same as performed at 10-year follow-up but excluding Means Ends Problem Solving procedure, administered by research assistants.

Biographical information also was collected.

RESULTS

5-Year Follow-up

At 5-year follow-up, the age range for the probands was 11 to 18 years. Some of the outcomes in the 5-year studies were evaluated relative to the hyperactive probands' own baseline, while others were evaluated relative to a control group, and several were evaluated in both ways (Figure 2.1). There was a significant decrease in hyperactive probands' parent-rated ADHD symptoms (hyperactivity, distractibility, aggressiveness, and excitability) over the 5-year follow-up (Minde, Weiss, & Mendelson, 1972; Weiss et al., 1971). The levels of ADHD symptomatology for the probands, however, were higher than for a group of matched controls (n = 20). Teacher ratings also confirmed higher levels of these ADHD-like symptoms in a subsample of 33 probands relative to a sample of 33 sex-matched classmates (Weiss et al., 1971). Notably, according to parent reports, hyperactivity was no longer the chief complaint, and distractibility and poor concentration became more of a concern. Classroom behavior observation of a subset of 24 probands and 24 age- sex- and IQ-matched controls in the same classroom by blinded raters revealed that, although they did not display higher levels of locomotion, the hyperactive probands engaged in more nonclassroom-related activity (e.g., playing with pencils) than controls and appeared more distractible and less focused. The probands' global psychiatric functioning, although improved relative to baseline, was also inferior to age-based norms (Minde et al., 1972), and clinical observation by interviewing psychiatrists indicated that many probands had markedly low self-esteem (Weiss et al., 1971). The latter was confirmed by a substudy in 15 of the hyperactive adolescents and 15 age- and IQ-matched controls that used formal measures of self-esteem (Hoy, Weiss, Minde, & Cohen, 1978). According to their parents, 25% of the probands had a history of antisocial behavior, with 10% having had court referrals. Teacher ratings indicated significantly higher levels of antisocial behavior in a subset of 33 probands than in 33 sex-matched classmates.

There was no change in probands' family function, or age-referenced cognitive function using the measures collected at baseline, but their age-referenced motor development standing had worsened (Minde et al., 1972; Weiss et al., 1971). In addition, a subsample of 15 hyperactive boys from this cohort performed more poorly on the visual–motor and motor tests and had poorer sustained attention than a sample of 15 age- and IQ-matched controls (Hoy et al., 1978). Another study in a subsample of

20 hyperactive probands (Cohen, Weiss, & Minde, 1972) showed that, relative to 20 matched controls, the probands were more speedy (impulsive) and made more errors of visual attention on the matching familiar figures paradigm (Kagan, 1964); they also showed higher field dependence on an imbedded figures test, which was only significant one-tailed (Witken, Dyk, & Goodenough, 1962). The probands performed equally well, however, on the Stroop paradigm. This finding is somewhat surprising given that meta-analyses of subsequent studies of Stroop performance in ADHD have reported medium effect sizes for at least some measures (Lansbergen, Kenemans, & van Engeland, 2007; van Mourik, Oosterlaan, & Sergeant, 2005).

Academic performance was markedly poor for the probands, with 70% repeating at least one grade (compared with 15% of controls), 35% repeating two grades or more, and 80% underachieving relative to class average. Ten percent had been placed in special classes and 5% had been expelled from school. Report cards indicated that a subset of 33 probands fared significantly worse on oral reading, arithmetic, and writing than 33 matched controls; notably, hyperactives' relative class standing had not changed in five years (Weiss et al., 1971). A study using formal testing in a subsample of 15 probands also showed that their spelling and word knowledge was significantly worse than that of matched controls (Hoy et al., 1978).

Variation in outcomes was examined by subdividing the probands into three groups based on the parental report of functioning across the following six areas: general adjustment, peer interactions, relationship to authority, antisocial behavior, interpersonal relationships, and sexual adjustment. Children with good adjustment in five of six areas made up the "good outcome" group (n = 28); children with poor adjustment in four of six areas made up the "poor outcome" group (n = 18); 41 children were classified as having neither good nor poor outcome. Relative to the "good outcome" group, the "poor outcome" group showed less improvement in distractibility, aggressiveness, family functioning (which actually deteriorated for poor outcome patients), and neurotic and psychopathic traits relative to baseline (Minde et al., 1972).

10-Year Follow-up

At 10-year follow-up probands' ages were 17 to 24 years. At that point, fewer hyperactive probands than controls were still living with parents (probands: 76% vs. controls: 95%), and more were living with a partner (probands: 8% vs. controls: 4.5%). In terms of ADHD symptoms, significantly more, though not all probands were restless by self-report and clinician observation compared with controls (Weiss, Hechtman, Perlman, Hopkins, & Wener, 1979). Hyperactive probands, however, were not rated at this point as more hyperactive by their parents than controls were rated by their respective parents. This suggests that, although still present, hyperactivity had substantially decreased, at least in its more easily observable forms.

Probands had poorer functional outcomes relative to the controls in several areas. Probands had more car accidents, more frequent changes of residence, and impulsive personality traits, all of which may be seen as illustrating continuing impulsivity (Weiss et al., 1979). There also was a trend for the probands to have had more court referrals in the previous five years, but not in the past year (Hechtman, Weiss, & Perlman, 1984a; Weiss et al., 1979). They had completed less education (a higher proportion of probands than controls was still in high school at the point of evaluation), with poorer academic performance, more failed grades, and more school expulsions/dropouts (Weiss et al., 1979). Fifty-three percent of controls and only 20% of probands were continuing full-time education (e.g., university studies). There was, however, no difference in job status, work satisfaction, terminations and lay-offs, or unemployment between the groups (Weiss & Hechtman, 1993; Weiss et al., 1979). Although teachers reported that probands' scholastic performance was inferior to that of controls, employers did not report that probands had a poorer occupational performance, based on employer reports regarding 31 hyperactive subjects and 24 controls who were working, and whose employers completed the questionnaire (Weiss, Hechtman, & Perlman, 1978). Thus, assuming that the subjects who were working were representative of the entire sample, it would appear that probands fared better occupationally than scholastically at the 10-year follow-up point.

Probands were also less psychologically well-adjusted than controls: they reported more problems during the interview, had more pathological scores on the Brief Psychiatric Rating Scale, and rated themselves lower on the measure of self-esteem and social integration, but not on SCL-90 (Weiss et al., 1978; Weiss et al., 1979). Lower self-esteem and poorer social skills in the probands were confirmed by a substudy in 18 probands and 18 matched controls focusing on self-esteem and social skills: probands scored more poorly than controls on two of the three self-esteem and one of the two social skills measures—suggesting problems in the area of social interactions, but not other social skills areas assessed. There was also a trend for probands to have fewer friends. Two probands (and none of the controls) were diagnosed as borderline psychotic (Weiss et al., 1979). Finally, a higher proportion of probands than controls abused alcohol and had used nonmedical drugs, especially cannabis and hallucinogens, in the past five years (Hechtman, Weiss, & Perlman, 1984c; Weiss et al., 1979).

A study in a subsample of 35 probands and 25 controls examined cognitive performance on matching familiar figures, embedded figures, and Stroop tests (Hechtman, Weiss, Finklestein, Werner, & Benn, 1976), which were administered five years earlier to a group of 20 probands (and 20 controls). Hyperactive probands no longer showed response speeds consistent with increased impulsivity on the matching familiar figures test (primarily due to more speedy responding by controls), but continued to be more inaccurate, which suggests persistent poorer attention to visual detail. The probands also continued to show greater field dependence on the embedded figures. There were no differences in Stroop performance between probands and controls.

15-Year Follow-up

At 15-year follow-up, subjects' age range was 21 to 33 years. At that time, there was no difference between the two groups in terms of living arrangements (i.e., single, married, common-law), but significantly more probands had children.

Sixty-six percent of the probands complained of at least one continuing symptom of the hyperactive syndrome (restlessness, poor concentration, impulsivity, explosiveness), compared with 7% of the control group, and their continuing symptoms had greater severity than those reported by controls. More probands than controls (44% vs. 9.7%) displayed motor restlessness during the interview based on clinician's observation (Weiss, Hechtman, Milroy, & Perlman, 1985).

Probands continued to have significantly less education (Weiss et al., 1985). Probands started work at an earlier age on average—18 years of age versus almost 20 years of age for controls—and had a significantly lower occupational status on the Hollingshead scale, as well as lower career aspirations. There was a trend for controls to report choosing jobs primarily based on the learning experience they offered, while probands tended to choose jobs based on the social environment of the job. Although probands were no more likely than controls to report difficulty concentrating on the job, more of them reported finding tasks too difficult. Probands both quit and were laid off (though not fired) more frequently than controls, and there was a trend for them to spend more time out of work but not in school. Thirty-seven probands and 33 controls permitted the researchers to obtain work performance ratings from their employers. At this point, the employers rated the hyperactive probands lower than controls on adequately fulfilling work, working independently, completing tasks, and getting along with supervisors. There was a trend for employers to report being less inclined to rehire probands than controls (Weiss & Hechtman, 1993).

Probands also continued to have poorer psychological adjustment than controls (Weiss et al., 1985). While 33% of controls had no psychiatric diagnosis, no significant symptoms, and a high level of functioning globally, only 11% of probands were functioning psychologically at this high level. Probands reported a more significant psychiatric history with a greater incidence of neurotic and interpersonal problems, more types of psychiatric symptoms endorsed, and more suicide attempts (six attempts in probands vs. none in controls; one proband had died by suicide). They now also reported significantly more symptoms of psychopathology than controls on the SCL-90, particularly in the areas of somatization and phobic anxiety (Hechtman & Weiss, 1986; Weiss et al., 1985). There was a trend for a higher proportion of probands to have a current DSM-III diagnosis, with significantly more probands meeting multiple diagnoses and having poorer global adjustment scores. The group difference was most pronounced for the diagnosis of antisocial personality disorder, with 23% of the probands versus 2.4% of controls meeting criteria. The authors note, however, that a third of the antisocial personality disorder diagnoses were mild and may not have been made by some investigators. Consistent with higher rates of this diagnosis, probands had higher severity of antisocial behavior (based on combined information from the interview, the SADS-L, and the SCL-90), engaged in marginally more acts of physical aggression, had marginally more court appearances in the past three years, and had committed significantly more law violations without police involvements (Hechtman & Weiss, 1986; Weiss & Hechtman, 1993). Notably, most offenses in the hyperactive group were committed by only a few individuals. There was also a nonsignificant trend for more probands than controls to have abused alcohol in the past year and to have tried heroin in the past three years, but no other differences in patterns of substance use (Hechtman & Weiss, 1986). Significantly more probands than controls reported having stopped using drugs in the past three years.

Finally, probands continued to rate themselves more negatively than controls on the California Psychological Inventory, which measures self-esteem and social integration, and the difference between probands and controls was more pronounced than at 10-year follow-up (although self-ratings became more positive for both groups). The relative worsening of social functioning in probands was also evident on the social skills measure: probands' social skills now fell short not only in the area of social interactions, but also in the areas of job interviews and assertion (Weiss & Hechtman, 1993). Note, however, that the 10-year assessment of social skills was carried out in a subsample, which, although well-matched with controls, had a higher IQ than the rest of the hyperactive sample.

Outcome Characterization

From their follow-up data (Table 2.1), the Montreal researchers concluded that adult outcomes of children with ADHD fell roughly into three categories: (1) about 30%–40% had fairly normal functioning in adulthood, similar to controls; (2) about 40%–50% had continuing symptoms of the original syndrome, as well as social, emotional, interpersonal, and occupational problems, in the absence of marked psychiatric or antisocial pathology; (3) about 10% had serious psychiatric disturbances, substance use problems, and/or antisocial behavior and criminality (Weiss & Hechtman, 1993). It is important to stress that these are not distinct categories and overlap to some degree.

TABLE 2.1

SUMMARY OF IMPAIRMENT AT THE 5-YEAR, 10-YEAR, AND 15-YEAR FOLLOW-UP POINTS

5-Year Follow-up		10-Year Follow-up		15-Year Follow-up	
Versus Previous Evaluation	Versus Controls	Versus Previous Evaluation	Versus Controls	Versus Previous Evaluation	Versus Controls
ADHD Sx ↓	↑	ADHD Sx? Hyperactivity ↓ Impulsiveness	↑ ↑	ADHD Sx? Hyperactivity	↑ ↑
Psychiatric function ↑	↓	Psychiatric function?	↓	Psychiatric function ↓	↓
Self-esteem	↓	Self-esteem ‖	↓	Self-esteem ‖	↓
		Social skills	↓	Social skills ↓	↓
Cognitive performance ‖	↓*	Cognitive performance ↑	↓		
Motor development ↓					
Academic performance ‖	↓	Academic performance?	↓		
		Educational attainment	↓	Educational attainment ↑	↓
Antisocial behavior ↑	↑				

TABLE 2.1

CONTINUED

5-Year Follow-up		10-Year Follow-up		15-Year Follow-up	
Versus Previous Evaluation	Versus Controls	Versus Previous Evaluation	Versus Controls	Versus Previous Evaluation	Versus Controls
Court referrals	?	Court referrals in the past five years ↑	↑†		
				Court appearances↓	↑†
				Law violations?	↑
		Court referrals in the past year (↓ vs. past five years)	||		
		Work functioning ||	||	Work functioning?	↓
		Substance use in the past five years	↑	Substance use in the past 3 years ↓	||
		Substance use in the past year	||		

Sx = symptoms; ↑ = higher than previously or higher than controls; ↓ = lower than previously or lower than controls; || = no difference, * = true only in certain areas; † = nonsignificant trend; ? = unclear from the available data. Note that for the outcome measures that are expected to improve with age (e.g., cognitive function, social skills) time-dependent improvement or worsening is determined based on level of functioning relative to the control group.

OUTCOME PREDICTORS

Predictors of Adolescent Outcome

In adolescence, all measures of baseline functioning jointly predicted whether a patient ended up in the "good outcome" or the "poor outcome" group described earlier (Minde et al., 1972). That is, better baseline functioning predicted better outcomes. Higher IQ and, to a lesser extent, lower levels of ADHD-type symptoms at baseline predicted better academic outcomes, whereas higher aggressiveness, parental psychopathology, poor mother–child relationship, and more punitive child-rearing practices at baseline predicted antisocial behavior (Weiss et al., 1971). All subjects who had antisocial behavior at 15-year follow-up had persistent histories of antisocial behavior dating back to initial assessment or 5-year follow-up; however, many probands with early antisocial behavior did not continue antisocial behavior into adulthood (Hechtman & Weiss, 1986). Long-term pharmacotherapy was not found to be a significant predictor of adolescent outcome (Weiss, Kruger, Danielson, & Elman, 1975).

Predictors of Adult Outcome

At the 10- to 12-year follow-up point, the authors undertook a study to evaluate a number of childhood variables (ages 6–12 years) as possible predictors of a host of outcomes in adulthood (ages 17–24 years) (Hechtman, Weiss, Perlman, & Amsel, 1984).

The predictor variables considered were: (1) Personal characteristics of the proband (e.g., IQ, hyperactivity, aggressiveness, emotional stability, frustration tolerance); (2) Social/academic parameters (e.g., school performance, peer relations, adult relations, antisocial behavior); and (3) Family parameters (e.g., socioeconomic status [SES], mental health of family members, emotional climate of the home, child-rearing practices, quality/stability of parents' relationship, age first worked).

The adult outcome variables examined were: (1) Emotional adjustment (e.g., Brief Psychiatric Rating Scale, personality disorders, peer relationships/friends; (2) School performance (e.g., grades completed, academic standing, grades failed); (3) Work record (e.g., number of full-time jobs, proportion of jobs fired from, proportion of jobs laid off from, longest full-time job); (4) Police involvement (e.g., number of offenses, severity of offenses); (5) Car accidents (e.g., number of accidents, accidents with bodily injury, cost of damage); (6) Alcohol and nonmedical drug use (e.g., present use, past use, extent of current use, extent of maximum use, number of drugs used).

For each set of outcome measures, a selection of the most theoretically relevant predictor variables was identified. Predictors and outcome measures were entered into a stepwise regression analysis (or a discriminant analysis for categorical outcomes) to determine which predictor variables best predicted a given outcome. The ability of single predictor variables to predict outcomes also was examined using correlation (or ANOVAs for categorical variables). For a summary of outcome predictors, see Table 2.2.

TABLE 2.2

PREDICTORS OF OUTCOMES IN ADOLESCENCE AND ADULTHOOD

Predictors	Outcomes
ADOLESCENT OUTCOMES	
All measures of baseline functioning (ADHD symptoms, family functioning, psychiatric functioning, cognitive functioning, academic functioning)	"Good outcome" vs. "poor outcome" group membership
IQ ADHD symptoms	Academic outcomes
Aggressiveness Parental psychopathology Mother–child relationship Child-rearing practices Baseline antisocial behavior	Antisocial behavior
ADULT OUTCOMES	
Personal characteristics: Baseline ADHD symptoms Emotional instability Low frustration tolerance IQ *Family Characteristics:* Mental health of family members Emotional climate at home Overall family rating	Emotional adjustment

(continued)

TABLE 2.2

CONTINUED

Predictors	Outcomes
Personal characteristics: IQ Hyperactivity Aggressiveness Initial school performance *Social characteristics:* Antisocial behavior at school *Family characteristics:* Socioeconomic status Child-rearing practices Mental health of family members Emotional climate at home Overall family rating	School performance
Personal characteristics: IQ Hyperactivity Antisocial behavior *Social characteristics:* Relationship with adults Peer relations Antisocial behavior *Family characteristics:* Socioeconomic status Age probands first worked	Work record
Personal characteristics: IQ Hyperactivity Aggressiveness Emotional instability Low frustration tolerance *Social characteristics:* Antisocial behavior Peer relations Adult relations	Police involvement

TABLE 2.2

CONTINUED

Predictors	Outcomes
Family characteristics: Socioeconomic status Mental health of family members Overall family rating Emotional climate at home Child-rearing practices	
Personal characteristics: Aggressiveness Emotional instability Low frustration tolerance *Family characteristics:* Mental health of family members Emotional climate at home	Car accidents (number, bodily injury) Car accidents (cost of damage)
Personal characteristics: Hyperactivity Aggressiveness IQ *Social characteristics:* Antisocial behavior *Family characteristics:* Overall family rating Mental health of family members	Alcohol and nonmedical drug use

The most important predictors of **emotional adjustment** in adulthood were baseline family parameters (mental health of family members, family rating, and emotional climate at home). **School performance** at the 10-year to 12-year follow-up was most strongly predicted by IQ, family SES, and child-rearing practices. Different aspects of **work record** were most strongly predicted by adult relations and family SES. The strongest predictors of **police involvement** were the emotional instability of the proband, family SES, family mental health, and child-rearing practices. For **car**

accidents, their overall number and the number of accidents with bodily injury were not associated with any predictor variables. Cost of damage, however, was most strongly predicted by the proband's low frustration tolerance, as well as by the emotional climate in the family home. Finally, the **extent of alcohol use** was most strongly predicted by baseline family rating; whether the proband was currently using **nonmedical drugs** was most strongly predicted by IQ, antisocial behavior, and family mental health.

A substudy also looked at adult outcomes of hyperactive children as a function of presence versus relative absence of sustained stimulant treatment in childhood (Hechtman, Weiss, & Perlman, 1984b). Probands followed by the Montreal group, who had only intermittent and largely nonstimulant treatment, were compared with a group of hyperactive children from a later cohort (late 1960s to early 1970s) who had received three to five years of sustained stimulant treatment. The stimulant-treated hyperactives were slightly older than the untreated subjects (21.8 years vs. 19.6 years), but were similar in terms of IQ and socioeconomic status. There were few differences in outcomes between stimulant-treated and relatively untreated hyperactives. Out of over 40 variables analyzed, treated hyperactives fared better in a few areas including fewer car accidents, seeing childhood more positively, stealing less in elementary school, and having better social skills and self-esteem. Overall, the Montreal study did not highlight pharmacotherapy as an important predictor of outcome, though it should be noted that sustained treatment did not continue into adulthood.

DISCUSSION

The findings of the Montreal group make it clear that although the symptoms of the original syndrome do tend to diminish as the child becomes older, in many cases they do not disappear completely. Two thirds of the hyperactive probands still complained of at least one disabling symptom of the original syndrome at 15-year follow-up. Motor hyperactivity showed the most improvement, though feelings of restlessness often remained.

Attentional symptoms became more of a concern, however, as the children entered adolescence.

More striking is the functional impairment of probands as they progressed through the various stages of their lives. In some areas, such as self-esteem and cognitive functioning, impairment stably persisted throughout development. In other areas, impairment evolved, and the areas of most significant impairment often coevolved with changing life priorities. In childhood (at baseline), hyperactivity and behavioral problems were the chief complaints. In adolescence, academic functioning appeared to be the most striking impairment, which is consistent with education being a major developmental goal at this stage. In late adolescence to young adulthood, hyperactive probands continued to have lower educational achievement and attainment, but some were working and performing at work as well as controls. This apparently unimpaired functioning at work, however, may have been partly an artifact of the sample of probands and controls examined at 10-year follow-up. More controls than hyperactives went on to pursue higher education, whereas more hyperactives than controls were still in high school at the time of the evaluation (likely due to having repeated grades). Thus, the 10-year sample evaluated for work performance may have over-represented lower-functioning controls (who did not go on to university) and higher functioning hyperactives (who completed school without delays). At the 15-year follow-up, significant work impairments among probands became apparent, as did social skills impairments related to work situations.

A major goal of conducting the 15-year follow-up was to evaluate the psychiatric outcomes of the probands, because it was felt that their age at 10-year follow-up (mean age 19.5 years) had not yet reached that of maximal risk for most psychiatric disorders. The 15-year data, indeed, showed significant impairment in psychological adjustment among probands that was overall more pronounced than at the 10-year follow-up. The area of psychiatric functioning that most distinguished hyperactives from controls was the prevalence of antisocial personality disorder. Antisocial behavior was a characteristic evident in the hyperactive sample from the start; as subjects grew older, however, it appeared to take on more criminal manifestations. It should be stressed, however, that only a few hyperactive subjects accounted for the majority of criminal acts committed and instances of police involvement, and the majority did not behave unlawfully. Finally, substance use seemed to have peaked in adolescence (the age of experimentation)—at which point hyperactive probands became heavier users than controls—but then subsided by mid-adulthood essentially to control group levels.

Most outcomes were predicted by a combination of baseline characteristics of the child (symptoms, IQ, emotional functioning), baseline family adjustment, and baseline social adjustment and status of the child. Many of the same characteristics (in similar combinations) predicted different types of outcomes (Table 2.2). One interpretation could be that a combination of child and family adjustment factors represents some measure of global functional adjustment, which can then predict multiple outcomes later on. One issue that the authors point out is multicollinearity: at least some predictor variables were highly mutually correlated, so there may have been some redundancy in the predictors (Weiss & Hechtman, 1993). A principal component analysis could have helped reduce the number of predictors by identifying latent factors. Another potential issue in examining outcome predictors in this case is the possibility of shared variance between certain predictors and outcomes. For example, family adjustment variables were significant predictors of all classes of outcomes. Family interviews, however, pointed to the possibility of family adjustment itself being affected by the proband (perhaps, especially if the proband is severely impaired), as family adjustment often improved when the proband left the home. Thus, it is possible that some of the variance in family adjustment that predicts the proband's functional outcomes is actually due to the proband's own level of impairment.

As pioneers of long-term follow-up in ADHD, the Montreal group had to contend with a few unique challenges that later groups did not encounter to the same degree. The first is the diagnostic criteria. At the start of the study, the only criteria available were the rather vague DSM-II criteria of Hyperkinetic Reaction of Childhood, so the authors relied on their own symptom rating system, which emphasized hyperactivity, distractibility, aggressiveness (which would now likely be linked with comorbid oppositional defiant or conduct disorders) and excitability. At the time of the final follow-up, the DSM-III diagnosis of attention deficit disorder with or without hyperactivity (ADD/H) was in use, which placed considerably more emphasis on inattention and impulsivity. The changes in the diagnostic criteria and the evolving understanding of the syndrome's key features over the course of the study make it difficult to estimate the degree of syndrome persistence from childhood into adulthood. It is clear, however, that two thirds of the probands complained of at least one continuing symptom that caused significant impairment. Another challenge was outcome selection—without any knowledge of what the syndrome might look like in adolescence and adulthood, it is difficult to know which outcomes are the important ones to measure. Thus, the measured outcomes evolved over the course of the study in a developmentally informed manner, with some outcomes introduced and others eliminated, and the findings represent a patchwork of cross-sectional and longitudinal data. Although there is imperfect continuity of outcomes, taken together the data provide a developmentally sensitive picture of the types of impairments that people who suffer from hyperactivity as children experience at different stages of their lives.

As is the case with many long-term follow-up studies, subject attrition over time represents a significant limitation. At 15-year follow-up only 60.5% of the original hyperactive sample was evaluated. Importantly, subjects lost to follow-up did not generally differ from the ones retained on baseline characteristics. Still, there is generally a tendency in longitudinal clinical research for more individuals with poorer outcomes to be lost to follow-up. The authors have observed, however, that a proportion of the probands who declined follow-up indicated that they were doing well and were declining to participate because they did not want to be reminded of their previous problems. Thus, it appears that a proportion of the probands lost to follow-up might have represented high-functioning individuals, which might have mitigated against the tendency for low-functioning individuals to be over-represented among those lost to follow-up. Another limitation is the number of outcomes measured without correction for multiple comparisons. In some cases, over 20 separate outcome components were evaluated, and few of the findings would have survived the correction for multiple comparisons. Uncorrected thresholds, however, are permissible in exploratory studies, which the Montreal studies were.

SUMMARY AND CONCLUSIONS

The Montreal studies have made a great contribution to our understanding of the developmental course of ADHD. Though earlier retrospective and cross-sectional studies had reached similar conclusions, the Montreal group was the first to demonstrate using a rigorous prospective design that childhood ADHD often leads to impairments in adolescent and adult functioning and to comprehensively examine the key areas of impairment. The findings indicate that the outcomes fall roughly into three categories: (1) about 30% –40% have fairly normal functioning in adulthood, similar to controls; (2) about 40%–50% have continuing symptoms of the original syndrome, as well as social, emotional, interpersonal, and occupational problems, in the absence of marked psychiatric or antisocial pathology; (3) about 10% have serious psychiatric disturbances, substance use problems, and/or antisocial behavior and criminality. Functional outcomes are predicted by a combination of initial personal, social, and family characteristics of the patient.

REFERENCES

Bakwin, H., & Bakwin, R. (1966). *Clinical Management of Behaviour Disorders in Children*. Philadelphia: W.B. Saunders.

Bender, L. (1938). *A Visual Motor Gestalt Test and its Clinical Use* (Research Monograph No. 3). New York: American Orthopsychiatric Association.

Clark, K. W. (1974). *Evaluation of a Group Social Skills Training Program with Psychiatric Inpatients: Training Vietnam Veterans in Assertion, Heterosocial and Job Interview Skills.* (Doctoral dissertation, ProQuest Information & Learning.).

Cohen, N. J., Weiss, G., & Minde, K. (1972). Cognitive styles in adolescents previously diagnosed as hyperactive. *Journal of Child Psychology and Psychiatry*, *13*(3), 203–209.

Davidson, H., & Lang, G. (1960). Children's perceptions of their teachers' feelings toward them related to self-perception, school achievement, and behavior. *The Journal of Experimental Education, 29*, 107–118.

Derogatis, L. R., Lipman, R. S., & Covi, L. (1973). SCL-90: an outpatient psychiatric rating scale—preliminary report. *Psychopharmacology Bulletin, 9*(1), 13–28.

Endicott, J., & Spitzer, R. L. (1978). A diagnostic interview: the schedule for affective disorders and schizophrenia. *Archives of General Psychiatry, 35*(7), 837–844.

Faraone, S. V., Sergeant, J., Gillberg, C., & Biederman, J. (2003). The worldwide prevalence of ADHD: Is it an American condition? *World Psychiatry: Official Journal of the World Psychiatric Association (WPA), 2*(2), 104–113.

Gough, H. (1975). *California Psychological Interview* (Rev. ed.). Palo Alto, CA: Consulting Psychologist Press.

Harris, D. B. (1963). *Children's Drawings as Measures of Intellectual Maturity: A Revision and Extension of the Goodenough Draw-a-Man Test.* New York: Harcourt, Brace.

Hechtman, L., & Weiss, G. (1986). Controlled prospective fifteen year follow-up of hyperactives as adults: non-medical drug and alcohol use and anti-social behaviour. *Canadian Journal of Psychiatry, 31*(6), 557–567.

Hechtman, L., Weiss, G., Finklestein, J., Werner, A., & Benn, R. (1976). Hyperactives as young adults: preliminary report. *Canadian Medical Association Journal, 115*(7), 625–630.

Hechtman, L., Weiss, G., & Perlman, T. (1984a). Hyperactives as young adults: past and current substance abuse and antisocial behavior. *American Journal of Orthopsychiatry, 54*(3), 415–425.

Hechtman, L., Weiss, G., & Perlman, T. (1984b). Young adult outcome of hyperactive children who received long-term stimulant treatment. *Journal of the American Academy of Child Psychiatry, 23*(3), 261–269.

Hechtman, L., Weiss, G., Perlman, T., & Amsel, R. (1984). Hyperactives as young adults: initial predictors of adult outcome. *Journal of the American Academy of Child Psychiatry, 23*(3), 250–260.

Hoy, E., Weiss, G., Minde, K., & Cohen, N. J. (1978). The hyperactive child at adolescence: Cognitive, emotional, and social functioning. *Journal of Abnormal Child Psychology, 6*(3), 311–324.

Kagan, J. (1964). Information processing in the child. Significance of analytic and reflective attitudes. *Psychological Monographs: General and Applied, 87*(1), 1–37.

Kessler, R. C., Adler, L., Barkley, R., Biederman, J., Conners, C. K., Demler, O., . . . Zaslavsky, A. M. (2006). The prevalence and correlates of adult ADHD in the United States: results from the National Comorbidity Survey Replication. *American Journal of Psychiatry, 163*(4), 716–723.

Lansbergen, M. M., Kenemans, J. L., & van Engeland, H. (2007). Stroop interference and attention-deficit/hyperactivity disorder: a review and meta-analysis. *Neuropsychology, 21*(2), 251–262.

Minde, K., Weiss, G., & Mendelson, N. (1972). A 5-year follow-up study of 91 hyperactive school children. *Journal of the American Academy of Child Psychiatry, 11*(3), 595–610.

Overall, J. E., & Gorman, D. R. (1962). The Brief Psychiatric Rating Scale. *Psychological Reports, 10*, 799.

Peterson, D. R., & Quay, H. C. (1967). *Factor-Analysed Problem Checklist*. Urbana: University of Illinois, Children's Research Center.

Platt, J. J., Spivack, G., & Bloom, N. (1971). *Means-ends Problem Solving Procedure (MEPS) Manual and Tentative Norms*. Philadelphia: Department of Mental Health Sciences, Hahnemann Medical College and Hospital.

Sloan, W. (1955). The Lincoln-Oseretsky motor development scale. *Genetic Psychology Monographs, 51*(2), 183–252.

van Mourik, R., Oosterlaan, J., & Sergeant, J. A. (2005). The Stroop revisited: a meta-analysis of interference control in AD/HD. *Journal of Child Psychology and Psychiatry, 46*(2), 150–165.

Weiss, G., & Hechtman, L. (1993). *Hyperactive Children Grown Up: ADHD in Children, Adolescents, and Adults* (2nd ed.). New York: Guilford Press.

Weiss, G., Hechtman, L., Milroy, T., & Perlman, T. (1985). Psychiatric status of hyperactives as adults: a controlled prospective 15-year follow-up of 63 hyperactive children. *Journal of the American Academy of Child Psychiatry, 24*(2), 211–220.

Weiss, G., Hechtman, L., & Perlman, T. (1978). Hyperactives as young adults: school, employer, and self-rating scales obtained during ten-year follow-up evaluation. *American Journal of Orthopsychiatry, 48*(3), 438–445.

Weiss, G., Hechtman, L., Perlman, T., Hopkins, J., & Wener, A. (1979). Hyperactives as young adults: a controlled prospective ten-year follow-up of 75 children. *Archives of General Psychiatry, 36*(6), 675–681.

Weiss, G., Kruger, E., Danielson, U., & Elman, M. (1975). Effect of long-term treatment of hyperactive children with methylphenidate. *Canadian Medical Association Journal, 112*(2), 159–165.

Weiss, G., Minde, K., Werry, J. S., Douglas, V., & Nemeth, E. (1971). Studies on the hyperactive child: VIII. Five-year follow-up. *Archives of General Psychiatry, 24*(5), 409–414.

Werry, J. S. (1968). Developmental hyperactivity. *Pediatric Clinics of North America, 15*(3), 581–599.

Witken, H. A., Dyk, R. B., & Goodenough, D. R. (1962). *Psychological Differentiation*. New York: Wiley.

Ziller, R. C., Hagey, J., Smith, M. D., & Long, B. H. (1969). Self-esteem: a self-social construct. *Journal of Consulting and Clinical Psychology, 33*(1), 84–95.

3

Long-Term Outcomes of Childhood Attention Deficit Hyperactivity Disorder

The New York Study

SYLVIANE HOUSSAIS, LILY HECHTMAN, AND RACHEL G. KLEIN

INTRODUCTION

This chapter summarizes the long-term clinical and functional outcomes of hyperactive children in the New York Study who were followed prospectively for 33 years. This time span marks the longest follow-up to date of children diagnosed with what is now termed Attention Deficit Hyperactivity Disorder (ADHD). No other prospective study of ADHD has followed the same cohort into the fourth and fifth decades of life, making its findings invaluable to a comprehensive understanding of the adult sequelae of childhood-diagnosed ADHD.

At the time of the study's inception, the analogue of ADHD was termed *hyperkinetic reaction of childhood (or adolescence)* and was defined by two short clauses in the second edition of the *Diagnostic and Statistical Manual of Mental Disorders* (DSM-II): "The disorder is characterized by overactivity, restlessness, distractibility, and short attention span, especially in young children; the behavior usually diminishes by adolescence" (American Psychiatric Association, 1968, p. 50). The vague nature of this definition belied the prevalence of the disorder at the time (Lange, Reichl, Lange, Tucha, & Tucha, 2010), and its lack of quantifiable diagnostic criteria underscored the need for empirical study. Moreover, although the definition acknowledged the possibility of the disorder's persistence into adolescence, it implied the rarity of such persistence, despite emerging evidence to the contrary (e.g., Anderson & Plymate, 1962; Laufer, 1962). Thus, the historical context provided scientific impetus for conducting controlled prospective research to understand better the disorder, its developmental course, and its outcomes. (Only one previous study had followed hyperactive children prospectively—the Montreal Study, described in the previous chapter.) The researchers also noted a public health impetus given then-growing evidence that hyperactive children disproportionately contribute to the pool of antisocial adults (e.g., Satterfield & Cantwell, 1975).

The study's original cohort consisted of children between 6 and 12 years of age (mean age 8 years) who were referred by schools to a psychiatric clinic between 1970 and 1978 for behavior problems. Subsequent funding from the National Institute of Mental Health (NIMH) and the National Institute on Drug Abuse (NIDA) allowed for three follow-up assessments of this cohort: 10 years later when participants were in late adolescence (mean age 18 years; FU18), 17 years later when they reached early adulthood (mean age 25 years; FU25), and 33 years later in mid-adulthood (mean age 41 years; FU41). This chapter will focus on outcomes from the last assessment point in mid-adulthood, but will also summarize adolescent and early adulthood findings that are important to understand the larger clinical and functional picture.

METHODOLOGY

Participants

Participants in the original cohort were identified from over one thousand children seen at a no-cost psychiatric research clinic at the Long Island Jewish Hillside Medical Center in Glen Oaks, New York. Their selection at the outset was for enrollment in treatment studies for their hyperactivity symptoms, wherein treatment mainly involved pharmacotherapy in one cohort, and pharmacotherapy and behavior therapy in a second cohort. These studies are described in Gittelman-Klein et al. (1976) and Gittelman et al. (1980). The childhood sample whose outcomes are summarized here comprised solely of white hyperactive boys. Although black children were initially included in the treatment studies, they were omitted from the longitudinal studies because they were insufficient in number (n = 14) to generate reliable data about their status as a social group, whose life outcomes were assumed to differ on the basis of other factors (e.g., discrimination) than those related to their hyperactivity. Moreover, although girls were also included in the treatment studies, there were only 19 in total, likely due to both their under-representation and the under-recognition of the disorder's prevalence among girls at the time (Nadeau, Littman, & Quinn, 1999). They were followed in adolescence (Mannuzza & Gittelman, 1984) and early adulthood but not beyond. Their outcomes at those time points did not differ from the boys but the sample size was too small to make any reliable generalizations about gender differences.

Thus, the outcomes reported are those of a cohort of 207 white hyperactive boys (hereafter, *probands*). This cohort represents two independent samples: one in which children, ages 6 through 12, were referred between 1970 and 1975, and one in which they were referred between 1971 and 1977. A minimum age criterion of 16 years was set for follow-up, therefore, each sample was followed separately in late adolescence (Gittelman, Mannuzza, Shenker, & Bonagura, 1985; Mannuzza et al., 1991) and early adulthood (Mannuzza, Klein, Bessler, Malloy, & LaPadula, 1993, 1998), with findings from the second sample being reported as replications of the same analyses done on the first sample. Findings from each sample were nearly identical and are, therefore, reported here as a single cohort in late adolescence and early adulthood for ease of communication, because no distinction between samples was made at the final time point (Klein et al., 2012). Readers are referred to the original reports cited above for further details. Comparison participants were recruited in late adolescence (total N = 178) and followed up in early adulthood and mid-adulthood. Table 3.1 shows the overall retention rates by group at each assessment point. Retention rates were slightly higher in the comparison group and decreased over time in both groups. Specifically, in late adolescence (mean age 18 years) when the comparison group was recruited, the overall retention rate of probands was 94%. In early adulthood (mean age 25 years), the retention rate of comparison participants was 94% and that of probands was 86%. In mid-adulthood (mean age 41 years), 76% of comparison participants versus 67% of probands were retained.

Selection Criteria for Probands

For initial entry into the treatment studies, the children had to meet the following criteria: (1) aged between 6 and 12 years; (2) referred by teachers because of behavior problems and had a previous history of behavior problems; (3) rated at least 1.8 out of 3 on the hyperactivity factor of the Conners Teacher Rating Scale (Conners, 1969); (4) rated

TABLE 3.1

PERCENT RETENTION AT THREE FOLLOW-UP ASSESSMENT POINTS

	Childhood	Late Adolescence (FU18)	Early Adulthood (FU25)	Mid-Adulthood (FU41)
Probands	N = 207 100%	N = 195 94%	N = 176 86%	N = 135 67%
Comparisons	—	N = 178 100%	N = 168 94%	N = 136 76%

at least 28 out of 44 on eleven items of the Parent Home Hyperactivity Scale, modified from the Werry-Weiss-Peters Activity Scale (Werry & Sprague, 1970); (5) obtained an IQ of 85 or above on the Wechsler Intelligence Scale for Children (Wechsler, 1949, 1974); (6) free of psychosis and neurological disorder; (7) living with English-speaking parents and have a home telephone; (8) received no prior pharmacological treatment.

With the goal of studying a relatively "pure" form of the hyperactivity disorder, and with the assumption that this disorder differed significantly from Conduct Disorder (CD), an attempt was made to screen out children who might have a comorbid CD. Thus, children were not accepted into the study if the school referral involved aggressive or other significant antisocial behaviors, or if the clinic evaluation suggested a pattern of antisocial activities. Although this process did not guarantee the exclusion of children with CD, parent and teacher ratings suggested considerable success in this regard: Among probands, the mean rating for conduct problem items was 0.7 (on a scale from 0 to 3), whereas the mean rating for inattention items was 2.55, the mean rating for hyperactivity items was 2.31, and the mean rating for impulsivity items was 2.34 (Mannuzza, Klein, Abikoff, & Moulton, 2004).

Because the recruitment of the original cohort antedated the development of diagnostic criteria, an important question is whether the children in this cohort would have been diagnosed with the equivalent of the contemporary conception of ADHD, combined-type (DSM-5) (American Psychiatric Association, 2013). Reasons to argue in favor of this include the following: (1) the children obtained elevated parent and teacher ratings on symptoms of hyperactivity, inattention, and impulsivity; (2) symptoms occurred both in school and at home; (3) the referrals indicated clear clinical impairment related to symptoms; (4) the children had a history of behavior problems; and (5) classroom ratings by blind observers showed significant differences between probands and "normal" children on measures of ADHD symptoms (Mannuzza et al., 1998). These reasons cannot categorically ensure diagnostic equivalence, but the clear overlap in criteria provides enough similarity to assume it for the purposes of reporting long-term outcomes of this single cohort.

Descriptions in Box 3.1 give a qualitative impression of the clinical cases presented at the time of referral. The same three boys will be revisited in mid-adulthood at the end of the chapter.

Selection Criteria for Comparison Participants

Comparison participants were recruited at the 10-year follow-up point in late adolescence, at mean age 18 years (FU18), from the Department of Adolescent Medicine of the same medical center from which the probands were recruited. Charts were reviewed to select boys who had reached the age of at least 16 years, had previously sought medical attention for routine physical examination or treatment of acute conditions (e.g., flu), had *not* sought treatment for accidental injuries (which were posited to be more frequent among hyperactive children) or serious chronic conditions (because of possible complications that might confound the intended comparisons), and had no recorded history indicating behavior problems in early school years. Once charts were identified, parents were called and provided with information about the study's protocol, and asked whether elementary school teachers had ever complained about the child's behavior. Any behavioral complaints ruled out recruitment. Only 5% of parents refused to participate.

Psychiatric Assessment Measures

At each assessment point, participants were administered a semistructured interview that included assessments of psychiatric disorders based on the DSM in use at the time (DSM-III at FU18, DSM-III-R at FU25, and DSM-IV-R at FU41). At FU18, participants' parents were also interviewed. The interviews were based on the NIMH Diagnostic Interview Schedule, modified to allow for clinical inquiry, for the participants and parents and

Box 3.1 CASE PRESENTATIONS FROM THE ORIGINAL CHILDHOOD COHORT

Rob, age 6 years, first grade

There have been complaints about Rob's behavior since nursery school, where the teacher reported not being able to control him, and where he once fell and sustained a concussion, because he "could not sit still." At the time of referral, Rob's behavior in school was described as "uncontrollable" and "disruptive." Teachers reported that he "will not sit still for a minute" and as a result, put him in isolation and did not allow him into the lunch area. At home, Rob is described as "very active" and "constantly moving and talking." His parents note: "He tries to behave, but he says he can't help it." During testing, Rob was in constant motion and had difficulty sustaining attention.

Francis, age 8 years, third grade

Francis "has always been a hyperactive kid, even as an infant." His parents and teachers complained about his hyperactivity and his pediatrician noted it. In nursery school, he was described as inattentive and overactive. At the time of referral, his school teachers noted: "He lacks self-control, has a short attention span, is disorganized, forgetful, impulsive, and constantly moving; other children are annoyed by his impulsivity." At home, "he can't seem to sit still, is extremely active, and constantly running and jumping." His parents also noted that he does not follow directions, must be told several times to do the same thing, and is difficult to discipline. During testing, Francis was restless and somewhat hyperactive.

Adam, age 10 years, fourth grade

Since kindergarten, Adam has had difficulty sitting still and has always had a short attention span. At the time of referral, his school teachers noted: "Adam is very restless, tends to clown, is an attention seeker, very energetic, active, disrupts, and is distractible. He gives up easily and frustrates easily." At home, Adam "cannot sit for more than a minute. He is constantly changing his activity, does not enjoy quiet activities, and is very distractible."

administered by trained clinicians who were blind to participants' group membership (i.e., probands vs. comparison). For more details on the interview design at each assessment point, see Gittelman et al. (1985), Mannuzza et al. (2011), Mannuzza et al. (1993), and Proal et al. (2011). To ensure that clinicians stayed blind to participants' group membership, the recruiting social worker explained the importance of the blind assessment and asked participants/parents not to discuss the participant's childhood during the interview. Moreover, interviews were limited to the period since the last assessment only (at FU18, since the age of 13), thereby precluding discussions of prior diagnoses. Disorders assessed included substance use disorder (SUD), conduct disorder (CD)[1] and antisocial personality disorder (APD),[1] mood disorders, and ADHD, among others. If disorders required symptoms to be present by a threshold age in childhood for diagnosis (e.g., ADHD), this criterion was suspended to preserve the blind assessment. At FU18, diagnoses were considered present if obtained from the participant or the parent.

Clinician interviewers formulated "definite" and "probable" diagnoses and wrote clinical narrative summaries describing functioning and justifying diagnoses. Definite diagnoses indicated that DSM criteria were fully met. Probable diagnoses indicated that the participant (or parent) reported fewer symptoms than required, but reported impairment related to the symptoms. ADHD, to err conservatively, was only established through definite diagnoses. For all other disorders, definite and probable diagnoses were combined in reported findings except when referring to ongoing diagnoses (only definite ongoing diagnoses were reported). Diagnoses were established as ongoing if participants met criteria within two months of the interview. Exceptions were SUD and CD/APD, for which ongoing diagnoses were established if participants met criteria within six months of the interview (for CD/APD, this time period was a DSM criterion; for SUD, a six-month period was

1. When referring to outcomes, the labels CD and APD are often combined as CD/APD because the difference in denominations reflects only the participants' age at follow-up.

established due to the chronic nature of SUDs). At FU41, rates of lifetime disorders were also established.

Functional Outcomes Measures

Educational Achievement

At FU25 and FU41, educational achievement consisted of the number of years of formal schooling completed, and by the type of educational experience and attainment (bachelor's degree, law degree, etc.).

Occupational Rank and Functioning

At FU25 and FU41, occupational rank was classified on a scale of 1 to 8 according to the Hollingshead and Redlich method (Hollingshead & Redlich, 1958), where 1 = higher executives, 8 = unemployed. Additional queries were made about work history (e.g., jobs held, job satisfaction, work relationships, lateness, job changes, and firings). At FU41, clinician interviewers also rated occupational functioning (among employed participants) during the previous six months, regardless of type of employment, on an anchored scale from 1 = superior to 6 = poor.

Social Functioning

Cohabitation and marital status were recorded at FU25 and FU41. Additionally at FU41, clinician interviewers rated social functioning on a 6-point scale, from 1 = superior to 6 = poor, based on participants' reports on friendships and social and leisure activities.

Criminality

Separate investigations into lifetime arrest records were carried out when participants were on average 22 years old (Mannuzza, Klein, Konig, & Giampino, 1989) and again when they were 38 years old (Mannuzza, Klein, & Moulton, 2008). Because the latter investigation presumably subsumed findings from the former, only the latter's results are summarized here (patterns were very similar in each). Participants were limited to those residing in New York State (93 probands and 93 comparisons at mean age 38 years) because of possible access and the accuracy of records from the New York State Division of Criminal Justice Services (although a wider analysis using online searches for arrest records for those participants living out of state yielded the same results). Outcomes analyzed included rates of arrests, convictions, incarcerations, types of charges of arrested participants, and age at first arrest.

Obesity

At FU41, 111 probands and 111 comparison participants self-reported their height and weight (Cortese, Ramos Olazagasti et al., 2013). Body Mass Index (BMI) was calculated and categorized as underweight (BMI < 18.5), normal weight (18.5 ≤ BMI < 25), overweight (25 ≤ BMI 30), or obese (BMI ≥ 30).

Risk-taking

Clinical interviews at FU41 contained questions about lifetime driving history and sexual history (Ramos Olazagasti et al., 2013). Structural Equation Modeling was used to analyze risky behaviors with latent variables constructed from interview indicators. Specifically, a latent variable called "risky driving" was constructed from indicators including license suspensions/revocations, speeding citations, reckless driving violations, DUI violations, and other moving violations. Risky driving in adulthood was defined as having occurred in the previous five years. A latent variable called "risky sex" included indicators of early sex (before age 15years), greater number of sexual partners (26 partners or more), and no or irregular birth control. Risky sex in adulthood was defined as having occurred during the past year.

Medical Outcomes, Hospitalizations, and Mortality

At FU41, interviews also contained questions about participants' medical history since the previous follow-up assessment (FU25) (Ramos Olazagasti et al., 2013). Questions were asked about 54 different medical conditions, grouped into four categories: neurological/neuromuscular (e.g., epilepsy, head injury), genitourinary (e.g., STDs), cardiovascular (e.g., heart attack, hypertension), and other. STDs, head injuries, hospitalizations (psychiatric and nonpsychiatric), and emergency department admissions were also examined individually. Mortality data were gathered through relatives' reports, Internet searches in LexisNexis Accurint services, the Social Security Death Index, and Google searches for obituaries.

Brain Imaging

At FU41, a number of participants consented to undergo brain scans. The purpose was to examine differences in gray and white matter deficits between groups. Specifically, 59 probands and 80 comparison participants underwent Magnetic Resonance Imaging (MRI) scans to test for group differences in cortical thinning and/or decreased gray matter in brain regions hypothesized to be related to ADHD (Proal et al., 2011). Additionally, 51 probands and 66 comparison participants underwent Diffusion Tensor Imaging (DTI) scans to test whether there were group differences in fractional anisotropy (FA, an index related to white matter structural properties) in white matter tracts that connect regions of the brain hypothesized to be related to ADHD (Cortese, Imperati et al., 2013).

RESULTS

Late Adolescence Outcomes (FU18)

In late adolescence, the ADHD syndrome persisted in approximately 41.5% of probands (Gittelman et al., 1985; Mannuzza et al., 1991). This is a noticeable improvement from childhood, but clearly demonstrates the persistence of the disorder in a substantial proportion of adolescents. In contrast, only 3.4% of comparison participants presented the disorder.

Probands also showed significantly higher rates of CD/APD than comparison participants (approximately 29.4% vs. 8%), and likewise, significantly higher rates of SUD than comparisons (approximately 13.1% vs.

2.1%). Drug abuse rather than alcohol abuse drove the difference in SUDs. No other significant differences in psychiatric disorders emerged between the groups.

The degree to which ADHD, CD/APD, and SUD occurred in the same cases was examined. Probands with persistent ADHD were significantly more likely to develop a CD/APD or SUD than probands who no longer met criteria for ADHD (i.e., remitted). Indeed, there were no significant differences between remitted probands and comparison participants in rates of CD/APD or SUD. Furthermore, probands (both persistent and remitted) who developed CD/APD at follow-up were much more likely to develop an SUD than probands who did not develop a CD/APD. Indeed, almost all cases of SUD among probands occurred among those who had developed a CD/APD. An examination of ages of onset to study the developmental sequence of the disorders showed that the occurrence of CD/APD almost entirely accounted for the added risk of SUD. For cases of concurrent CD/APD and SUD, CD/APD always either preceded or coincided with the age of onset of SUD.

Thus, outcomes in late adolescence showed a worrisome pattern of negative outcomes among probands, despite a marked overall improvement in ADHD symptoms. The pattern aggregated persistent ADHD, CD/APD, and SUD in a predictable developmental sequence. Notably, the sequence did not suggest a direct link between ADHD and SUD, but rather an indirect link mediated by the development of CD/APD.

On a more positive note, there were no significant group differences in mood or anxiety disorders between probands and comparison participants.

Early Adulthood Outcomes (FU25)

In early adulthood, the rate of ADHD among probands dropped to approximately 5.7% (Mannuzza et al., 1993, 1998). As expected, the rate significantly differed from comparison participants (among whom ADHD was almost nonexistent, with approximately 0.6% prevalence).

The drop in both groups from rates in early adolescence is notable. The researchers pointed out that reliance on self-report in early adulthood possibly underestimated prevalence (diagnoses in late adolescence were established on the basis of self *or* parent report, i.e., criteria met on one or the other report was sufficient). The prevalence of ADHD at each follow-up point will be addressed further in the discussion.

As in late adolescence, probands also showed significantly higher rates of APD (approximately 14.8% vs. 2.4%) and SUD (approximately 14.2% vs. 4.2%) than comparison participants. Again, differences in SUDs were driven by drug rather than alcohol abuse.

Significant comorbidity occurred between APD and SUD. Probands with an APD were significantly more likely to develop an SUD, and there were no differences in rates of SUDs among probands who did *not* develop an APD vs. comparison subjects (who had a low rate of APD at approximately 2.5%). The rate of ADHD among probands was too low for meaningful analyses of persistent vs. remitted subgroups, but the data did show that probands with at least one continuing ADHD symptom were significantly more likely to have an APD or SUD than probands without any ADHD symptoms. This suggests that the association among persistent ADHD, APD, and SUD identified in late adolescence remains to some degree in adulthood. However, the fact that rates of APD and SUD were more than double the rate of ADHD in probands, also suggests that the negative outcomes of APD and SUD tend to develop in individuals with childhood-diagnosed ADHD regardless of the persistence/remittance of ADHD in adulthood.

Functional outcomes were also affected at FU25. Specifically, the educational and occupational achievements of probands appeared significantly compromised (Mannuzza, Klein, Bessler, Malloy, & Hynes, 1997; Mannuzza et al., 1993). Controlling for age and IQ, probands completed a little over two years *less* formal schooling than comparison participants. Moreover, only 3% of probands were enrolled in graduate school, whereas over 15% of comparison participants were enrolled. These disadvantages in education translated to disadvantages in occupational rank. Probands had significantly lower occupational rankings than comparisons, with significantly fewer probands holding professional positions, such as lawyers, scientists, accountants, and stockbrokers. A large proportion of probands were owners of small businesses. In contrast, the largest proportion of comparison participants were accountants and stockbrokers (Mannuzza et al., 1993). It could be argued that the prevalence of APD among probands might account for deficits in educational and occupational outcomes, given that individuals with APD are more likely to drop out of school and attain lower-ranking positions. Indeed, there was a significant negative correlation between APD and educational outcomes (formal schooling) and between APD and occupational rank. When a subgroup of probands without APD was examined alongside comparison participants, however, significant group differences remained in both educational and occupational outcomes, suggesting that childhood-diagnosed ADHD contributed to these disadvantages independent of the development of APD.

Overall, outcomes in early adulthood pointed to a continuation of the clinical patterns that emerged in adolescence, with accompanying functional deficits, despite a marked reduction in ADHD symptoms. The absence of group differences in mood or anxiety disorders between probands and comparison participants was also sustained.

Mid-adulthood Outcomes (FU41)

Psychiatric Disorders

In mid-adulthood, patterns of findings related to ongoing psychiatric disorders were similar to those in adolescence and early adulthood. ADHD was significantly more prevalent in probands (22.2%) than in comparison participants (5.1%) (Klein et al., 2012). Likewise, rates of APD significantly differed by group: 16.3% of probands but no comparison participant had APD. Alcohol disorders did not differ by group, but drug disorders did: Probands were three times more likely to have a nonalcoholic SUD than comparison participants. No group differences emerged in mood or anxiety disorders.

Ongoing ADHD was not significantly related to APD (unlike in adolescence and early adulthood), but was related to ongoing SUD—probands with ongoing ADHD were three times more likely to have a drug use disorder than probands without ADHD. Ongoing ADHD was also significantly associated with a co-occurrence of APD and SUD in probands.

Lifetime psychiatric disorders were examined in mid-adulthood. During their lifetime, probands had significantly higher rates of APD, nonalcoholic SUD, and nicotine dependence than comparison participants, but did not differ on lifetime alcohol use disorder or lifetime mood and anxiety disorders.

Notably, although the researchers had expected that childhood ADHD would be associated with an overall increased risk of adult-onset (age 21 years and over) psychiatric disorders (other than ADHD and APD, which required childhood onset), this was not the case. Probands were no more likely than comparison participants to incur new mental disorders as of age 21 years, although a trend ($p < .09$) was found for elevated mood disorders in probands (Klein et al., 2012). This excess in depressive disorders in probands was accounted for by the presence of SUD (unpublished data).

Educational, Occupational, and Social Outcomes

At FU41, probands had on average two and a half fewer years of schooling than comparison participants. Significantly more probands (31.1% vs. 4.4%) than comparisons failed to complete high school, and significantly fewer probands had bachelor's degrees (15.6% vs. 34.6%) and master's degrees or higher (3.7% vs. 29.4%) (Klein et al., 2012).

The group differences seen in educational attainment were also seen in occupational attainment: Probands showed significantly lower attainment on the Hollingshead occupational scale than comparison participants. Although most probands (83.7%) were employed, significantly fewer were employed than comparisons (94.9%), and their median salary was a striking $40,000 less than that of comparisons. Finally, although employed probands were evaluated as performing well ("average-to-good") on an occupational functioning scale, comparison participants had significantly superior evaluations ("good-to-very-good"). All of the above contributed to an overall lower socioeconomic status for probands (Klein et al., 2012).

Similarly, probands' mean overall social functioning was relatively worse than comparison participants: probands' ratings fell in the "average-to-good" range whereas comparison participants had "good-to-very-good" ratings. In terms of marital status, most probands and most comparisons participants were cohabitating with a spouse, but significantly more probands were currently divorced (9.6% vs. 2.9%) and had ever been divorced (31.1% vs. 11.8%) than comparison participants (Klein et al., 2012).

It could be argued that the greater prevalence of ongoing psychiatric disorders among probands explains their inferior occupational and social outcomes. Analyses among probands who did not meet criteria for any psychiatric disorders (32.6%), however, showed that they nevertheless had significantly worse social functioning but not worse occupational functioning (though there was a trend in that direction, $p < .07$). Thus, it seems that childhood ADHD predicts inferior adult outcomes in these functional domains even in the absence of current psychiatric disorders.

Criminality

There were significant differences in indicators of criminality between probands and comparison participants at mean age 38 years. Controlling for age, SES at FU25, and IQ at FU25, significantly more probands than comparison participants had been arrested (once, multiple times, because of an aggressive offense), charged with a felony, convicted, and incarcerated (Mannuzza et al., 2008). Age at first arrest did not differ.

Analyses were carried out on rates of multiple arrests to examine whether CD/APD and SUD identified at either FU18 or FU25 were significantly associated with criminality at or before FU25 (excluding criminality post-FU25 in order to equate the interval covered by psychiatric assessment and criminal history). Rates of multiple arrests were significantly greater in probands with APD than without (37% vs. 8%). Probands without APD did not differ from comparisons. The same relationship was found for SUD. Rates of multiple arrests were greater in probands with SUD than without (37% vs. 8%). Probands without SUD did not differ from comparisons. Regression analyses showed that APD and SUD were independent predictors of multiple arrests (i.e., APD stayed significant after controlling for SUD and vice versa).

Further analyses were carried out on the 29 probands who had all the negative outcomes of interest: APD, SUD, and had been arrested. Based on the ages at onset of APDs and SUDs and on the age at first arrest, three different developmental sequences were observed. APD preceded[2] SUD, which preceded first arrest in the majority of the cases (69%). In the remaining cases, the following patterns appeared: APD developed around the same time as SUD, and both preceded the first arrest; APD preceded SUD, which developed around the time as the first arrest; or APD preceded the first arrest, which preceded SUD. Notably, in no cases did APD develop after SUD.

In sum, considering the above with findings from adolescence and early adulthood, the previously identified pattern of childhood ADHD leading to the development of CD/APD and SUD can be extended to lead to the more serious outcome of criminal behavior.

Obesity

At FU41, probands had significantly higher mean BMIs (30.1 vs. 27.6) and obesity rates (41.1% vs. 21.6%) than comparison participants (Cortese, Ramos Olazagasti et al., 2013). These differences remained significant after adjusting for SES and lifetime mental disorders. Persistent (N = 24) versus remitted (N = 87) probands did not differ significantly in BMI or obesity rates. However, after adjusting for SES and lifetime mental disorders, contrary to expectations, remitted probands had significantly higher BMI (30.4 vs. 27.6) and obesity rates (44.8% vs. 29.2%). Thus, children diagnosed with ADHD are at increased risk of obesity as adults, even if their ADHD symptoms eventually normalize.

Risk-taking

Over their lifetime, probands engaged in significantly more risky driving and risky sex than comparison participants (Ramos Olazagasti et al., 2013). Moreover, at FU41, probands engaged in significantly more risky driving in the past five years, but not more risky sex in the past year.

2. In all these sequences, "preceded" signifies the event (onset of disorder or first arrest) occurred at least 1 year earlier.

Probands were more likely to have been judged at fault in two or more driving accidents, and to have been involved in two or more accidents resulting in injury.

Structural Equation Modeling (SEM) was used to test for the direct effect of ADHD on risky behaviors (risky driving and risky sex), the direct effect of CD/APD on risky behaviors, and the indirect effect of ADHD on risky behaviors through the development of CD/APD. As expected, lifetime CD/APD had a direct effect on risky behaviors. There was also a significant *indirect* effect of childhood ADHD on risky behaviors through the development of CD/APD. Importantly, there was no direct effect of ADHD on risky behaviors once CD/APD was accounted for (Ramos Olazagasti et al., 2013).

Medical Outcomes, Hospitalizations, and Mortality

Significantly more probands had three or more emergency department admissions (37% vs. 21%) and reported having had a head injury (9% vs. 3%) than comparison participants (Ramos Olazagasti et al., 2013). Emergency admissions were related to risky driving reported above, but head injuries were not. Rates of STDs were also significantly higher in probands than in comparisons (15% vs. 7%). Further analyses showed that use of birth control did not predict STDs, but greater number of sexual partners did.

Other medical conditions did not significantly differ between groups. Importantly, for probands who had been included in stimulant treatment studies in childhood (N = 182 of 207), no association was found between total cumulative stimulant dosage and cardiovascular disease (Ramos Olazagasti et al., 2013).

Significantly more probands than comparison participants (24.4% vs. 6.6%) had been hospitalized in psychiatric facilities (Klein et al., 2012). Moreover, of those hospitalized, probands had more repeated psychiatric hospitalizations than comparison participants. In both groups, most psychiatric hospitalizations were related to substance abuse. There was no difference between groups in rates of nonpsychiatric hospitalizations (Ramos Olazagasti et al., 2013).

A significantly greater proportion of probands were deceased (N = 15 of 207 or 7%) than comparisons (N = 5 of 178, or 3%) (Klein et al., 2012). Deaths of probands were less often related to identified medical conditions than deaths of comparison participants (Ramos Olazagasti et al., 2013). Of the 15 deaths of probands, only four were related to identified physical conditions: two died of cancer, one of cardiac arrest, and one of diabetic coma. Of the 11 remaining, three died of suicide, one of alcohol/drug overdose, two of homicide, two of occupational deaths, one was hit by a car, one fell from a roof, and one cause of death was unknown. Of the 5 deaths of comparison participants, three were related to identified medical conditions: two died of cancer, one of AIDS. Of the remaining two, one died of alcohol/drug overdose, and one died in the 9/11 terrorist attacks.

Brain Imaging

At FU41, gray matter and white matter deficits were tested in a number of participants who consented to undergo brain scans. Findings indicated that the cortex was significantly thinner in probands than in comparison participants in the dorsal attentional network and limbic areas (Proal et al., 2011). In addition, gray matter was significantly decreased in probands in the right caudate, right thalamus, and bilateral cerebellar hemispheres. These regions underpin top-down control of attention and regulation of emotion and motivation. Probands with persistent ADHD in adulthood (N = 17) did not differ significantly from those with remitted ADHD in adulthood (N = 26) when results were corrected using a false discovery rate. At uncorrected $p < .05$, remitters had thicker cortex relative to persisters in the medial occipital cortex, insula, parahippocampus, and prefrontal regions, suggesting that diagnostic remission may result from compensatory maturation of these regions.

Probands also exhibited significantly lower fractional anisotropy (FA) than comparisons in the right superior and posterior corona radiata, right superior longitudinal fasciculus, and in a left cluster including the posterior thalamic radiation, the retrolenticular part of the internal capsule, and the sagittal stratum (Cortese, Imperati et al., 2013). These white matter tracts connect regions involved in high-level as well as sensorimotor functions, suggesting that both types of processes are involved in the pathophysiology of ADHD. Persisting and remitted probands did not differ significantly in FA related to any of the above white matter tracts. These findings were argued to support the interpretation that changes in white matter might represent a stable neurobiological trait independent of remission.

PREDICTORS

The findings summarized above outline the lifelong disadvantages that can stem from a childhood diagnosis of ADHD, even in the case of eventual syndromic remittance. However, the findings also show that not all children diagnosed with ADHD grow up to experience these disadvantages. Box 3.2 contains excerpts from clinical case summaries at FU41 of the same three probands described earlier in Box 3.1.

In childhood, Rob, Francis, and Adam's parents and teachers described them in very similar ways, presenting symptoms of distractibility, inattention, hyperactivity, and impulsivity across settings. In adulthood, however, there appeared clear variability in functioning and impairment. Rob seemed to have gotten by adequately, achieving relative success in educational, occupational, and social domains. However, residual symptoms of inattention, impulsivity, and hyperactivity continued to hamper him—to the point of his seeking renewed treatment for them. Francis appeared fully remitted, showing no signs of his earlier symptoms or impairment, and functioning at superior levels in the educational, occupational, and social domains. His case illustrates an optimal developmental course despite his early childhood symptoms and impairment. In contrast, the case of Adam illustrates a particularly detrimental developmental course. Symptoms of inattention, distractibility, and impulsivity clearly persisted and impaired both his personal and professional functioning. Frequent interpersonal conflicts indicated antisocial tendencies, which spiraled into heavy alcohol and drug use, and criminality. His course incurred negative outcomes both for himself and those around

Box 3.2 **CASE PRESENTATIONS AT THE FINAL ADULT FOLLOW-UP (FU41)**

Rob, age 39 years

Rob has a Bachelor's of Science in Education and Psychology. He has had a stable work history in business, has been promoted consistently, and is now a regional manager. He has been married nine years, spends his free time with his wife and two children, and has maintained contact with close friends. He enjoys sporting events and golf. His work and marriage are very good.

Rob states that he is "addicted" to nicotine (30/day), and has experienced difficulty with tasks requiring concentration. Because of his poor concentration, he has to write everything down. His family complains that he does not listen, leading to arguments. "I have difficulty organizing." He frequently loses things and is very distractible and impatient. "I want people to get to the point . . . I have little tolerance for bullshit." He argues frequently with people who do not do their job. He always likes to be on the go, "I'm hyper; I can't sit still." He has had complaints that he talks too much. At age 34, he decided to seek treatment for "my ADHD."

Francis, age 41 years

According to Francis, his problems with hyperactivity, inattention, and impulsivity remitted at age 14. His academic performance was superb in junior high and high school; he was a member of the honor society, obtained science awards, attended advanced placement courses, and so on. His social functioning was also excellent; he had several friends, had an exclusive relationship, was a member of sports teams, and so forth. Francis was accepted to several colleges. After college, he completed medical training at prestigious institutions. He was considered a "model employee" and never had any problems with patients or coworkers.

At age 41, Francis has been happily married for 14 years, has two children, and is working as a physician at a medical center. Francis spends most of his leisure time with his wife and children; they regularly entertain in their home. He is a member of a tennis team, and serves as a coach for one of his children's team. He reports liking his job and the people he works with, and he feels very satisfied with his life.

Adam, age 46 years

Adam completed 3.5 years of college as an accounting major. He started a business, which he sold four years later. He worked in his father's business for 18 years but was fired for stealing large sums. He spent the money on drugs and travel for two years. Since then, he has held numerous jobs as a cook, typically staying an average of six months, then "I get sick of working."

Adam has been married for 18 years and has three sons. He states that he has no close friends, that his wife is his best friend. He has great difficulty staying on tasks: "My mind wanders . . . I can't read books, only magazines." He does not follow through on instructions, which he forgets. He fails to complete tasks, starts 10 things at the same time and cannot finish one: "I start one thing and my brain jumps to something else." He has a tendency to act impulsively, going on trips "out of the blue," and buying things: "I like it, I'm buying it." He is very impatient; for example, when others are speaking, he interrupts, talks out of turn, and acts exasperated, which leads to conflicts at home and work.

Adam started drinking daily at age 22. From ages 31 to 36, he drank heavily through the day. This led to multiple problems related to alcohol and alcohol withdrawal. His alcohol use then escalated to cocaine use. He became depressed and attempted suicide. He was selling drugs, failed to pay his mortgage, which led to his home being foreclosed. He stole money from his father. He stole and sold his wife's ring to get money for drugs and has written bad checks. He has been arrested six times (including for driving with a suspended license, possession of marijuana, spousal abuse, and grand theft). He has thrown things at his wife and many people complained that he placed his children in dangerous situations (e.g., having them where he got and used drugs).

At age 43, he and his wife (also a drug abuser) went to a rehabilitation program. He has not used drugs in the past two years. He now lives in his parents' or friends' homes.

him, and a substantial cost to society given his unemployment, criminal record, and need for rehabilitation.

Longitudinal studies have attempted to identify early childhood factors that can help predict developmental courses, but this has proven difficult because of the multiplicity of genetic and environmental factors that can influence outcome, and because of the large power required to identify stable predictors while controlling for multiple comparisons. In the New York Study, Mannuzza et al. (1990) analyzed various childhood factors (childhood IQ, childhood parental SES, etc.) to see if they could significantly predict outcomes at FU18, but none remained significant after controlling for multiple comparisons.

The most salient predictive pathway that emerged over the course of the study involves the development of Conduct Disorder and/or Antisocial Personality Disorder (CD/APD). In late adolescence, the persistence of ADHD was related to the development of CD/APD, which, in turn, was related to Substance Use Disorder (SUD). The development of CD/APD almost entirely accounted for the relationship between ongoing ADHD and SUD. In early adulthood, despite a drop in ongoing ADHD, probands still showed high rates of (often comorbid) APD and SUD. Thus, CD/APD and SUD developed while ADHD persisted in adolescence, and then continued in adulthood even as ADHD remitted. Analyses of ages of onset confirmed that the most common developmental sequence in comorbid cases was ADHD → CP/APD → SUD. In later adulthood, criminality was added as a negative outcome to that developmental chain. That is, probands were at increased risk of criminal behavior, but only if they developed APD or SUD in adolescence. Similarly, probands showed increased propensity for risk-taking behaviors (risky driving and risky sexual behavior), but the development of APD fully mediated that effect.

The finding that children with ADHD are at increased risk for developing conduct and antisocial personality disorders has been supported by many other follow-up studies (Barkley, Fischer, Smallish, & Fletcher, 2004; Biederman et al., 1996; Weiss & Hechtman, 1993).

The particular effect of CD/APD as a mediator of the development of SUD has also been supported by several population studies (August et al., 2006; Cadoret & Stewart, 1991; Elkins, McGue, & Iacono, 2007; Fergusson, Horwood, & Ridder, 2007; Flory & Lynam, 2003). In these latter studies, and in the New York Study at FU18, ADHD did not significantly predict SUD once CD/APD was accounted for. Other studies, however, find both a direct and indirect effect (through APD) of ADHD on later SUD (see review in Molina & Pelham, 2014). In the New York Study at FU41, there was a weak but significant direct association between ongoing ADHD and SUD. The researchers cautioned, however, that interpretation of associations between ongoing adult ADHD and SUD is not always straightforward given the behavioral effects of some recreational drugs that can mimic ADHD symtoms (Klein et al., 2012).

Overall, the consistency of findings showing the detrimental effects of the development of CD/APD for children diagnosed with ADHD highlights the importance of early intervention to interrupt the cascade of symptoms into a negative developmental course. The fact that most children with ADHD who had developed CD/APD at FU18 did not have APD at FU41 (only about one quarter persisted into adulthood) shows that earlier dysfunctions can attenuate, and, thus, developmental courses can change.

DISCUSSION

Conduct Disorder/Antisocial Personality Disorder Comorbidity

A major issue that has undermined other studies' (e.g., Barkley et al., 2004; Satterfield & Schell, 1997) conclusions about the mediating role of CD/APD in the development of downstream negative outcomes for children with ADHD, is whether the children already had CD in childhood, which later developed into APD, which then produced the other negative outcomes. This possible confound was largely circumvented in the New York

Study by screening out children with potential CD at referral. Evidence for the success of this screening process is presented in Mannuzza et al. (1993). The authors argued that two important implications follow. The first is that “relatively pure” childhood ADHD (i.e., uncomplicated by childhood CD) predisposes to the outcomes summarized in this chapter. The second implication is that this study’s conclusions may actually represent an underestimation of the downstream difficulties encountered by “typical” children with ADHD; both community and clinic studies have shown that the rate of comorbid CD among children with ADHD can be quite high (August & Stewart, 1982; Szatmari, Boyle, & Offord, 1989). Thus, the children in this study may have had a “milder form” of dysfunction than most children with ADHD. However, a recent follow-up study—the Multimodal Treatment Study of Children with ADHD (MTA)—found lower rates of comorbid childhood CD and ADHD, around 14% (The MTA Cooperative Group, 1999), and the teacher-rated hyperactivity factor score for that study was 1.82 whereas the same score in the New York Study was 2.11. Thus, the New York sample may be somewhat comparable to other samples. Nonetheless, the screening out of CD at referral in this study substantiates the argument that ADHD itself predisposes to later CD/APD, SUD, and other negative outcomes. The early and sustained treatment of ADHD itself should thus be the locus of intervention when possible.

Attention Deficit Hyperactivity Disorder Prevalence

As with other long-term follow-up studies of ADHD, perhaps the most important finding concerned the persistence of the disorder well past adolescence into adulthood. Each type (combined, predominantly inattentive, and predominantly hyperactive/impulsive) was equally prevalent in adulthood, though it has been argued that types in adulthood are less clinically meaningful (Barkley, Murphy, & Fischer, 2008). However, the rates at FU18, FU25, and FU41 followed an unexpected pattern—dipping to a low at FU25, and then surging again at FU41. Several explanations for this are possible. First, as mentioned earlier, the sharp decrease from FU18 to FU25 might partially be attributed to the change in assessment procedure from using two informants at FU18 (self and parent, using an either/or rule for diagnosis) to using self-report only at FU25. The two-informant (using either/or rule) procedure is liable to yield higher rates of pathology because of the greater opportunity to prompt reports of dysfunction from separate informants. Nevertheless, an actual decrease in dysfunction also likely contributed to the decrease in prevalence from FU18 to FU25. More surprising was the resurgence in prevalence from FU25 (5.7% in probands vs. 0.6% in comparisons) to FU41 (22.2% in probands vs. 5.1% in comparisons). The researchers pointed to the change from DSM-III-R at FU25 to DSM-IV at FU41 as a possible reason, given evidence that higher rates of ADHD have been reported using DSM-IV than DSM-III-R (Faraone, Sergeant, Gillberg, & Biederman, 2003), but downplayed this possibility based on analyses that showed that the rate at FU25 would have increased by only about 2% in probands if DSM-IV criteria had been used (Klein et al., 2012). More likely factors may be the increased media coverage of ADHD leading to either incorrect self-identification or accurate recognition/recall of childhood dysfunction (Hallowell & Ratey, 1994), or the fact that levels of inattention, hyperactivity, and impulsivity increase in acuteness later in life with increasing expectations of responsibility, wherein these adults might reinterpret their earlier histories in light of their ongoing difficulties. Comparisons of prevalence rates in other follow-up studies, should they eventually follow participants into their forties and fifties, will be informative on this account. Increases in self-reported ADHD over time in younger adults have also been reported by Barkley et al. (2008).

Strengths of the Study

The New York Study had many design strengths as an outcomes study in that it was prospective, included appropriate controls, employed specific selection criteria, had an adequate sample size at its origin, showed minimal attrition in the first two follow-up intervals, obtained data from multiple sources in childhood and late adolescence, and relied on assessments that were conducted blind to group membership. The outcomes assessed were selected to be informative, valid, and sensitive to the developmental stages of the participants. The replication of findings at FU18 and FU25 from independent samples is also a strength, given the multitude of factors beyond an investigator's control that could invalidate findings from a single sample (e.g., cohort effects, interviewer effects, comparison group characteristics, etc.).

Limitations of the Study

The sample was limited to white men of average intelligence who were referred to a psychiatric clinic because of a presentation that corresponded to combined-type ADHD. Thus, the findings should not be generalized to women, other ethnic groups, and predominantly inattentive ADHD presentations.

Limitations in terms of retention and characteristics of comparison participants could have inflated the relative dysfunction of adult probands. Specifically, comparison participants lost to follow-up at FU41 had lower IQs than those assessed, and tended to have lower SES and more previous drug-related disorders (Klein et al., 2012).

Also at FU41, 31.8% of living probands were lost to follow-up. Those lost did not seem to differ from those retained in terms of previously measured characteristics, but it is always possible that the group lost to follow-up fared better or worse on outcomes at FU41 than the group retained (e.g., they did not want to participate to avoid reporting how badly they were doing, or perhaps were doing very well and did not want to be reminded of previous difficulties).

Finally, as mentioned earlier, the shift in procedure from using two informants at FU18 to using only self-report at FU25 and FU41 is a limitation given the well-documented weaknesses of self-report-based assessments of ADHD (Barkley et al., 2008).

SUMMARY AND CONCLUSIONS

This prospective study followed white male boys diagnosed with ADHD at a mean age of eight years and free of Conduct Disorder into their fourth and fifth decades of life. Compared with peers without ADHD, probands showed greater persistence of ADHD, along with greater prevalence of CD/APD and SUD in late adolescence. These dysfunctions continued into early adulthood, even when ADHD remitted for the majority of the sample, and were associated with deficits in educational and occupational attainment, leading to a relative economic disadvantage. Furthermore, the disproportionally high rate of CD/APD and SUD in probands versus comparison participants translated to significantly higher rates of criminality, risk-taking behavior, and risk-related medical outcomes in adulthood. Probands also showed elevated obesity rates in relation to comparison participants, but no differences in mood or anxiety disorders. Brain imagery studies extended the group differences to the neurobiological level—showing differences in areas of the brain related to both top-down control of attention, regulation of emotion, motivation, and bottom-up sensorimotor functions.

There is heterogeneity in the clinical and functional outcomes of children with ADHD. This study's findings show that childhood ADHD does not preclude superior functioning in various life domains. It does predispose, however, to maladjustment in adolescence and adulthood in a subset of these children, particularly those who develop CD/APD early on.

REFERENCES

American Psychiatric Association. (2013). *Diagnostic and Statistical Manual of Mental Disorders: DSM-5*. Washington, DC: American Psychiatric Association.

American Psychiatric Association. (1968). *Diagnostic and Statistical Manual of Mental Disorders* (2nd ed.). Washington, DC: The Association.

Anderson, C. M., & Plymate, H. B. (1962). Management of the brain-damaged adolescent. *American Journal of Orthopsychiatry*, *32*(3), 492–500.

August, G. J., & Stewart, M. A. (1982). Is there a syndrome of pure hyperactivity? *The British Journal of Psychiatry: The Journal of Mental Science, 140*, 305–311.

August, G. J., Winters, K. C., Realmuto, G. M., Fahnhorst, T., Botzet, A., & Lee, S. (2006). Prospective study of adolescent drug use among community samples of ADHD and non-ADHD participants. *Journal of the American Academy of Child and Adolescent Psychiatry, 45*(7), 824–832.

Barkley, R. A., Fischer, M., Smallish, L., & Fletcher, K. (2004). Young adult follow-up of hyperactive children: antisocial activities and drug use. *Journal of Child Psychology and Psychiatry, and Allied Disciplines, 45*(2), 195–211.

Barkley, R. A., Murphy, K. R., & Fischer, M. (2008). *ADHD in Adults: What the Science Says*. New York: Guilford Press.

Biederman, J., Faraone, S. V., Milberger, S., Jetton, J. G., Chen, L., Mick, E., . . . Russell, R. L. (1996). Is childhood oppositional defiant disorder a precursor to adolescent conduct disorder? Findings from a four-year follow-up study of children with ADHD. *Journal of the American Academy of Child and Adolescent Psychiatry, 35*(9), 1193–1204.

Cadoret, R. J., & Stewart, M. A. (1991). An adoption study of attention deficit/hyperactivity, aggression and their relationship to adult antisocial personality. *Comprehensive Psychiatry, 32*(1), 73–82.

Conners, C. K. (1969). A teacher rating scale for use in drug studies with children. *The American Journal of Psychiatry, 126*(6), 884–888.

Cortese, S., Imperati, D., Zhou, J., Proal, E., Klein, R. G., Mannuzza, S., . . . Castellanos, F. X. (2013). White matter alterations at 33-year follow-up in adults with childhood attention-deficit/hyperactivity disorder. *Biological Psychiatry, 74*(8), 591–598.

Cortese, S., Ramos Olazagasti, M. A., Klein, R. G., Castellanos, F. X., Proal, E., & Mannuzza, S. (2013). Obesity in men with childhood ADHD: a 33-year controlled, prospective, follow-up study. *Pediatrics, 131*(6), e1731–e1738.

Elkins, I. J., McGue, M., & Iacono, W. G. (2007). Prospective effects of attention-deficit/hyperactivity disorder, conduct disorder, and sex on adolescent substance use and abuse. *Archives of General Psychiatry, 64*(10), 1145–1152.

Faraone, S. V., Sergeant, J., Gillberg, C., & Biederman, J. (2003). The worldwide prevalence of ADHD: Is it an American condition? *World Psychiatry: Official Journal of the World Psychiatric Association (WPA), 2*(2), 104–113.

Fergusson, D. M., Horwood, L. J., & Ridder, E. M. (2007). Conduct and attentional problems in childhood and adolescence and later substance use, abuse and dependence: results of a 25-year longitudinal study. *Drug and Alcohol Dependence, 88* (Suppl 1), S14–S26.

Flory, K., & Lynam, D. R. (2003). The relation between attention deficit hyperactivity disorder and substance abuse: what role does conduct disorder play? *Clinical Child and Family Psychology Review, 6*(1), 1–16.

Gittelman-Klein, R., Klein, D. F., Katz, S., Saraf, K., & Pollack, E. (1976). Comparative effects of methylphenidate and thioridazine in hyperkinetic children. I. Clinical results. *Archives of General Psychiatry, 33*(10), 1217–1231.

Gittelman, R., Abikoff, H., Pollack, E., Klein, D. F., Katz, S., & Mattes, J. A. (1980). A controlled trial of behavior modification and methylphenidate in hyperactive children. In *Hyperactive Children: The Social Ecology of Identification and Treatment* (pp. 221–243). Orlando, FL: Academic Press, Inc.

Gittelman, R., Mannuzza, S., Shenker, R., & Bonagura, N. (1985). Hyperactive boys almost grown up. I. Psychiatric status. *Archives of General Psychiatry, 42*(10), 937–947.

Hallowell, E. M., & Ratey, J. J. (1994). *Driven to Distraction: Recognizing and Coping with Attention Deficit Disorder from Childhood through Adulthood.* New York: Pantheon.

Hollingshead, A., & Redlich, F. (1958). Social Class and Mental Illness: A Community Study. New York: John Wiley & Sons, Inc.

Klein, R. G., & Mannuzza, S. (1991). Long-term outcome of hyperactive children: a review. *Journal of the American Academy of Child and Adolescent Psychiatry, 30*(3), 383–387.

Klein, R. G., Mannuzza, S., Olazagasti, M. A. R., Roizen, E., Hutchison, J. A., Lashua, E. C., & Castellanos, F. X. (2012). Clinical and functional outcome of childhood attention- deficit/hyperactivity disorder 33 years later. *Archives of General Psychiatry, 69*(12), 1295–1303.

Lange, K. W., Reichl, S., Lange, K. M., Tucha, L., & Tucha, O. (2010). The history of attention deficit hyperactivity disorder. *Attention Deficit and Hyperactivity Disorders, 2*(4), 241–255.

Laufer, M. W. (1962). Cerebral dysfunction and behavior disorders in adolescents. *The American Journal of Orthopsychiatry, 32*, 501–506.

Mannuzza, S., Castellanos, F. X., Roizen, E. R., Hutchison, J. A., Lashua, E. C., & Klein, R. G. (2011). Impact of the impairment criterion in the diagnosis of adult ADHD: 33-year follow-up study of boys with ADHD. *Journal of Attention Disorders, 15*(2), 122–129.

Mannuzza, S., & Gittelman, R. (1984). The adolescent outcome of hyperactive girls. *Psychiatry Research, 13*(1), 19–29.

Mannuzza, S., Klein, R. G., Abikoff, H., & Moulton, J. L. (2004). Significance of childhood conduct problems to later development of conduct disorder among children with ADHD: a prospective follow-up study. *Journal of Abnormal Child Psychology, 32*(5), 565–573.

Mannuzza, S., Klein, R. G., Bessler, A., Malloy, P., & Hynes, M. E. (1997). Educational and occupational outcome of hyperactive boys grown up. *Journal of the American Academy of Child and Adolescent Psychiatry, 36*(9), 1222–1227.

Mannuzza, S., Klein, R. G., Bessler, A., Malloy, P., & LaPadula, M. (1993). Adult outcome of hyperactive boys. Educational achievement, occupational rank, and psychiatric status. *Archives of General Psychiatry, 50*(7), 565–576.

Mannuzza, S., Klein, R. G., Bessler, A., Malloy, P., & LaPadula, M. (1998). Adult psychiatric status of hyperactive boys grown up. *The American Journal of Psychiatry, 155*(4), 493–498.

Mannuzza, S., Klein, R. G., Bonagura, N., Malloy, P., Giampino, T. L., & Addalli, K. A. (1991). Hyperactive boys almost grown up. V. Replication of psychiatric status. *Archives of General Psychiatry, 48*(1), 77–83.

Mannuzza, S., Klein, R. G., Konig, P. H., & Giampino, T. L. (1989). Hyperactive boys almost grown up. IV. Criminality and its relationship to psychiatric status. *Archives of General Psychiatry, 46*(12), 1073–1079.

Mannuzza, S., Klein, R. G., & Moulton, J. L. (2008). Lifetime criminality among boys with attention deficit hyperactivity disorder: a prospective follow-up study into adulthood using official arrest records. *Psychiatry Research, 160*(3), 237–246.

Mannuzza, S., Konig, P. H., & Giampino, T. L. (1990). Childhood predictors of psychiatric status in the young adulthood of hyperactive boys: a study controlling for chance associations. In *Straight and Devious Pathways from Childhood to Adulthood* (pp. 279–299). New York: Cambridge University Press.

Molina, B. S. G., & Pelham, W. E. (2014). Attention-deficit/hyperactivity disorder and risk of substance use disorder: developmental considerations, potential pathways, and opportunities for research. *Annual Review of Clinical Psychology, 10,* 607–639.

Nadeau, K. G., Littman, E. B., & Quinn, P. O. (1999). *Understanding Girls with AD/HD.* Silver Spring, MD: Advantage Books.

Proal, E., Reiss, P. T., Klein, R. G., Mannuzza, S., Gotimer, K., Ramos-Olazagasti, M. A., . . . Castellanos, F. X. (2011). Brain gray matter deficits at 33-year follow-up in adults with attention-deficit/hyperactivity disorder established in childhood. *Archives of General Psychiatry, 68*(11), 1122–1134.

Ramos Olazagasti, M. A., Klein, R. G., Mannuzza, S., Belsky, E. R., Hutchison, J. A., Lashua- Shriftman, E. C., & Castellanos, F. X. (2013). Does childhood attention-deficit/hyperactivity disorder predict risk-taking and medical illnesses in adulthood? *Journal of the American Academy of Child and Adolescent Psychiatry, 52*(2), 153–162.e4.

Satterfield, J., & Cantwell, D. (1975). Psychopharmacology in the prevention of antisocial and delinquent behavior. In *Recent Advances on Child Psychopharmacology* (pp. 227–237). New York: Human Sciences Press.

Satterfield, J. H., & Schell, A. (1997). A prospective study of hyperactive boys with conduct problems and normal boys: adolescent and adult criminality. *Journal of the American Academy of Child and Adolescent Psychiatry, 36*(12), 1726–1735.

Sibley, M. H., Pelham, W. E., Molina, B. S. G., Coxe, S., Kipp, H., Gnagy, E. M., . . . Lahey, B. B. (2014). The role of early childhood ADHD and subsequent CD in the initiation and escalation of adolescent cigarette, alcohol, and marijuana use. *Journal of Abnormal Psychology, 123*(2), 362–374.

Szatmari, P., Boyle, M., & Offord, D. R. (1989). ADDH and conduct disorder: degree of diagnostic overlap and differences among correlates. *Journal of the American Academy of Child and Adolescent Psychiatry, 28*(6), 865–872.

The MTA Cooperative Group. Multimodal Treatment Study of Children with ADHD. (1999). A 14-month randomized clinical trial of treatment strategies for attention- deficit/hyperactivity disorder. *Archives of General Psychiatry, 56*(12), 1073–1086.

Wechsler, D. (1949). *Wechsler Intelligence Scale for Children.* New York: The Psychological Corporation.

Wechsler, D. (1974). *Manual for the Wechsler Intelligence Scale for Children—Revised.* New York: The Psychological Corporation.

Weiss, G., & Hechtman, L. T. (1993). *Hyperactive Children Grown Up: ADHD in Children, Adolescents, and Adults.* New York: Guilford Press.

Werry, J., & Sprague, R. (1970). Hyperactivity. In *Symptoms of Psychopathology* (pp. 397–417). New York: John Wiley & Sons.

4

The Milwaukee Longitudinal Study of Hyperactive (ADHD) Children

RUSSELL A. BARKLEY AND MARIELLEN FISCHER

At the time the Milwaukee study was initiated, attention deficit hyperactivity disorder (ADHD) was known as hyperactive child syndrome, hyperkinesis, or hyperkinetic disorder of childhood (in *Diagnostic and Statistical Manual of Mental Disorders* [DSM-II], American Psychiatric Association, 1968; see Barkley, 2015—History). Despite the term focusing on excessive motor activity, the diagnosis also included symptoms of inattention, distractibility, and impulsiveness. Children so identified, in most cases, would today meet DSM-5 criteria for ADHD-Combined Presentation (American Psychiatric Association, 2013). Begun in 1979 with grant funding from the National Institute of Mental Health, the study initially was not intended to be a follow-up study of hyperactive children but rather an intensive study of mother–child interactions and the effects of age and stimulant medication (methylphenidate) on those interactions (see Barkley, Karlsson, Strzelecki, & Murphy, 1984; Barkley, Karlsson, & Pollard, 1985; Barkley,

Karlsson, Pollard, & Murphy, 1985). By the time the studies were completed, however, several factors led to it becoming such a longitudinal study: (1) the sample sizes were substantial enough to warrant doing so, allowing for attrition; (2) there were no follow-up studies of hyperactive children into adolescence that had so intensively studied parent–child interactions and how they may have contributed to the adolescent outcome of these children; (3) no prior study had utilized such rigorous research diagnostic criteria for case identification; and (4) only three prior longitudinal studies of sizeable samples of North American children with hyperactivity and control children had been published by the early 1980s (New York, Iowa, and Montreal). Those were in addition to the Swedish longitudinal study by Gillberg and colleagues of children with disorders of attention, motor, and perceptual abilities (DAMP) that had some relevance to understanding the adolescent outcomes of hyperactive children (Rasmussen & Gillberg, 2001). There was thus ample need in the field for further study of the life course risks and outcomes of hyperactive children.

This chapter discusses the most important results of this project, including efforts to identify predictors of outcomes for the hyperactive (ADHD) children. It is largely adapted from the book, which provides a more thorough presentation and discussion of these findings from the age of 27 years (and final) follow-up (Barkley, Murphy, & Fischer, 2008). That book permitted us to contrast the results for ADHD children followed to adulthood with large samples of clinically referred adults subsequently diagnosed with ADHD in adulthood and two control groups (clinical, community) where both studies had used the same or similar measures. Because of the numerous measures collected and the number of follow-up points in the longitudinal study, it is impossible to present all of our findings within the page limitations required for this chapter. We have, therefore, selected for emphasis here only results from the last follow-up point and even then for the most important domains of functioning in major life activities.

FOLLOW-UP TIMELINE AND PARTICIPATION

This study initially evaluated a group rigorously diagnosed as hyperactive in childhood (N = 158) along with a matched community control group (N = 81) followed concurrently. These two groups were originally evaluated in 1979–1980 when they were ages 4 to 12 years. The majority of these participants (Hyperactive N = 123, or 78%; Normal N = 66, or 81%) were then re-evaluated in 1987–1988 when they were 12 to 20 years of age, having a mean age of 15 (see Barkley, Fischer, Edelbrock, & Smallish, 1990, 1991; Fischer, Barkley, Edelbrock, & Smallish, 1990; Fischer, Barkley, Fletcher, & Smallish, 1993a; Fischer et al., 1993b; Fletcher, Fischer, Barkley, & Smallish, 1996). The participants were reassessed in 1992–1996 when they were at least 19 years of age or older (ages 19–25 years of age, mean = 21 years) (see Barkley, Fischer, Smallish, & Fletcher, 2002, 2004, 2006; Barkley, Smith, Fischer, & Navia, 2006; Fischer & Barkley, 2006; Fischer, Barkley, Smallish, & Fletcher, 2002, 2005, 2007; Smith, Bauer, Fischer, Barkley, & Navia, 2005). The participation rate at that follow-up was 93% (147 of 158) for the hyperactive group and 90% (73 of 81) for controls. For the final follow-up (at a mean age of 27), 135 of the original hyperactive participants agreed to participate (85%), as did 75 of the original 81 control participants (93%); an excellent rate of participation across an 18+ year span (see Barkley et al., 2008). Two control and three hyperactive participants had died by the final follow-up.

PARTICIPANT SELECTION CRITERIA

At childhood entry into the study, all participants were required to: (1) have an IQ greater than 80, (2) be free of gross sensory or motor abnormalities, and (3) be the biological offspring of their current mothers or have been adopted by them shortly after birth. The original sex composition was 91% male and 9% female. The racial composition was 94% White, 5% Black, and 1% Hispanic. The hyperactive group originally was recruited from consecutive referrals to a child neuropsychology service specializing in the treatment of hyperactive children at Milwaukee Children's Hospital. The community control children were recruited using a "snowball" technique in which the parents of the hyperactive children were asked to provide the names of their friends who had children within the age range of interest to the study. These friends of the parents then were contacted about the study, further screened, and finally selected for evaluation. At that time, the parents were asked about other friends of theirs who had children and these families then were contacted to participate and so on.

Empirically based diagnostic criteria were not available at the time these children were recruited; just the DSM-II. Based upon research and conceptual statements in the field at the time, Barkley developed research criteria for identifying hyperactive children and these were employed at the study entry (see Barkley, 1982). To be considered hyperactive, the children had to: (1) have scores on both the Hyperactivity Index of the Revised Conners Parent Rating Scale—Revised (CPRS-R; Goyette, Conners, & Ulrich, 1978) and the Werry-Weiss-Peters Activity Rating Scale (WWPARS, see Barkley, 1981) that met or exceeded two standard deviations above the mean for severity for same age, same sex normal children; (2) have scores on the Home Situations Questionnaire (HSQ; Barkley, 1990) indicating significant pervasiveness of behavioral problems in at least 6 or more of the 14 problem situations on this scale (a score exceeding +1 SD); (3) have parent and/or teacher complaints (as reported by parent) of poor sustained attention, poor impulse control, and excessive activity level; (4) have developed their behavior problems prior to 6 years of age; (5) have had their behavioral problems for at least 12 months; and (6) have no indication of autism, psychosis, thought disorder, epilepsy, gross brain damage, or mental retardation. The use of the Conners and Werry scales made this study the first to include quantitatively based diagnostic criteria in follow-up research on hyperactive children. Supporting the fact that such criteria currently would select children with ADHD according to DSM criteria, over 70% of the hyperactive cases met those criteria for ADHD 8–10 years later at the adolescent follow-up (Barkley, Fischer et al., 1990). Therefore, we will regard these participants as ADHD in childhood for this chapter.

Eligibility for the community control group was based on: (1) no history of referral to a mental health professional; (2) no current parental or teacher complaints of significant behavioral problems; (3) scores within 1.5 standard deviations of the mean for normal children on both the Hyperactivity Index of the CPRS-R and the WWPARS; and (4) no evidence of any other psychiatric disorder.

Dependent Measures

Several hundred scores from numerous measures of outcomes have been collected on these cases across all follow-up points. For the final follow-up all participants completed a battery of measures that assessed psychiatric disorders, history of mental health treatments, outcomes in major life activities (education, occupation, dating, sexual activity, driving, money management, etc.), antisocial activities and drug use, and medical history. Structured interviews were the primary means of evaluating these domains but some psychological tests and rating scales also were collected. Participants provided the name of another adult who could best describe their current functioning, typically current spouse/partners or parents. Those others also completed interviews and scales. For a complete inventory of measures collected at this follow-up, see the book by Barkley et al. (2008).

OUTCOMES AND PREDICTORS

Determining Current Attention Deficit Hyperactivity Disorder in Adulthood

Deciding who continued to be ADHD at this adult follow-up was not as straightforward as it might first appear. Applying the DSM-IV criteria available at that time was problematic for several reasons not least of which was because its development was not based on adults and required some adjustments for use with them (Barkley et al., 2008; McGough & Barkley, 2004) and that the age of onset was invalid and unreliable (Barkley & Biederman, 1997). Also, the choice of whose reports to use in determining the diagnosis was an issue (parents as used at study entry and earlier follow-ups or self-reports). Using self-report, only 30% of the hyperactive group would meet the threshold of having at least six of nine symptoms on either symptom DSM list by self-report. If we added the additional impairment requirement the figure falls to 24%. If the reports of others (the collaterals) were used instead, these figures would be 26% and 25%, respectively.

ADHD is conceptualized in the DSM as a neurodevelopmental disorder as evident by having "developmentally inappropriate" symptoms. Holding to that view, we employed a developmental reference criterion to determine persistence of disorder at follow-up to contrast against the above results for the DSM-IV criteria. In this case, we used a threshold of four self-reported symptoms from either list in the DSM-IV as that represented the same threshold of developmental deviance we had used to select these cases as hyperactive (or ADHD) in childhood (+2SDs). Using this threshold along with imposing an impairment requirement resulted in 44% (N = 55) being ADHD at follow-up. Notice that an additional 20% of participants would now be viewed as ADHD, nearly double the initial rate of 24% noted above had strict DSM-IV guidelines been employed. This illustrates the problem with DSM-IV when applied to adults and why DSM-5 needed to make some adjustments to the thresholds applied to adults. Henceforth, we refer to this group as being H+ADHD, or hyperactive with current ADHD. The remaining 80 members of the original hyperactive group were termed H−ADHD. These two groups then were compared against each other and the control group (N = 75) for analyzing all dependent measures collected in this project. Note that the H−ADHD group does not comprise only cases of complete remission. Many are subsyndromic or borderline cases of ADHD that fall just shy of being ADHD by these criteria; for instance, 32% of this group would be classified as ADHD had other reports been used.

What percentage of the original ADHD group could be said to have remitted or recovered from their disorder? We considered cases to be completely recovered if they had five or fewer *total* ADHD symptoms and had one or no impaired domains indicated in the interview (both falling within +1SD of the control group means). We found that 36% of the hyperactive group met these two criteria for recovery. None of the H+ADHD group had recovered while 60% of the H−ADHD group had. Considering the entire hyperactive group, 44% met criteria for having ADHD by the mean age of 27, 36% would be considered to be recovered, and 20% would, therefore, be considered *subsyndromic* or symptomatic but *not* within the normal range. Using other reports, the results would be 41%, 35%, and 24%, respectively. If the criteria for recovery had to be met using *both* self *and* other-reports, just 14% did so. Thus, the rate of remission is between 14% and 36% depending on how rigorous one wishes to be in defining recovery.

Demographic Information at Follow-up

The categorical demographic information for our groups is shown in Table 4.1. Our findings largely reflect the outcomes of boys, which is true for all other prior longitudinal studies tracking participants to this age in adulthood. Fortunately, more recent follow-up studies discussed in this text have recruited sufficient females to study any sex differences in outcomes. The small ethnic minority representation across these groups prevented us from examining specific ethnic groups within our data for any reliable or meaningful differences. The groups did not differ in the percentage as to who were currently single, married, or separated/divorced. But fewer members of the H+ADHD group were currently employed compared with the H−ADHD and Control group. The dimensional measures are displayed in Table 4.2. Both of the H groups had less education, a lower IQ, lower Hollingshead Job Index, and hence lower socioeconomic status (Hollingshead, 1975) than our control group.

TABLE 4.1

DEMOGRAPHIC CHARACTERISTICS FOR HYPERACTIVE AND CONTROL GROUPS FOR CATEGORICAL MEASURES

Group:	H+ADHD		H−ADHD		Control				Pair-wise
Measure	**N**	**%**	**N**	**%**	**N**	**%**	X^2	*p*	**Contrasts**
Sex (Males)	46	83.6	70	87.5	70	93.3	3.09	NS	
Ethnic Group (White)	46	83.6	65	81.2	73	97.3	10.32	.006	1,2<3
MARITAL STATUS									
Single (Not Married)	37	67.3	52	65.0	41	54.7	4.58	NS	
Married Now	16	29.6	26	32.9	32	42.7			
Divorced/Separated	2	3.8	2	2.6	2	2.7			
LIVING ARRANGEMENTS									
Live Alone	4	7.3	11	13.9	8	10.7	18.85	NS	
Live with Spouse	16	29.6	27	34.2	33	44.0			
Live with Parents	9	16.7	15	19.0	8	10.7			
Live with Others	26	48.1	27	33.7	26	34.7			
Currently Employed	41	74.5	73	91.3	68	90.7	9.49	.009	1<2,3

Sample sizes are H+ADHD = 55, H−ADHD = 80, and Controls = 75. N = sample sizes that fell into each categorical measure; % = the percentage of the entire group sample that fell into each categorical measure. X^2 = results for the Pearson omnibus chi-square. *P* = probability value for the chi-square result. H+ADHD = Hyperactive group that currently has a diagnosis of ADHD at follow-up. H−ADHD = Hyperactive group that does not have a diagnosis of ADHD at follow-up. From Barkley, R. A., Murphy, K. R., & Fischer, M. (2008). *ADHD in Adults: What the Science Says*. New York: Guilford Press.

TABLE 4.2

DEMOGRAPHIC CHARACTERISTICS BY GROUP FOR DIMENSIONAL MEASURES

Group:	(1) H+ADHD		(2) H–ADHD		(3) Community				Pair-wise
Measure	Mean	SD	Mean	SD	Mean	SD	*F*	*p*	Contrasts
Age (years)	26.8	1.4	27.2	1.4	27.0	0.9	1.83	NS	
Education (years)	12.2	2.2	12.8	2.1	15.8	2.3	51.49	<.001	1,2 <3
Verbal IQ (Vocabulary)	10.5	3.4	10.6	3.3	14.1	2.6	29.55	<.001	1,2<3
Nonverbal IQ (Blocks)	11.6	3.2	11.6	3.4	13.0	2.9	4.85	.009	1,2<3
Hollingshead Job Index	32.3	19.8	40.1	20.6	56.0	27.0	18.11	<.001	1,2<3
Hollingshead SES	28.4	11.2	33.2	12.7	45.4	15.1	28.80	<.001	1,2<3

SD = standard deviation, F = F-test results of the analysis of variance (or covariance), p = probability value for the F-test, NS = not significant. H+ADHD = Hyperactive group that currently has a diagnosis of ADHD at follow-up. H–ADHD = Hyperactive group that does not have a diagnosis of ADHD at follow-up. Verbal IQ is from the WAIS-III Vocabulary subtest, Nonverbal IQ is from the Block Design subtest; Hollingshead = Hollingshead Job Index; SES (socioeconomic status) = Hollingshead Index of Social Position. Sample sizes are H+ADHD = 55, H–ADHD = 80, Controls = 75 for Age, Education, and Hollingshead measure. For WAIS IQ Subtests, they are H+ADHD = 52, H–ADHD = 79, and Controls = 73. From Barkley, R. A., Murphy, K. R., & Fischer, M. (2008). *ADHD in Adults: What the Science Says*. New York: Guilford Press. Copyright by Guilford Press. Reprinted with permission.

TABLE 4.3

PSYCHIATRIC EVALUATION AND TREATMENT HISTORY SINCE LAST FOLLOW-UP (AGE 21) BY GROUP

Group:	(1) H+ADHD		(2) H−ADHD		(3) Community				Pair-wise
Measure	**N**	**%**	**N**	**%**	**N**	**%**	X^2	p	**Contrasts**
Evaluated in Interim	25	45.5	14	17.5	11	14.7	19.42	<.001	1>2,3
Dx of Any Psych Disorder in Interim	17	30.9	3	3.8	9	12.0	20.52	<.001	1>2,3
Outpatient Treatment in Interim	19	34.5	11	13.8	11	14.7	10.72	.005	1>2,3
Ever in Residential Treatment	10	18.2	10	12.5	3	4.0	6.86	.032	1>3
Ever Psychiatrically Hospitalized	10	18.2	6	7.5	2	2.7	9.94	.007	1>3
Ever Treated with Psychiatric Drugs	22	40.0	17	21.3	10	13.3	12.93	.002	1>2,3
Currently in Therapy	5	9.1	3	3.8	6	8.2	1.88	NS	
Currently on Meds	8	14.5	6	7.5	5	6.7	2.77	NS	

Sample sizes were: H+ADHD = 55, H−ADHD = 80, and Community = 75.

N = sample sizes that fell into each categorical measure; % = the percentage of the entire group sample that fell into each categorical measure. X^2 = results for the Pearson omnibus chi-square. *P* = probability value for the chi-square result. Pair-wise contrasts = results for the paired comparisons of the groups with each other, if the omnibus chi-square was significant ($p<.05$). [S] = significant main effect for sex. H+ADHD = Hyperactive group that currently has a diagnosis of ADHD at follow-up. H−ADHD = Hyperactive group that does not have a diagnosis of ADHD at follow-up. Dx = Diagnosis; Psych = psychiatric; Meds = psychiatric medication. From Barkley, R. A., Murphy, K. R., & Fischer, M. (2008). *ADHD in Adults: What the Science Says.* New York: Guilford Press.

Treatment Received in Adulthood

The percentages of each group that had received various types of psychiatric treatment between ages 21 and 27 appear in Table 4.3. More of the H+ADHD group had sought a psychiatric or psychological evaluation, had received some form of outpatient treatment, or were currently in some type of psychological therapy. Only a small percentage of each group was currently taking a psychiatric medication (7%–14%) and the groups did not differ in this respect. As these figures suggest, the vast majority of individuals in the two H groups were not currently receiving any form of treatment.

GLOBAL IMPAIRMENT RATINGS

Participants rated themselves on global ratings of impairment in a variety of domains of major life activities; we also obtained those ratings from others who knew them well. Those findings appear in Table 4.4. More members of the H+ADHD group are rated as being "Often" impaired than of the community control group in every domain assessed here, currently and in childhood, by self or by other reports. The H+ADHD group also rated them selves as being more likely to be impaired in all but one domain of current and childhood functioning than the H−ADHD group, the exception being in sports and similar activities during childhood. The reports of others largely agreed with this pattern of results but not entirely. Others rated more of the members of both H groups as being impaired in each of these domains of current functioning than was the case in self-reports and they rated these two H groups as being similarly likely to be impaired in six of the ten domains assessed on the rating scale. In short, others perceive more of these H cases to be impaired in adulthood than do the H cases themselves and view the groups as equivalently so in most domains. Whereas the H+ADHD group self-reported more impairment than the H−ADHD group in most domains of childhood functioning, others did not see it that way. They viewed both H groups

TABLE 4.4

DOMAINS OF MAJOR LIFE ACTIVITIES RATED AS OFTEN IMPAIRED BY GROUP (FROM RATING SCALES)

Group: Measure	(1) H+ADHD N	%	(2) H−ADHD N	%	(3) Community N	%	X^2	*p*	Pair-wise Contrasts
CURRENT SELF-RATINGS									
Home Life	19	35.2	7	9.0	1	1.4	31.83	<.001	1>2>3
Work or Occupation	15	29.3	4	5.2	9	13.0	13.95	.001	1>2,3
Social Interactions	17	31.5	4	5.1	3	4.3	26.84	<.001	1>2,3
Community Activities	11	20.4	3	3.8	2	2.9	15.56	<.001	1>2,3
Educational Activities	22	40.7	15	19.2	5	7.2	20.77	<.001	1>2>3
Dating or Marital Activities	24	44.4	4	5.2	4	5.8	44.54	<.001	1>2,3
Money Management	34	63.0	15	19.5	3	4.3	56.86	<.001	1>2>3
Driving	15	28.3	2	2.6	4	5.9	24.31	<.001	1>2,3
Leisure Activities	11	20.4	1	1.3	1	1.4	23.59	<.001	1>2,3
Daily Responsibilities	20	30.7	8	10.3	2	2.9	30.00	<.001	1>2,3
Any Domain	43	79.6	30	37.5	16	21.3	45.00	<.001	1>2>3
CHILDHOOD SELF-RATINGS									
Home Life	39	72.2	29	36.3	15	20.3	35.86	<.001	1>2>3
Social Interactions	41	75.9	27	33.8	12	16.2	48.24	<.001	1>2>3
Community Activities	28	51.9	19	23.8	6	8.1	31.67	<.001	1>2>3
School	40	74.1	51	63.8	23	31.1	27.49	<.001	1,2>3
Sports, Clubs, Organizations	25	46.3	14	17.5	14	18.9	16.68	<.001	1>2,3
Self-care	27	50.0	19	23.8	8	10.8	25.27	<.001	1>2>3
Daily Chores/ Responsibilities	39	72.2	29	36.3	14	18.9	37.69	<.001	1>2>3
Any Domain	50	92.6	55	68.8	22	29.3	56.16	<.001	1>2>3
CURRENT OTHER-RATINGS									
Home Life	29	53.7	25	32.5	8	11.6	25.24	<.001	1>2>3
Work or Occupation	19	36.5	19	24.4	6	8.7	13.72	.001	1,2>3
Social Interactions	26	48.1	20	25.6	1	1.4	37.23	<.001	1>2>3
Community Activities	14	26.9	12	15.4	1	1.4	16.77	<.001	1,2>3

TABLE 4.4

CONTINUED

Group:	(1) H+ADHD		(2) H−ADHD		(3) Community				Pair-wise
Measure	N	%	N	%	N	%	X^2	*p*	Contrasts
Educational Activities	19	35.2	17	21.8	4	5.8	16.70	<.001	1,2>3
Dating or Marital Activities	28	53.8	27	34.6	5	7.2	31.79	<.001	1>2>3
Money Management	33	61.1	38	48.7	8	11.6	35.87	<.001	1,2>3
Driving	19	35.8	18	23.1	3	4.4	19.04	<.001	1,2>3
Leisure Activities	15	27.8	12	15.4	5	7.2	9.57	.008	1>3
Daily Responsibilities	28	51.9	22	28.2	5	7.2	30.37	<.001	1>2>3
Any Domain	39	72.2	47	60.3	17	22.7	36.36	<.001	1,2>3
CHILDHOOD OTHER-RATINGS									
Home Life	40	74.1	49	64.5	4	5.7	73.18	<.001	1,2>3
Social Interactions	36	66.7	39	50.6	3	4.1	60.23	<.001	1,2>3
Community Activities	23	43.4	35	45.5	3	4.2	24.97	<.001	1,2>3
School	46	85.2	62	80.5	12	17.1	81.14	<.001	1,2>3
Sports, Clubs, Organizations	22	40.7	29	37.7	2	2.9	30.73	<.001	1,2>3
Self-care	14	25.9	19	24.7	0	0.0	21.13	<.001	1,2>3
Play and Leisure	29	53.7	25	32.5	3	4.3	37.68	<.001	1>2>3
Daily Chores/ Responsibilities	37	68.5	47	61.0	9	12.9	48.94	<.001	1,2>3
Any Domain	50	92.6	66	84.6	16	21.3	92.54	<.001	1,2>3

N = sample size endorsing this item; % = percent of group endorsing this item; X^2 = results of the omnibus chi-square test; *p* = probability value for the chi-square test; Pair-wise Contrasts = results of the chi-square tests involving pair-wise comparisons of the three groups. H+ADHD = Hyperactive group that currently has a diagnosis of ADHD at follow-up. H−ADHD = Hyperactive group that does not have a diagnosis of ADHD at follow-up. Sample sizes for self-ratings of current impairments were H+ADHD = 53, H−ADHD = 77, and Controls = 69. Sample sizes for self-ratings of childhood impairment were H+ADHD = 54, H−ADHD = 80, and Controls = 74. Sample sizes for other ratings of current impairments were H+ADHD = 54, H−ADHD = 78, and Controls = 69. Sample sizes for other ratings of childhood impairment were H+ADHD = 54, H−ADHD = 76, and Controls = 70. From Barkley, R. A., Murphy, K. R., & Fischer, M. (2008). *ADHD in Adults: What the Science Says*. New York: Guilford Press. Copyright by Guilford Press. Reprinted with permission.

as being more likely to be impaired in seven of the eight domains (play being the exception) than the control group and to be equivalently so. So as to be sure that impairment was likely a consequence of ADHD, we correlated ratings of ADHD symptoms with those of impairment. Severity of current ADHD, variously measured, was significantly and moderately related to severity of impairment, variously measured, whether using ratings of current functioning or retrospectively recalled functioning in childhood.

We examined a set of variables from earlier follow-up points for their value in predicting current impairment. Self-rated current impairment was linked to severity of childhood hyperactivity, persistence of ADHD to age 21 years, and severity of oppositional defiant disorder (ODD) symptoms self-reported at age 21. These results imply that current impairment is not being driven solely by severity of earlier ADHD or its persistence over time. Yet these three predictors accounted for approximately 19% of the variance in current self-rated severity of impairment, suggesting that other factors are playing a role in current impairment. We also found that the severity of ADHD symptoms at childhood, at adolescence, and early adulthood predicted more severe impairment at age 27 as rated by others. Such findings show that impairment is not simply associated with current ADHD but with severity of the disorder at earlier developmental periods.

Some clinicians and advocates for the adult ADHD community have claimed that ADHD conveys gifts, positive traits, or special abilities individuals would not otherwise possess. "People with ADD have special gifts, even if they are hidden. The most common include originality, creativity, charisma, energy, liveliness, and unusual sense of humor, areas of intellectual brilliance, and spunk." (Hallowell & Ratey, 2005, p. 6). Others have claimed different benefits from the disorder (Hartmann, 2005; Shelley-Tremblay & Rosen, 1996). We wish we could say there is evidence in our study supporting such an idealistic view of this disorder. But none have been found on hundreds of measures we collected across development (see Barkley et al., 2008) or in any other longitudinal study to our knowledge.

Comorbidity

Both children and adults diagnosed with ADHD have high rates of comorbidity with other disorders, rising to over 80% for another disorder, and over 50% for two other disorders when clinic-referred samples are studied, either children followed to adulthood or adults with the disorder (Barkley et al., 2008). Oppositional defiant disorder (ODD), conduct disorder (CD), learning disabilities (LD), and eventually, antisocial personality disorder (ASPD) and substance use disorders are among the more common disorders that are reliably linked to ADHD across development (Angold, Costello, & Erkanli, 1999; Brown, 2000; Pliszka, 2009). To a lesser extent, anxiety disorders and depressive disorders have been documented in some follow-up studies but not in others. Recently, these disorders were more strongly linked to the attention disorder known as sluggish cognitive tempo (SCT) or concentration deficit disorder than to ADHD (Barkley, 2014). SCT can overlap with ADHD in up to half or more cases of each disorder; a finding that could partially explain this comorbidity with internalizing disorders (Barkley, 2012, 2013).

The comorbid disorders for which our participants were at significant risk, both currently and over their lifetimes, are shown in Table 4.5. As noted there, most of these were based on using the Structured Clinical Interview for DSM Disorders (SCID; Spitzer, Williams, Gibbons, & First, 1995). In keeping with several other longitudinal studies of children with ADHD grown up, we failed to find any elevated risks specifically for major depressive disorder (MDD) or dysthymia. This is quite surprising given that major depression was found to be more prevalent in the hyperactive group (27%) at the last follow-up (age 21) than in the Community group. Yet even though the risk for MDD or dysthymia specifically was not found here, the risk for any mood disorder was elevated, as was the specific risk for depressive personality disorder, both of which are in keeping with some linkage between ADHD and depression (Faraone & Biederman, 1997).

We found a greater occurrence of generalized anxiety disorder in the H+ADHD than in the Community group. Unlike prior research of either clinic-referred adults or children grown up, we also found a significantly

TABLE 4.5

SIGNIFICANT CURRENT AND PAST SCID DIAGNOSES AND CURRENT AND CHILDHOOD ODD AND CD BY SELF-REPORT BY GROUP

Group:	(1) H+ADHD		(2) H−ADHD		(3) Community				Pair-wise
Measure	N	%	N	%	N	%	X^2	p	**Contrasts**
AXIS I DISORDERS—CURRENT									
Alcohol Abuse	11	20.4	6	7.6	6	8.0	6.44	.040	1>2,3
Alcohol Dependence	6	11.1	2	2	3	4	5.10	NS	
Cannabis Abuse	5	9.3	5	6.3	5	6.7	0.46	NS	
Cannabis Dependence	2	3.7	0	0.0	4	5.3	4.03	NS	
PTSD	10	18.5	5	6.3	1	1.3	13.39	.001	1>2,3
Social Phobia	7	13.0	5	6.3	1	1.3	7.25	.027	NS
Specific Phobia	9	16.7	11	14.1	3	4.0	6.23	.044	1,2>3
Generalized Anxiety	6	11.5	1	1.3	2	2.7	8.66	.013	1>2,3
Any Mood Disorder	13	24.5	5	6.3	3	4.0	16.40	<.001	1>2,3
Any Drug Disorder	14	25.9	8	10.3	10	13.3	6.40	.041	1>2
Any Anxiety Disorder	24	46.2	17	22.7	7	9.3	23.06	<.001	1>2>3
AXIS I DISORDERS—PAST									
Any Mood Disorder	7	13.2	2	2.6	3	4.0	7.23	.027	1>2
Any Drug Disorder	28	53.8	41	53.2	30	40.0	3.50	NS	
Any Anxiety Disorder	4	7.7	8	10.7	3	4.0	2.43	NS	
PERSONALITY DISORDERS—CURRENT									
Avoidant	8	14.8	1	1.3	1	1.2	15.96	<.001	1>2,3
Obsessive–Compulsive	9	16.7	4	5.1	2	2.7	10.07	.006	1>2,3
Passive Aggressive	18	33.3	5	6.3	1	1.3	34.88	<.001	1>2,3
Depressive	8	14.8	4	5.1	0	0.0	12.79	.002	1>2>3
Paranoid	9	16.7	4	5.1	3	4.0	8.33	.015	1>2,3
Borderline	13	24.1	3	3.8	1	1.3	24.88	<.001	1>2,3

TABLE 4.5

CONTINUED

Group:	(1) H+ADHD		(2) H–ADHD		(3) Community				Pair-wise
Measure	N	%	N	%	N	%	X^2	p	Contrasts
Antisocial	21	38.9	13	16.5	6	8.0	19.92	<.001	1>2,3
Any Personality Disorder	36	66.7	22	27.8	9	12.0	44.08	<.001	1>2>3
DISRUPTIVE DISORDERS									
ODD Current	26	47.3	13	16.3	3	4.0	38.27	<.001	1>2>3
ODD Childhood	41	74.5	38	47.5	6	8.0	60.97	<.001	1>2>3
CD Childhood	33	61.1	41	51.3	22	29.7	13.73	.001	1,2>3

Disorders were established using the *Structured Clinical Interview for DSM-IV Disorders* (SCID) (Spitzer, Williams, Gibbon, & First, 1995) except for ODD and CD, which were documented using a DSM-IV based interview constructed for this project. N = sample size endorsing this item; % = percentage of group endorsing this item; X^2 = results of the omnibus chi-square test; p = probability value for the chi-square test; Pair-wise Contrasts = results of the chi-square tests involving pair-wise comparisons of the three groups. PTSD = Post Traumatic Stress Disorder. H+ADHD = Hyperactive group that currently has a diagnosis of ADHD at follow-up. H–ADHD = Hyperactive group that does not have a diagnosis of ADHD at follow-up. ODD = Oppositional Defiant Disorder, CD = Conduct Disorder. From Barkley, R. A., Murphy, K. R., & Fischer, M. (2008). *ADHD in Adults: What the Science Says*. New York: Guilford Press. Copyright by Guilford Press. Reprinted with permission.

higher risk for specific phobias and post-traumatic stress disorder (PTSD). But the H+ADHD and H–ADHD groups differed only in their rates of generalized anxiety disorder (GAD) and PTSD. Thus, growing up as a hyperactive (ADHD) child conveys a greater risk for specific phobias by adulthood. But persistent ADHD into adulthood further elevates the risk for GAD and PTSD beyond that conveyed by childhood hyperactivity status alone. Why PTSD would be elevated in the H+ADHD group and not in the other two groups when this has not been reported in any prior studies is not immediately evident. Perhaps it was never specifically evaluated in the earlier literature—an issue we cannot readily discern from the methods published for other studies. These findings contradict those of several prior follow-up studies of ADHD children into adulthood where no such elevated risk was evident (Mannuzza et al., 1993, 1998; Rasmussen & Gillberg, 2001; Weiss & Hechtman, 1993). Why this should be so is not immediately obvious to us. But consistent with most other follow-up studies, we did not find elevated rates of obsessive–compulsive disorder (OCD) or tic disorders in either hyperactive group relative to the control group. Nor did we find any elevated rates of bipolar disorder over the control group.

More of the H+ADHD groups (20%) had a current alcohol abuse disorder than either the H−ADHD or Community control groups, who did not differ from each other (8% each). Many prior follow-up studies have found such an association of ADHD with alcohol use problems in adults. In contrast, risks for cannabis abuse or dependence disorders were not elevated. But the H+ADHD group did show a marginally significant risk for having at least one or more drug use disorders relative to the H−ADHD group. Such findings imply that drug use disorders may be generically more likely to occur in conjunction with ADHD at adult outcome for children with the disorder even if no link to a specific drug use disorder is evident.

Our groups did not differ in their likelihood of having any past specific disorders as self-reported. But when we looked at risk for the larger categories of disorders (mood, anxiety, and drug-use disorder clusters), we found a significant elevation of risk for any mood disorder in the H+ADHD group compared with the H−ADHD group. Yet the difference between these two groups and the community control group was only marginally significant. The risk for any anxiety disorder in their histories remained low and not significant across all three groups, while the risk for any prior drug use disorder was quite high (40%–54%), though again not different among the groups largely because it was also quite high in our control group.

The risk for any personality disorder was more than twice as great in the H+ADHD than H−ADHD group (67% vs. 28%) and was more than five times greater than in the Community control group (12%). Therefore, persistent ADHD into adulthood has a high comorbidity with personality disorders. Consistent with most prior longitudinal studies, the most common was antisocial personality disorder. This was followed by passive–aggressive and borderline personality disorders. OCD, paranoid, depressive, and avoidant disorders were also elevated to a small but significant extent in the H+ADHD group relative to the H−ADHD and control groups. Quite consistent with past research, we, too, found a higher occurrence of ODD and CD in the histories of both the H groups here compared with the control group, with the H+ADHD group having the highest risk for past and current ODD. We found a similar pattern of results when the reports of others were used for determining these SCID disorders but the rates of occurrence were lower than found here for self-reports.

We examined the degree of agreement between self and other-reported disorder *categories* in the SCID (i.e., if the disorder was self-reported, was it also other-reported?). The greatest agreement was for the risk for any personality disorder (72%, Kappa = .46) and for any drug use disorder (71%, Kappa = .60). The risk for any anxiety disorder showed moderate-to-low agreement (45%; Kappa = .39) and that for any mood disorder was quite low (18%; Kappa = .12). Again, the lower agreements for the latter two disorders may have to do with the lessened visibility of mood states to others.

In general, we found that the mean number of SCID disorders based on self-reports was significantly greater in the H+ADHD group (Mean = 3.4, SD = 3.5) than in the H−ADHD (Mean = 0.9, SD = 1.5) or control groups (Mean = 0.8, SD = 1.9) ($F = 22.39$, $p<.001$), with the latter two groups not differing from each other. It, therefore, appears that the persistence of ADHD into adulthood is associated with an elevated risk of comorbidity more generally than is the case for hyperactive children who no longer qualify for an ADHD diagnosis or the Community control cases by adult follow-up. We found no differences among the groups in their risk for a past history of any self-reported SCID disorders, however. Overall, we found that more than 84% of the H+ADHD group had at least one other disorder, a level nearly twice that for the H−ADHD group and nearly four times that for the control group. Nearly 61% of the currently ADHD group had at least two other disorders, while 45% had three or more disorders all of which were higher than in either control group.

Educational History

At the age 21 follow-up (Barkley, Fischer et al., 2006) we found that more than three times as many H than control group members had been retained in grade at least once (42% vs. 13%) during their schooling or had been suspended from high school at least once (60% vs. 18%). The H group members had completed fewer years of education and had a lower grade point average (1.69 vs. 2.56 out of a possible 4.0) and class ranking in their last year of schooling (69th percentile vs. 49th percentile) than those in the control group. More of the H group also had received special educational services while in high school relative to the control group. Most alarming was that 32% of the H group had failed to complete high school compared with almost none of the members of the control group. Substantially fewer H than control children had ever enrolled in college (21% vs. 78%) or were currently attending at this follow-up point (15% vs. 66%). In the Montreal follow-up study, approximately 20% attempted a college program yet only 5% completed a university degree program as compared with over 41% of control children (Weiss & Hechtman, 1993). These findings demonstrate that the educational domain is a major one for impaired functioning and reduced attainment for children growing up with ADHD.

By the age 27 follow-up, these results had not changed much. Both of the hyperactive groups, regardless of having current ADHD, were less likely to have graduated from high school (62%–67%) than were members of the Community control group (99%), and far fewer members of the hyperactive groups had attended college (9%–20%) than had the control adults (68%). We found that both H groups had attained fewer years of education (M = 12.2 for H+ADHD and 12.8 for H−ADHD, respectively vs. 15.8 for Controls), had been suspended more times from school (16.5 and 14.5 vs. 1.3), and had been truant from school (93.2 and 71.9) more than our control group (23.5). Yet the two H groups did not differ from each other on these outcomes.

On academic achievement tests, both hyperactive groups scored lower in reading skills, but members of the H+ADHD group were even more impaired in spelling and math ability than were those in the H−ADHD group. All this implies that whether or not ADHD persists to adulthood, growing up with it as a child substantially predisposes one to significant educational risks and overall to less attainment.

We chose two categorical outcomes that were significantly more impaired in the H than control group: having ever been retained in grade and having graduated high school. We used 14 predictors from childhood study entry, and teen and young adult (age 21) follow-up points to study predictors of high school graduation. Just three predictors were related to this outcome, namely, pervasiveness of childhood ADHD (HSQ scores), the severity of teen ADHD symptoms as reported by parents, and the severity of CD symptoms self-reported at age 21. That the CD symptoms only enter the equation after the age at which one typically graduates high school suggests it may not be so much a predictor as an outcome associated with or interacting with not completing high school. We say this because the severity of conduct problems in childhood and specifically the severity of ODD and CD at teen follow-up were not predictive of high school graduation in this analysis. This makes it clear that the likelihood of graduating from high school is largely related to ADHD especially in high school, but may become associated with an increased risk for CD symptoms thereafter.

We also found that the number of years of education attained was predicted by 6 of the 14 predictors. Those from childhood were severity of hyperactivity (WWPARS), IQ, and pervasiveness of behavioral problems (HSQ). From the teen follow-up measures, an additional three predictors were significant, namely, teen math achievement (WRAT) and the number of teen CD and ODD symptoms as reported by parents. Once more, teen ODD symptoms surprised us by being associated with *more* years of education once teen CD symptoms had been controlled in the equation. This suggests that teen ODD symptoms that are independent of CD may actually make positive contributions to educational success. In total, these predictors accounted for nearly 44% of the variance in educational attainment.

Occupational Functioning

We found that significantly fewer of the H+ADHD group were currently employed compared with both the H−ADHD and Community control adults. The H+ADHD group also reported themselves to be more likely to have problems with others at work as well as difficulties with their behavior and workplace performance more generally as compared with these other two groups. Table 4.6 shows the results for most of our measures of occupational history and functioning. There we see that it is the H+ADHD group that is the most impaired in these various indices of occupational adjustment relative to the control groups. Although both H groups held lower status jobs relative to our control group at this follow-up, the H+ADHD group rated themselves as having lower workplace performance quality than the other two groups. The groups did not differ in their current annual salary or in the length of time they had held their current position. But the two H groups reported working fewer hours per week than did the Community group.

The H+ADHD group also had held more jobs since leaving high school. Given such a higher job turnover rate, we adjusted for this difference across groups in the questions dealing with workplace adjustment by computing the percentage of jobs held in which these problems had been reported to occur. The H+ADHD group experienced a greater percentage of jobs in which they had trouble getting along with others, behavior problems, had been fired or dismissed from the job, or had been disciplined formally by their supervisors compared with both the H−ADHD and control groups. The currently ADHD group also reported quitting more jobs due to hostility with others than the Community group. The H−ADHD group placed between these two extremes but did not differ significantly from either of the other groups. Apparently, children growing up with persistent ADHD may experience even more workplace adjustment problems than do those whose ADHD does not persist. Even so, being ADHD in childhood predisposes toward lower occupational status regardless of the persistence of ADHD to age 27, most likely due to its adverse effects noted above on educational success and eventual years attained. But persistent ADHD to adulthood appears to have a far more adverse impact on current job functioning than does simply being ADHD in childhood.

We analyzed a number of potential predictors of current work performance and the number of jobs from which the participant had been fired. Work performance was predicted only by the number of current ADHD

TABLE 4.6

OCCUPATIONAL FUNCTIONING FOR EACH GROUP ON DIMENSIONAL MEASURES IN THE MILWAUKEE STUDY

Group:	(1) H+ADHD		2) H–ADHD		(3) Community				Pair-wise
Measure	**Mean**	**SD**	**Mean**	**SD**	**Mean**	**SD**	*F*	*p*	**Contrasts**
Hollingshead Job Index[IQ]	35.2	19.8	42.4	20.6	51.7	27.3	7.05	.001	1,2<3
Time at Current Job (months)	22.7	22.8	27.0	29.7	30.8	26.5	1.20	NS	
Number of Jobs since High School	4.9	5.4	3.5	2.0	2.5	1.4	8.92	<.001	1>2,3
Hours Worked Per Week	43.3	14.0	44.4	9.6	49.2	12.8	4.23	.016	1,2<3
Annual Salary (K)[IQ]	26.3	14.4	30.7	19.4	35.1	18.1	2.83	NS	
Self-Rated Work Quality	2.0	0.7	1.6	0.6	1.5	0.6	7.17	.001	1>2,3
% Jobs Trouble with Others	25.7	30.8	6.9	16.2	6.2	21.0	13.58	<.001	1>2,3
% Jobs Behavior Problems	26.5	36.6	6.0	15.4	2.1	9.2	20.94	<.001	1>2,3
% Jobs Fired (dismissed)	43.2	39.1	30.0	34.4	14.0	30.3	11.45	<.001	1>2>3
% Jobs Quit for Hostility	31.1	34.6	21.3	35.7	14.8	29.9	3.61	.029	1>3
% Jobs Quit for Boredom	30.5	40.1	25.1	38.8	25.8	37.6	0.33	NS	
% Jobs Disciplined	28.1	34.0	8.1	22.2	3.1	15.6	17.77	<.001	1>2,3

SD = standard deviation, *F* = *F*-test results of the analysis of variance (or covariance), *p* = probability value for the *F*-test, NS = not significant, K = thousands of dollars, Work Quality rated 1–5 (1 = excellent, 5 = poor). [IQ] = WAIS-3 vocabulary and block design scores were used as covariates on these measures. Where covariates were used, means are marginal means. Work quality was rated from 1 (excellent) to 5 (poor). From Barkley, R. A., Murphy, K. R., & Fischer, M. (2008). *ADHD in Adults: What the Science Says.* New York: Guilford Press. Copyright by Guilford Press. Reprinted with permission.

symptoms (self-reported) and by nonverbal IQ (WAIS-III block design subtest). The percentage of jobs from which participants had been fired was predicted by years of education and by the number of self-rated current ODD symptoms.

Substance Use

At the age 21 follow-up (Barkley et al., 2004) we subdivided the H group into those who did and did not have lifetime CD by young adulthood (self-reported) and compared them to the control group for their frequency of use of 11 different drugs. In all cases, it was the hyperactive group having CD that accounted for these differences, with there being no significant differences between the hyperactive alone and control groups in any form of drug use.

By age 27, the H children were at greater risk of being a current tobacco or alcohol user or of ever having gotten drunk. Whether their ADHD had persisted to age 27 made little difference here. While the H+ADHD group included a significantly greater percentage of individuals who had ever smoked tobacco than did the Community group, the H–ADHD group placed between these two extremes and did not differ significantly from either of them. Noteworthy here is that the groups did not differ in the percentage of individuals who had ever tried any of the other illegal drugs we surveyed except that the H+ADHD group included significantly more members who had illegally used a prescription drug compared with the other two groups.

As for frequency of substance use, the number of years that participants had been smoking and their frequency of cigarette use per day did not differ among our three groups. Nor did the frequencies differ for marijuana, cocaine, or speed. This latter result is likely due to the small sample sizes compounded by the substantially skewed and kurtotic distributions for these frequencies, in which there were high-use outliers in each group causing standard deviations to be as large or larger than mean scores. Nevertheless, we did not find a greater use of marijuana in the H+ADHD group specifically or in the hyperactive group more generally, yet that has been found in clinic-referred adults with ADHD (Barkley et al., 2008). We did find that the H+ADHD group consumed more alcoholic drinks per week than either the H−ADHD or control group, in keeping with their greater incidence of alcohol use disorders found above (see Comorbidity). Both hyperactive groups also used caffeinated beverages more often each day than the Community group. Noteworthy is that risk for and frequency of drug use in the hyperactive group was not found to be related to stimulant medication use as a child, in keeping with results from our earlier age 21 follow-up (Barkley, Fischer, Smallish, & Fletcher, 2003) or with other studies on this issue (Wilens, Faraone, Biederman, & Gunawardene, 2003). In contrast, those who had *never* been treated with a stimulant were *more* likely to have tried speed (9% vs. 1%) (p = .045) or to have used a prescription drug illegally (23% vs. 2%) (X^2 = 11.70, p = .001). This supports the meta-analytic review by Wilens et al. (2003) that treatment of ADHD with stimulants in childhood and adolescence may have a protective effect against some types of drug use or abuse later in life. At the very least, childhood medication treatment does not increase the risk for later substance use, dependence, or abuse.

Antisocial Activities

A number of prior follow-up studies show that children with ADHD are at greater risk for antisocial activities, arrests, and even antisocial personality disorder by adulthood. The percentages of each group that had ever committed each form of criminal activity are shown in Table 4.7. As is evident here, both H groups were more likely to have committed acts of breaking and entering, assaulting others with their fists, and carrying illegal weapons. Both had been arrested and jailed more often than the Community control group. Clearly, as they grow up, children with ADHD are at significant risk for these forms of criminal activity and their legal consequences, regardless of whether their ADHD has persisted to age 27. In other instances, however, the H+ADHD group was the only one to

TABLE 4.7

CRIME CATEGORIES FOR EACH GROUP IN THE MILWAUKEE STUDY

Group:	(1) H+ADHD		(2) H−ADHD		(3) Community				Pair-wise
Measure	N	%	N	%	N	%	X^2	p	Contrasts
Stolen other's property	41	74	46	58	34	45	11.11	.004	1>2,3
Stolen other's money	26	47	33	42	21	28	5.65	NS	
Robbed someone of money	4	7	2	2	1	1	3.72	NS	
Breaking and entering	8	14	12	15	2	3	7.69	.021	1,2>3
Assaulted with fists	23	42	26	33	12	16	11.09	.004	1,2>3
Assaulted with a weapon	16	29	5	6	2	3	25.46	<.001	1>2,3
Set fires intentionally	6	11	7	9	4	5	1.41	NS	
Carried a weapon illegally	22	40	16	20	6	8	19.60	<.001	1>2>3
Forced someone to have sex	1	2	0	0	0	0	2.81	NS	
Possessed illegal drugs	37	67	48	61	36	48	5.26	NS	
Sold drugs illegally	22	40	21	27	14	19	7.31	.026	1>3
Engaged in disorderly conduct	26	47	27	34	18	24	7.66	.022	1>3
Arrested	40	73	41	52	25	33	19.77	<.001	1>2>3
Jailed	32	58	36	46	18	24	16.33	<.001	1,2>3

Sample sizes for these comparisons were H+ADHD = 55, H−ADHD = 79, and Community = 75.

N = sample size endorsing this item; % = percentage of group endorsing this item; X^2 = results of the omnibus chi-square test; p = probability value for the chi-square test; Pair-wise Contrasts = results of the chi-square tests involving pair-wise comparisons of the three groups. H+ADHD = Hyperactive group that currently has a diagnosis of ADHD at follow-up. H−ADHD = Hyperactive group that does not have a diagnosis of ADHD at follow-up. From Barkley, R. A., Murphy, K. R., & Fischer, M. (2008). *ADHD in Adults: What the Science Says*. New York: Guilford Press. Copyright by Guilford Press. Reprinted with permission.

differ from the other two groups. This was the case for stealing property, assaulting others with a weapon, selling drugs, or engaging in disorderly conduct. Thus, ADHD that persists until age 27 seems to convey additional risks for these forms of antisocial behavior beyond that linked to just childhood ADHD status.

The most common forms of criminal activity associated with persistent ADHD by adulthood were stealing property (74%) followed by illegal drug possession (67%), assaulting others with fists (42%), engaging in disorderly conduct (47%), selling drugs (40%), and carrying illegal weapons (40%). Nearly three quarters of the H+ADHD group had been arrested and more than half had served some time in jail. These figures were only somewhat lower for the H−ADHD group (52% and 46%, respectively).

We then created a measure reflecting Criminal Diversity that represented the number of different crime categories in which an individual had committed crimes, formed by summing across the 10 crimes in Table 4.7, with the exception of being arrested or jailed. The H+ADHD group (M = 4.25, SD = 2.83) had committed significantly more types of crime than either the H−ADHD (M = 3.07, SD = 2.47) or the Community group (M = 2.03, SD = 2.33; $F = 18.17$, $df = 2/203$, $p = .041$), which did not differ from each other. In sum, our impression is that as children with ADHD grow up, they are at considerably higher risk for various antisocial activities, more so than are self-referred adults seen in clinics at adulthood (Barkley et al., 2008). Both means of studying adult ADHD reveal that they have more antisocial activity than control groups in many instances, but childhood ADHD conveys more risk in this respect, especially if it persists to age 27.

We examined a set of 17 variables as potential predictors of two measures of criminality: crime diversity and arrest frequency. For crime diversity, we found that five predictors were able to account for an impressive 48% of the variance in lifetime criminal diversity scores. These were pervasiveness of childhood ADHD and behavior problems generally (HSQ), the number of teen CD symptoms, the number of different illegal drugs the teen had reported trying by teen follow-up, the number of CD symptoms reported at age 21, and years of education obtained by age 21. That educational attainment is significantly associated with lifetime criminal diversity is hardly surprising. Our sense is that this is much like teen drug use in that these factors are interactive or produce a spiraling effect over time. We base this on the fact that earlier levels of antisocial activity in childhood and adolescence already were statistically controlled in these equations by the time years of education entered as a significant predictor. This would indicate to us that lower levels of education are making an independent contribution to crime diversity beyond that accounted for by earlier crime diversity.

Seven significant predictors for the number of arrests self-reported by age 27 accounted for 41% of the variance. Many, not surprisingly, are the same as those predicting criminal diversity above. Several are not and require additional comment. Childhood hyperactivity (WWPARS scores) made an independent contribution to lifetime arrests independently of that contribution made by childhood conduct problems (CPRS-R scores). Others have found the same (Loeber, Burke, Lahey, Winters, & Zera, 2000) in that severity of childhood hyperactivity makes some contribution to later antisocial activities and arrest rates. And level of ODD symptoms (this time at age 21) makes a positive or protective contribution to risk of being arrested once severity of CD currently and earlier in development is controlled in these equations. We found the same thing for predicting high school graduation above. As we noted then, severity of ODD that is *independent* of severity of CD may not be an adverse characteristic of a teen or young adult but a healthy one. We believe this may show that argumentativeness, stubbornness, and even defiance that is *not* associated with antisocial behavior may not be an adversity during development. Instead, it may be a sign of healthy independence from others and authority more generally and a willingness to openly reason, debate, argue, and otherwise reasonably challenge parental authority.

Health and Lifestyle Domains

A major aim of our age 27 follow-up was to conduct a more in-depth exploration of health and medical status and medical histories in our groups. As a global measure of health concerns, we used the Skinner Computerized Lifestyle Assessment (Skinner, 1994), but we also collected detailed information on health and medical illnesses and conducted lab work on blood and urine samples. This gives the most complete picture to date of the health risks that may be associated with children growing up with ADHD. The H+ADHD group had a higher percentage of its cases having concerns or risks about eating habits, sleep problems, social relations, tobacco use, nonmedical drug use, and emotional health than did the Community group. This H+ADHD group differed specifically from its sister group without ADHD (H−ADHD) in the domains of eating habits, sleep, and emotional health. Even the H group that was no longer considered to be ADHD had more concerns in the areas of sleep and tobacco use than did the Community group. We can conclude from this that childhood ADHD predisposes to a wider array of health concerns and risks regardless of whether it persists to age 27, but that persistent ADHD carries even higher risks than nonpersistent ADHD. Other studies have likewise shown elevated rates of various health problems among children and adults with ADHD (Barkley, 2015).

We questioned participants as to whether they, their parents, their siblings, or their grandparents ever had experienced any of 32 medical problems. Just six of these medical history problems reached significance: (1) Mental health problems in parents were more common in the H+ADHD group (31%) than in parents of the other two groups (14% each); (2) Peptic ulcers were more common in the parents of both H groups (11% and 10%) than in the parents of the control group (0). Siblings had greater peptic ulcer risk, but this was only siblings of the H+ADHD group (24%) compared with those of the H−ADHD group (12%) and the control group (1%); (3) Bronchitis was significantly more common ($p = .04$) in the grandparents of the H+ADHD group (20%) compared with the grandparents of the H−ADHD and control groups (6% and 9%); (4) Arthritis was significantly more common ($p = .003$) in the parents of the H+ADHD group (20%) than in the parents of either control group (5% and 4%); (5) Cancer in grandparents was significantly *less* common in the H−ADHD group (33%) than in the grandparents of the other two groups (50%–54%); and

(6) Arthritis was significantly more common (p = .003) in the parents of the H+ADHD group (20%) than in the parents of either control group (5% and 4%). Great caution must be used in evaluating these results, however, given the large number of statistical tests done here relative to the few findings of significance, because the latter could be due to chance. Concerning just the participants and not their relatives, no differences were found among the groups in the number of illnesses they endorsed in their own history (H+ADHD = 2.3, SD = 1.5; H−ADHD = 1.8, SD = 1.5, and Community = 2.3, SD = 1.6; F = 2.08, p = NS).

We also asked whether participants had ever had surgery, broken bones, allergies, a chronic medical problem, or been hospitalized for nonsurgical reasons. The groups did not differ in the first four areas, but the H+ADHD group was nearly twice as likely to have been hospitalized for nonsurgical reasons (53%) compared with the H−ADHD and control groups (29% and 21%, respectively). A significantly greater percentage in both hyperactive groups had ever experienced a serious injury (60% and 59%) and an accidental poisoning (11% and 14%) than had the control group (42% for injury, 3% for poisoning) The groups did not differ in the percentage currently taking prescription drugs (23%–40%) or using over-the-counter medications (71%–80%). These findings are consistent with earlier research showing hyperactive/ADHD children carry a substantially higher risk for accidental injuries and poisonings as well as nonpsychiatric hospitalizations and emergency room admissions (Barkley, 2015).

We then used a standard interview common to the life insurance industry to evaluate our participants for their *current* medical or general health concerns. This interview covered 59 medically related complaints. Both of the H groups differed from the Community group in 26 of these concerns. In general, the group with persistent ADHD into adulthood has a greater percentage of individuals voicing such concerns than either the H−ADHD or Community groups. This was true for: significant weight changes in the past year, night sweats, heat or cold intolerance, dental problems, pain or ringing in the ears, throat irritation, shortness of breath, sleeping with bed elevated, concerns about moles, painful or burning urination, bruising easily, other bleeding problems, headaches, and depression or anxiety.

The H+ADHD group differed from just the Community control group in several additional complaints; namely, throat hoarseness, pain in the legs when walking, weak urine stream, and numbness or loss of feeling. In a few areas, the hyperactive group that was no longer ADHD at age 27 (H−ADHD) complained more than Community control adults about sinus problems, problematic cough, difficulty swallowing, nighttime urination, back pain, and unusual hair growth. But the H+ADHD group also had more members making such complaints than the control group with the two hyperactive groups not differing in this respect.

We computed the sum of these 59 problems as an index of global health concerns and found that the H+ADHD group had significantly more such complaints (M = 12.3, SD = 7.0) than the H−ADHD group (M = 8.4, SD = 4.7) who had more such concerns than the Community group (M = 6.1, SD = 5.9; $F = 24.75$, $df = 2/204$, $p < .001$). Being a child with ADHD in this study is, therefore, associated with a greater diversity of current medical complaints than with control cases, but those with persistent ADHD have more such complaints than those no longer ADHD by age 27. These findings are consistent with more recent cross-sectional studies showing elevated health complaints in children (Giacobo, Jane, Bonillo, Arrufat, Araujo, 2014) and teens with ADHD (Brook, Brook, Zhang, Seltzer, & Finch, 2012). Not surprisingly, we found that the somatization scale from the Symptom Checklist-90-R (Derogatis, 1986) explained 37% of the variance in these total problem scores. We also found that fewer of the H+ADHD (44%) group reported exercising regularly compared with the other groups (65% and 69%, respectively). If all of these patterns continue forward in life we can hypothesize a greater likelihood of later-life health problems being associated with ADHD, especially in those individuals having persistent ADHD.

Our groups did not differ in height or weight at age 27, similar to the findings of Weiss and Hecthman (1993). And childhood treatment with stimulant medication was not significantly associated with either of these measures. These data provide no evidence of long-term suppression of growth into adulthood in height, weight, or body mass index in children treated with stimulants regardless of treatment duration. They are in complete agreement with the Weiss and Hechtman (1993) longitudinal study of hyperactive children who likewise found no such effects. But we did find that the persistently ADHD group had a significantly greater body mass index than the community control group with the H−ADHD group placing between these two and not differing significantly from either of them. As a result, twice as many (40%) of the two ADHDs group qualified as being obese (BMI ≥ 30) than did the control group (20%), which replicates the findings in the New York longitudinal study (Cortese, Olazagasti, Klein, Castellanos, Proal, & Mannuzza, 2013).

Both hyperactive groups had significantly lower HDL cholesterol than the Community group, while only the H+ADHD group had a greater HDL-to-Total cholesterol ratio, both of which are risk factors for future cardiovascular disease (Devroey, Vantomme, Betz, Vandevoorde, & Kartounian, 2004). We found no important differences among these groups in the results of their urine, blood, and routine physical examinations.

Finances and Money Management

To our knowledge, no previous follow-up studies of ADHD had examined this domain in any detail. In all but one of the 13 financial problem areas we explored, the H+ADHD group had a significantly larger percentage of cases having that problem than in the Community control group. The exception was for writing checks with insufficient funds, where no group differences were found. In seven of these problem areas, the H+ADHD group also had a higher risk than the H−ADHD group, these being trouble managing their money, buying on impulse, missing rent and credit card payments, exceeding credit card limits, not having a savings account, and having a poor credit rating (self-reported). In some areas, the two hyperactive groups had more participants with problems than the Community group but did not differ from each other, suggesting that having been a hyperactive/ADHD child carried some risk for financial problems even if ADHD had not persisted to this follow-up. These areas were: difficulty saving money, having utilities turned off for nonpayment, having a vehicle repossessed, declaring bankruptcy, and not saving for retirement. This was also evident in other problem areas where the H−ADHD group fell below the level of risk for the H+ADHD group yet remained at higher risk than the Community controls, such as in: managing money, buying on impulse, missing rent payments, and having a poor credit rating. In summation, both hyperactive groups had a higher percentage of many of these financial problems than did the control group suggesting that growing up with ADHD from childhood is a risk factor for financial difficulties even if that ADHD does not persist to age 27. But where it does persist, it increases the risks of financial difficulties even more.

As for gambling, we found little evidence of gambling activities associated with ADHD other than an increased likelihood of betting on card games, which seemed fairly trivial. For several reasons, this finding should not surprise us. First, the New York follow-up study (Mannuzza et al., 1993, 1998) reported that their hyperactive group was no more likely to be diagnosed with pathological or addictive gambling related disorders than was the control group. Second, research conducted while this study was underway found that excessive gambling is related principally to antisocial personality and not to ADHD (Raylu & Oei, 2002). We found such an association in our ADHD groups between those with and without ASPD on seven of our gambling issues, replicating this relationship. So it is ASPD rather than ADHD that is driving any links with gambling.

We focused on 13 possible predictors from childhood, adolescence, and young adulthood (age 21) in a regression analysis predicting the number of different money problems. Five predictors were significant (24% of the variance). These were severity of childhood hyperactivity, pervasiveness of childhood ADHD and behavior problems, the number of CD symptoms at adolescent follow-up, and the number of ADHD symptoms (self-reported) and years of education at the age 21 follow-up.

Driving Risks

We believe that Weiss and Hechtman (1993) may have been the first to note an association of hyperactivity in children with increased car accidents by adolescents and adults. This led us to do a detailed survey of driving problems and adverse outcomes at the age 21 follow-up (Fischer et al., 2007), which replicated this initial finding as well as a number of other driving problems. At the age 27 follow-up, we also found that more members of the hyperactive groups were likely to have experienced many of these adverse outcomes than were members of the Community control group, thus replicating and extending our results from the age 21 follow-up. Fewer members of the H groups were likely to have a current license, probably owing to the fact that more members of both groups had their license suspended or revoked at some time in their driving careers. More of them were also likely to have had their license suspended at least two or more times. Although the groups did not differ in the percentage that had ever had a crash in their driving history, more members of both H groups had been involved in at least two or more such crashes. Of interest was the finding that more than twice as many of the H+ADHD group had been cited for reckless driving as in the other two groups, and more of these individuals had been cited at least two or more times for this infraction. Where driving risks were found, as in crashes and license revocations, it was growing up as a child with ADHD that posed the risk factor here regardless of its persistence to this last follow-up. But persistent ADHD is more likely to be associated with reckless driving and its repeated occurrence. This was evident as well in the total number of different driving problems, where we found that the H+ADHD group had significantly more problems (M = 5.2, SD = 2.7) than the Community group (M = 3.8, SD = 2.4) with the H−ADHD group falling between these two groups and not differing from either of them (M = 4.6, SD = 2.3; $F = 5.28$, $df = 2/205$, $p = .006$).

We studied predictors of two major outcomes here: crash frequency and diversity of adverse driving outcomes. Out of 12 possible predictors, we found that the best ones for predicting crash frequency were, not surprisingly, severity of ADHD, older age, the number of self-reported speeding tickets one had received, a poorer credit rating (self-reported), and higher levels of hostility. The best predictors for the number of different driving problems reported by participants were: severity of childhood hyperactivity (CPRS-R), severity of teen ADHD, and years of education received by age 21, but these accounted for only 8% of the variance.

Numerous studies have documented further the greater and multilevel risks that teens and adults with ADHD encounter in driving (Aduen, Korfler, Cox, Sarver, & Lunsford, 2015; Barkley, 2015; Barkley & Cox, 2007). These span the levels of basic cognitive abilities necessary for driving (slower and more variable reaction time, motor incoordination, inattention, impulsivity, and limited self-awareness and monitoring) to operation of the vehicle (variable steering, erratic braking for possible threats, etc.) to risky driving (less use of seat belts, speeding, road rage) to diminished use of safe driving habits to adverse outcomes (more citations, crashes, and license suspensions).

Risky Sexual Behavior

At the time our 27-year follow-up was underway, only two prior studies had examined this domain of psychosocial functioning; our 21-year follow-up (Barkley, 1998; Barkley, Fischer, Smallish, & Fletcher, 2006) and later the Pittsburgh longitudinal study (Flory, Molina, Pelham, Gnagy, & Smith, 2006). We reported a pattern of early initiation of intercourse (one year earlier on average) and riskier sexual activity (more partners, less use of contraception) in the hyperactive group (Barkley, 1998; Barkley, Fischer, Smallish, & Fletcher, 2006). This riskier pattern of conduct led to a markedly increased risk for teen pregnancy (38% vs. 4%) and sexually transmitted diseases (STDs) (17% vs. 4%) among the hyperactive as opposed to the control group. Later, Flory and colleagues (Flory, Molina, Pelham, Gnagy, & Smith, 2006) demonstrated a similar pattern of sexual conduct in young male adults with a history of childhood ADHD. They found that childhood ADHD was associated with earlier initiation of sexual activity and intercourse, more sexual partners, more casual sex, and more partner pregnancies. Both longitudinal studies found that these risks were further elevated by the co-occurrence of higher levels of conduct problems, but such problems did not account for the separate contribution made by ADHD. By the age-27 follow-up, we found that the groups differed in the number of lifetime sex partners with the H+ADHD group (M = 17, SD = 22) having more such partners than the control group (M = 8, SD = 9) but not differing from the H−ADHD group (M = 13, SD = 19). This was not related to the age of the participant. The groups did not differ in the number of sex partners they had during the past year (1–2), or in the frequency of intercourse in the past year (about monthly). But, we found that significantly more members of both hyperactive groups had either gotten pregnant, in the case of females, or gotten someone else pregnant, in the case of males. The percentages were more than triple that of the Community group. As one might guess, more members of the H groups were the biological parents of offspring than was true for the control group. The H+ADHD group, however, had more children (M = 1.1, SD = 1.4) than the H−ADHD group (M = 0.8, SD = 1.0), who had more offspring than the control group (M = 0.2, SD = 0.6) Thus, degree of ADHD is clearly related to not just early parenthood but to having more children. These initial findings of heightened risky sexual behavior in those with elevated ADHD symptoms have now been replicated in community samples (Donahue, Lichtenstein, Lundstrom, Anckarsater, Gumpert et al., 2013; Fontaine, Carbonneau, Barker, Vitaro, Herbert et al., 2008; Galera, Messiah, Melchior, Chastang, Encrenaz et al., 2010).

DISCUSSION

We explored other areas of risk and deficit in our ADHD groups (social relations, dating, marriage, neuropsychological deficits, etc.), but space precludes reviewing those findings here (see Barkley et al., 2008). Instead, we have tried to focus here on those we consider of greatest importance, many of which either had not been explored in much detail in prior longitudinal studies or had not been studied at all. The totality of our results show that growing up with ADHD (hyperactive child syndrome) poses risks across virtually every domain of major life activities studied to date, including psychiatric comorbidity, educational and occupational functioning, driving, health, finances, sexual activities, and social relationships, among others. ADHD is clearly not a developmentally benign disorder. Although some of our findings essentially replicated earlier such studies, such as global educational and occupational risks and comorbidity, they also extended prior studies to a group of more rigorously diagnosed cases of hyperactivity/ADHD than had been the case in prior studies. And we explored new domains of impairment not previously investigated.

We also found that for some domains of impairment, such as the educational domain, whether ADHD had persisted to the 27-year follow-up did not matter much concerning the elevated risks posed by growing up with the disorder. Yet in other areas, such as current occupational functioning and adjustment, those in whom ADHD had persisted were more impaired on various measures than were those whose ADHD had not persisted. But even the nonpersistent group typically had higher levels of problems in these areas than did the control children as young adults. And so, although the longer ADHD had persisted into adulthood the greater were the present impairments, recovering from ADHD or being subsyndromic by young adulthood did not leave these cases unscarred.

Where we were able to examine predictors of outcome, it was clear that ADHD in childhood and its persistence over time contributed some variance to most of the outcomes reported here. For some domains, such as driving, finances, drug use, and some aspects of adult comorbidity, the presence of conduct problems in childhood, CD by adolescence, and CD symptoms at age 21 also were associated with adversities at outcome. For most outcomes, however, the amount of variance explained by these predictors was relatively modest, suggesting that impairments at age 27 also are linked to other factors not explored in our study. All of this suggests that the pathway from childhood ADHD to likely impairments experienced in adulthood is neither an easily predicted nor straightforward one.

Not mentioned above because it was not significant in our analyses was the finding that the extent of psychiatric, psychological, or special educational treatment in childhood had no detectable impact on the adult outcomes of these children, probably owing largely to the fact that it was principally limited to childhood. For instance, the average time on medication was a mere three years by the adolescent follow-up and the vast majority were no longer taking medication during high school or at the age-21 follow-up. Klein and colleagues (Klein, Mannuzza, Olazagasti,

Roizen, Hutchison et al., 2012) at their 33-year follow-up of the New York study samples reported that most of the problems evident at that point had begun in adolescence. Coupled with our results one can see a reasonable inference here: The time of greatest risk for the emergence of comorbidity and impairments in major life activities is the time in development when children growing up with ADHD are less likely to be receiving treatment—adolescence. By extension, treatments that are not sustained through adolescence and into adulthood are unlikely to alter the life course outcomes of children growing up with ADHD.

A broad conclusion from our research and the other longitudinal studies is quite evident to us: ADHD needs to be considered as largely a chronic neurodevelopmental disorder that poses numerous and serious risks for the adult outcomes of these children. Those risks not only make ADHD a serious mental health condition but a serious public health condition as well. As long as it persists, ADHD requires management, much like the chronic medical condition of diabetes. Like that condition, ADHD requires a package of multiple interventions that should be instituted as early as the disorder is detected, and, more importantly, should be sustained throughout adolescence and into young adulthood. It is reassuring to see now that not only has adult ADHD been increasingly accepted as a valid and serious disorder since the early 1990s, thanks largely to the findings of the longitudinal studies reviewed in this text, but that it is being increasingly treated. Yet there is far more work to be done given that the majority of adults with ADHD still go undiagnosed and untreated despite promising gains in these services. The substantial social, emotional, educational, occupational, and financial costs, among others, that this disorder is now known to pose to both the afflicted and to society demand nothing less.

REFERENCES

Aduen, P. A., Korfler, M. J., Cox, D. J., Sarver, D. E., & Lunsford, E. (2015). Motor vehicle driving in high incidence psychiatric disability: Comparison of drivers with ADHD, depression, and no known psychopathology. *Journal of Psychiatric Research*, *64*, 59–66.

American Psychiatric Association. (1968). *Diagnostic and Statistical Manual of Mental Disorders* (2nd ed.). Washington, DC: Author.

American Psychiatric Association. (2013). *Diagnostic and Statistical Manual of Mental Disorders* (5th ed.). Washington, DC: Author.

Angold, A., Costello, E. J., & Erkanli, A. (1999). Comorbidity. *Journal of Child Psychology and Psychiatry*, *40*, 57–87.

Barkley, R. A. (1981). *Hyperactive Children: A Handbook for Diagnosis and Treatment*. New York: Guilford Press.

Barkley, R.A. (1982). Guidelines for defining hyperactivity in children (Attention Deficit Disorder with Hyperactivity). In B. Lahey & A. Kazdin (Eds.), *Advances in Clinical Child Psychology (Vol. 5)* (pp. 137–180). New York: Plenum.

Barkley, R. A. (1990). *Attention Deficit Hyperactivity Disorder: A Handbook for Diagnosis and Treatment*. New York: Guilford Press.

Barkley, R. A. (1998). *Attention Deficit Hyperactivity Disorder: A Handbook for Diagnosis and Treatment* (2nd ed.). New York: Guilford Press.

Barkley, R. A. (2012). Distinguishing sluggish cognitive tempo from attention deficit hyperactivity disorder in adults. *Journal of Abnormal Psychology*, *121*, 978–990.

Barkley, R. A. (2013). Distinguishing sluggish cognitive tempo from ADHD in children and adolescents: executive functioning, impairment, and comorbidity. *Journal of Clinical Child and Adolescent Psychology*, *42*, 161–173.

Barkley, R. A. (2015). *Attention Deficit Hyperactivity Disorder: A Handbook for Diagnosis and Treatment* (4th ed.). New York: Guilford Press.

Barkley, R. A. (2014). Sluggish cognitive tempo (concentration deficit disorder?): current status, future directions, and a plea to change the name. *Journal of Abnormal Child Psychology*, *42*, 117–125.

Barkley, R. A., & Biederman, J. (1997). Towards a broader definition of the age-of-onset criterion for attention deficit hyperactivity disorder. *Journal of the American Academy of Child and Adolescent Psychiatry*, *36*, 1204–1210.

Barkley, R. A., & Cox, D. J. (2007). A review of driving risks and impairments associated with Attention-Deficit/Hyperactivity Disorder and the effects of stimulant medication on driving performance. *Journal of Safety Research*, *38*, 113–128.

Barkley, R.A., Fischer, M., Edelbrock, C.S., & Smallish, L. (1990). The adolescent outcome of hyperactive children diagnosed by research criteria, I: An 8-year prospective follow-up study. *Journal of the American Academy of Child and Adolescent Psychiatry*, *29*, 546–557.

Barkley, R. A., Fischer, M., Edelbrock, C. S., & Smallish, L. (1991). The adolescent outcome of hyperactive children diagnosed by research criteria, III: Mother-child interactions, family conflicts, and maternal psychopathology. *Journal of Child Psychology and Psychiatry*, *32*, 233–256.

Barkley, R. A., Fischer, M., Smallish, L., & Fletcher, K. (2002). The persistence of attention-deficit/hyperactivity disorder into young adulthood as a function of reporting source and definition of disorder. *Journal of Abnormal Psychology*, *111*, 279–289.

Barkley, R. A., Fischer, M., Smallish, L., & Fletcher, K. (2003). Does the treatment of ADHD with stimulant medication contribute to illicit drug use and abuse in adulthood? Results from a 15-year prospective study. *Pediatrics*, *111*, 109–121.

Barkley, R. A., Fischer, M., Smallish, L., & Fletcher, K. (2004). Young adult follow-up of hyperactive children: Antisocial activities and drug use. *Journal of Child Psychology and Psychiatry, 45*, 195–211.

Barkley, R. A., Fischer, M., Smallish, L., & Fletcher, K. (2006). Young adult follow-up of hyperactive children: Adaptive functioning in major life activities. *Journal of the American Academy of Child and Adolescent Psychiatry, 45*. 192–202.

Barkley, R. A., Smith, K., Fischer, M., & Navia, B. (2006). An examination of the behavioral and neuropsychological correlates of three ADHD candidate gene polymorphisms (DRD4 7+, DBH TaqI A2, and DAT1 40bp VNTR) in hyperactive and normal children followed to adulthood. *American Journal of Medical Genetics: Neuropsychiatric Genetics, 141B* (5), 487–498.

Barkley, R., Karlsson, J., & Pollard, S. (1985). Effects of age on the mother-child interactions of hyperactive boys. *Journal of Abnormal Child Psychology, 13*, 631–637.

Barkley, R., Karlsson, J., Pollard, S., & Murphy, J. (1985). Developmental changes in the mother-child interactions of hyperactive boys: Effects of two dose levels of Ritalin. *Journal of Child Psychology and Psychiatry, 26*, 705–715.

Barkley, R., Karlsson, J., Strzelecki, E., & Murphy, J. (1984). The effects of age and Ritalin dosage on the mother-child interactions of hyperactive children. *Journal of Consulting and Clinical Psychology, 52*, 750–758.

Barkley, R. A., Murphy, K. R., & Fischer, M. (2008). *ADHD in Adults: What the Science Says*. New York: Guilford Press.

Brook, J. S., Brook, D. W., Zhang, C., Seltzer, N., & Finch, S. J. (2012). Adolescent ADHD and adult physical and mental health, work, and financial stress. *Pediatrics*. Advance online publication.

Brown, T. E. (2000). *Comorbidity in Attention Deficit Disorders in Children, Adolescents, and Adults* (pp. 125–170). Washington, DC: American Psychiatric Press.

Cortese, S., Olazagasti, M. A. R., Klein, R. G., Castellanos, F. X., Proal, E., & Mannuzza, S. (2013). Obesity in men with childhood ADHD: a 33-year controlled, prospective follow-up study. *Pediatrics. Advance online publication*. doi: 10.1542/peds.2012-0540.

Devroey, D., Vantomme, K., Betz, W., Vandevoorde, J., & Kartounian, J. (2004). A review of the treatment guidelines on the management of low levels of high-density lipoprotein cholesterol. *Cardiology, 102*, 61–66.

Derogatis, L. (1986). *Manual for the Symptom Checklist 90 Revised (SCL-90-R)*. Baltimore, MD: Author.

Faraone, S. V., & Biederman, J. (1997). Do attention deficit hyperactivity disorder and major depression share familial risk factors? *Journal of Nervous and Mental Diseases, 185*, 533–541.

Fischer, M., & Barkley, R. A. (2006). Young adult outcome of hyperactive children: Leisure, financial and social activities. *International Journal of Disability, Development, and Education, 53*, 229–245.

Fischer, M., Barkley, R. A., Edelbrock, C. S., & Smallish, L. (1990). The adolescent outcome of hyperactive children diagnosed by research criteria, II: Academic, attentional, and neuropsychological status. *Journal of Consulting and Clinical Psychology, 58*, 580–588.

Fischer, M., Barkley, R. A., Fletcher, K., Smallish, L. (1993a). The stability of dimensions of behavior in ADHD and normal children over an 8-year period. *Journal of Abnormal Child Psychology, 21*, 315–337.

Fischer, M., Barkley, R. A., Fletcher, K., & Smallish, L. (1993b). The adolescent outcome of hyperactive children diagnosed by research criteria, V: Predictors of outcome. *Journal of the American Academy of Child and Adolescent Psychiatry, 32*, 324–332.

Fischer, M., Barkley, R. A., Smallish, L., & Fletcher, K. (2002). Young adult follow-up of hyperactive children: Self-reported psychiatric disorders, comorbidity, and the role of childhood conduct problems. *Journal of Abnormal Child Psychology, 30*, 463–475.

Fischer, M., Barkley, R. A., Smallish, L., & Fletcher, K. (2007). Hyperactive children as young adults: Driving ability, safe driving behavior, and adverse driving outcomes. *Accident Analysis and Prevention, 39*, 94–105.

Fletcher, K., Fischer, M., Barkley, R. A., & Smallish, L. (1996). A sequential analysis of the mother-adolescent interactions of ADHD, ADHD/ODD, and Normal teenagers neutral and conflict discussions. *Journal of Abnormal Child Psychology, 24*, 271–298.

Flory, K., Molina, B. S., Pelham, W. E., Jr., Gnagy, E., & Smith, B. (2006). Childhood ADHD predicts risky sexual behavior in young adulthood. *Journal of Clinical Child and Adolescent Psychology, 35*, 571–577.

Donahue, K. L., Lichtenstein, P., Lundstrom, S., Anckarsater, H., Gumpert, C. H., Langstrom, N., & D'Onofrio, B. M. (2013). Childhood behavior problems and adolescent sexual risk behavior: Familial confounding in the child and adolescent twin study in Sweden (CATSS). *Journal of Adolescent Health, 52*, 606–612.

Fontaine, N., Carbonneau, R., Barker, E. D., Vitaro, F., Herbert, M., Cole, S. M., ,. . .Tremblay, R. E. (2008). Girls' hyperactivity and physical aggression during childhood and adjustment problems in early adulthood. A 15-year longitudinal study. *Archives of General Psychiatry, 65*, 320–328.

Galera, C., Messiah, A., Melchior, M., Chastang, J. F., Encrenaz, G., Lagarde, E., ,. . .Fombonne, E. (2010). Disruptive behaviors and early sexual intercourse: The GAXEL Youth Study. *Psychiatry Research, 177*, 361–363.

Giacobo, R. S., Jane, M. C., Bonillo, A., Arrufat, F. J, & Araujo, E. (2014). ADHD and functional somatic symptoms: Structural equations of a conceptual model. *Child and Adolescent Mental Health, 19*, 83–89.

Goyette, C.H., Conners, C.K., & Ulrich, R.F. (1978). Normative data for Revised Conners Parent and Teacher Rating Scales. *Journal of Abnormal Child Psychology, 6*, 221–236.

Hallowell, R. M. & Ratey, J. J. (2005). *Delivered from distraction:Getting the most out of life with attention deficit disorder*. New York: Ballantine Books.

Hartmann, T. (1993). *The Edison gene: ADHD and the gift of the hunter child*. Rochester, VT: Park Street Press.

Hollingshead, J. (1975). A four-factor index of social position. Author.

Loeber, R., Burke, J. D., Lahey, B. B., Winters, A., Zera, M. (2000). Oppositional defiant and conduct disorder: A review of the past 10 years, Part I. *Journal of the American Academy of Child and Adolescent Psychiatry, 39*, 1468–1484.

Klein, R. G., Mannuzza, S., Olazagasti, M. A., Roizen, E., Hutchison, J. A., Lashua, E. C., . . . et al. (2012). Clinical and functional outcome of childhood attention-deficit/hyperactivity disorder 33 years later. *Archives of General Psychiatry, 69*, 1295–1303.

Mannuzza, S., Gittelman-Klein, R., Bessler, A., Malloy, P., & LaPadula, M. (1993). Adult outcome of hyperactive boys: Educational achievement, occupational rank, and psychiatric status. *Archives of General Psychiatry, 50*, 565–576.

Mannuzza, S., Klein, R., Bessler, A., Malloy, P., & LaPadula, M. (1998). Adult psychiatric status of hyperactive boys grown up. *American Journal of Psychiatry, 155*, 493–498.

McGough, J. J., & Barkley, R. A. (2004). Diagnostic controversies in adult ADHD. *American Journal of Psychiatry, 161*, 1948–1956.

Pliszka, S. R. (2009). *Treating ADHD and Comorbid Disorders: Psychosocial and Psychopharmacological Interventions*. New York: Guilford Press.

Rasmussen, P., & Gillberg, C. (2001). Natural outcome of ADHD with developmental coordination disorder at age 22 years: A controlled, longitudinal, community-based study. *Journal of the American Academy of Child and Adolescent Psychiatry, 39*, 1424–1431.

Raylu, N., & Oei, T. P. S. (2002). Pathological gambling: a comprehensive review. *Clinical Psychology Review, 22*, 1009–1061.

Shelley-Tremblay, J. F., & Rosen, L. A. (1996). Attention deficit hyperactivity disorder: An evolutionary perspective. *Journal of Genetic Psychology: Research and Theory in Human Development, 157*, 443–453.

Skinner, H. A. (1994). *Computerized Lifestyle Assessment*. North Tonawanda, NY: Multi-Health Systems, Inc.

Smith, K. M., Bauer, L., Fischer, M., Barkley, R. A., & Navia, B. (2005). Identification and characterization of human NR4A2 polymorphisms in attention deficit hyperactivity disorder. *American Journal of Medical Genetics, Part B: Neuropsychiatric Genetics, 133B*(1), 57–63.

Spitzer, R. L., Williams, J., Gibbon, M., & First, M. B. (1995). *The Structured Clinical Interview for DSM-IV (SCID)*. New York: Biometric Research Department, New York State Psychiatric Institute.

Weiss, G., & Hechtman, L. (1993). *Hyperactive Children Grown Up* (2nd ed.). New York: Guilford Press.

Wilens, T. E., Faraone, S. V., Biederman, J., & Gunawardene, S. (2003). Does stimulant therapy of Attention Deficit/Hyperactivity Disorder beget later substance abuse? A meta-analytic review of the literature. *Pediatrics, 11*(1), 179–185.

5

The Pittsburgh ADHD Longitudinal Study (PALS)

BROOKE S. G. MOLINA, MARGARET H. SIBLEY, SARAH L. PEDERSEN, AND WILLIAM E. PELHAM, JR.

INTRODUCTION

The Pittsburgh ADHD Longitudinal Study (PALS) is a large prospective study of children diagnosed with attention deficit hyperactivity disorder (ADHD) and a demographically similar group of youth without ADHD recruited for comparison purposes. The study was designed to test hypotheses regarding the onset, course, and consequences of problematic alcohol and other substance use for children with ADHD. For this purpose, assessments conducted over the past 20 years have been designed for their sensitivity to developmental progression of alcohol and drug use and for their comprehensive coverage of theoretically important predictors, mediators, and moderators of outcome. As such, the PALS has contributed substantially to the empirical literature on both alcoholism and other substance use disorder (SUD) risk for children with ADHD and to our understanding of the long-term course of ADHD. At the time of this chapter's writing, the PALS remains ongoing with most participants between 28 and 35 years old.

Historical Context

When the PALS was initially launched in the 1990s, little was known about the extent of risk for alcohol and other SUDs for children with ADHD. Studies had suggested the possibility of increased risk (e.g., Barkley et al., 1990; Gittelman et al., 1985; Hartsough & Lambert, 1987; Loney, 1993; Weiss & Hechtman, 1993), but the findings were variable. For example, Barkley and colleagues (1990) reported an increased risk of cigarette, alcohol, and marijuana use for adolescents with childhood hyperactivity, but Bonferroni corrections relegated two findings to statistical nonsignificance. Gittelman and colleagues (1985) found ADHD to be a long-term risk factor for drug, but not alcohol, use disorder (Gittelman et al., 1985; Mannuzza et al., 1991) while Loney (1993) and Weiss and Hechtman (1993) reported group differences for certain alcohol outcomes.

At the time, longitudinal studies of children with ADHD were only just beginning to characterize the long-term course of ADHD into adolescence and emerging adulthood, and the assessment of alcohol and other SUDs was incidental to the broader category of adjustment. Standard, developmentally informed protocols for the longitudinal assessment of substance use and SUDs were underdeveloped in longitudinal studies of ADHD (but not in the addiction literature). For example, extant studies of ADHD did not include adolescent reports of frequency and quantity of consumption or age when substances were first used; these are important variables known in the SUD literature to capture risky consumption patterns with prognostic utility, particularly among adolescents. These indicators facilitate the identification of additional factors, such as parental monitoring, that have prevention and intervention implications (rather than waiting until SUD has fully developed in adulthood to intervene, perhaps with less effect). Thus, the PALS was designed to measure these variables. It was also designed with ample power to test hypotheses about mediating and moderating factors. The samples of most longitudinal studies of children diagnosed with ADHD were small for this purpose, with approximately one hundred or so probands, which, when combined with limited SUD and risk factor assessments, left many questions unanswered regarding the extent and the reasons behind risk of SUDs for children with ADHD.

Many other questions regarding long-term outcome for children with ADHD existed and have been important to address alongside SUD risk. These included, for example, extent of vulnerability to other risky or otherwise health-endangering behaviors, the unfolding of comorbidities including conduct problems and depression, and the extent to which childhood ADHD persisted into adolescence and adulthood and what measurement approaches were needed to understand this outcome. The PALS has sought to address many of these questions.

METHOD

Overview

The PALS has included three phases of individuals with ADHD: (1) a preliminary one-time assessment of children with ADHD as adolescents (n = 142 ADHD, n = 100 non-ADHD, aged 13–18 years); (2) a large, ongoing study of individuals with childhood ADHD followed prospectively, some through adolescence, and all through adulthood (n = 364 ADHD, n = 240 non-ADHD, aged 11–28 years at the first follow-up assessment); and (3) additional adult participants with childhood ADHD from resumed recruitment efforts begun in 2012. (Analyses making use of data from these additional participants, 45 to date, are not included in the current chapter.) Over half of the children who participated in the first study as adolescents are participants in the ongoing PALS study with recurring assessments. Below we describe the methods for recruitment and interviewing of the ongoing longitudinal sample.

Participants

PALS ADHD Group. The ADHD group, n = 364, was recruited from a pool of 516 study-eligible participants diagnosed with *Diagnostic and Statistical Manual of Mental Disorders* (DSM-III-R or DSM-IV) ADHD in childhood and treated at the Attention Deficit Disorder clinic at Western Psychiatric Institute and Clinic (WPIC) in Pittsburgh, Pennsylvania from 1987 to 1996. Of the 516 study-eligible participants, 493 were recontacted an average of 8.35 years later (*SD* = 2.79) to participate in annual interviews. Of those contacted, 364 (70.5%) enrolled in the PALS and their data are described in many of our publications. At the first follow-up interview, the ADHD group ranged in age from 11 to 28 years with 99% falling between 11 and 25 years of age. They were admitted to the follow-up study on a rolling basis between the years 1999 and 2003 and completed their first follow-up interview immediately upon enrollment.

All of these probands participated in the Summer Treatment Program (STP) for children with ADHD, an eight-week intervention that included behavioral modification, parent training, and psychoactive medication trials where indicated (Pelham & Hoza, 1996; Pelham et al., 2010). Diagnostic information for the probands was collected at initial referral to the clinic in childhood (baseline) using parent and teacher DSM- III- R and DSM-IV symptom ratings scales Disruptive Behavior Disorders Rating Scale (DBD); (Pelham, Evans, Gnagy, & Greenslade, 1992) and a semistructured diagnostic interview administered to parents by a PhD-level clinician. The interview consisted of the DSM-III-R or DSM-IV descriptors for ADHD, oppositional defiant disorder (ODD), and conduct disorder (CD) with supplemental probe questions regarding situational and severity factors. It also included queries about other comorbidities to determine whether additional assessment was needed. Following DSM guidelines, diagnoses of ADHD, ODD, and CD were made if a sufficient number of symptoms were endorsed (considering information from both parents and teachers) to result in diagnosis. Two PhD-level clinicians independently reviewed all ratings and interviews to confirm DSM diagnoses, and when disagreement occurred, a third clinician reviewed the file and the majority decision was used. Exclusion criteria for probands were assessed in childhood (baseline) and included a full-scale IQ < 80, a history of seizures, neurological problems, pervasive developmental disorder, schizophrenia, and/or other psychotic or organic mental disorders.

Participants in the follow-up study were compared with the eligible individuals who did not enroll on demographic (i.e., age at first treatment, race, parental education level, and marital status) and diagnostic (i.e., parent and teacher ratings of ADHD and related symptomatology) variables collected at baseline in childhood. Only 1 in 14 comparisons was statistically significant at the $p < .05$ significance level. Participants had a slightly lower average Conduct Disorder symptom rating on a four-point scale as indicated by a composite of parent and teacher ratings (participants $M = 0.43$, $SD = .31$; nonparticipants $M = 0.53$, $SD = .39$, Cohen's $d = .30$).

PALS Comparison Group. The non-ADHD group participants numbered 240 without ADHD. They were recruited from the greater Pittsburgh community between 1999 and 2001 from several sources including pediatric practices in Allegheny County (40.8%), advertisements in local newspapers (27.5%), local universities and colleges (20.8%), and other methods (10.9%) such as Pittsburgh Public Schools and word of mouth. Comparison group recruitment lagged three months behind the ADHD group enrollment in order to obtain demographic similarity (discussed below). A telephone screening interview was administered to parents of potential comparison group participants to gather basic demographic characteristics, history of diagnosis or treatment for ADHD and other behavior problems, presence of exclusionary criteria as previously listed for the ADHD group, and a checklist of ADHD symptoms. Young adults also provided self-report of ADHD symptoms (see *Measures*). ADHD symptoms were counted as present if reported by either the parent or the young adult. Participants who met DSM-III-R criteria for ADHD, either currently or historically, were excluded from study consideration.

If a potential comparison group participant passed the initial phone screen, senior research staff members met to determine whether he/she was demographically appropriate for the study. Each potential participant was examined on four demographic characteristics: (1) age, (2) gender, (3) race, and (4) parent educational level. He or she was deemed study-eligible if his/her enrollment increased the comparison group's demographic similarity to the participants diagnosed with ADHD. At the end of the recruitment process, the two groups were equivalent on the four demographic variables noted above. Because the age range is wide, analyses are sometimes conducted within age group subsamples (see Table 5.1) or in interaction with age.

Procedure

Baseline (childhood) diagnostic information was gathered for the ADHD group at initial referral to the clinic during childhood. Follow-up interviews are conducted by postbaccalaureate research staff. All questionnaires (paper and pencil or web-based) are completed privately. During informed consent, participants are assured of the confidentiality of disclosed materials. This privacy is reinforced by a Certificate of Confidentiality from the National Institute on Alcohol Abuse and Alcoholism. In cases where distance prevents participant travel to the research offices, information is collected through mail, telephone correspondence, and home visits. PALS follow-up interviews were conducted yearly beginning in the year of enrollment until 2008 when the assessment schedule was revised to age-targeted assessments (annually to age 23, followed by assessments at ages 25, 27, 30, and every five years thereafter). Participants always have been permitted to take any prescribed psychoactive medications on the day of their follow-up visits; however, increasingly small numbers of the sample have been medicated as age has increased. At the first follow-up interview, at the mean age of 17, only 23.9% were taking psychotropic medication (Kuriyan et al., 2014), and this number reflected an averaging of a higher percentage in adolescence with a lower percentage in adulthood.

Guiding Principles

Due to the well-established under-reporting of symptoms and impairment by children with ADHD (Owens et al., 2007), the PALS always has included

TABLE 5.1

DEMOGRAPHIC CHARACTERISTICS OF THE PITTSBURGH ADHD LONGITUDINAL STUDY (PALS) SAMPLE

	Non-ADHD n = 240	ADHD n = 364
Age (M, SD) at initial follow-up assessment*		
Adolescent Subsample (n = 120 non-ADHD; n = 163 ADHD)	14.52 (1.78)	14.74 (1.73)
Adult Subsample (n = 120 non-ADHD; n = 201 ADHD)	19.77 (1.73)	20.20 (2.19)
Full Sample	17.17 (3.16)	17.74 (3.38)
Gender (% male)	88.7	89.6
Race		
% European American	84.6	80.8
% African American	9.2	11.0
% Other	6.2	8.2
Ethnicity		
% Not Hispanic or Latino	99.2	99.2
% Hispanic Latino	0.8	0.8
Highest Parent Education**	7.41 (1.65)	7.14 (1.62)
Parental Income (Median)	$67,318	$62,959
Single Parent Household (%)	23.6	33.2
Age at Childhood Assessment (years)	NA	9.40 (2.27)
Co-occurring DBDs in Childhood	NA	
% ODD		47.2
% CD		35.9
Follow-Up Interval (M, SD)	NA	8.35 (2.79)

NOTE: *Age range at initial follow-up assessment was 11 to 28 years old with 3 participants older than 25; the adolescent subsample was 11–17 years old. *Parent education: Scale of 1 (< 7th grade education) to 9 (graduate professional training), with 7 = Associate's or two-year degree. Group differences were statistically significant at $p < .05$ or less for parental income and percentage single parent household. Probands newly recruited since 2012, n = 45, reflecting resumed recruitment from the original pool of children with ADHD, are excluded from this table. DBD= Disruptive Behavior Disorder.

additional informant reports of functioning. These included teacher and school reports of symptoms, behavior, and academic performance during adolescence; parent reports of multiple indicators of functioning through adolescence and adulthood; and recently, romantic partner and friend reports of symptoms and functioning beginning at age 30. Moreover, physician records of prescribed psychoactive medications have been collected to confirm this type of treatment (Kuriyan et al., 2014).

Our assessment battery has included a wide range of domains selected to reflect the putative predictors, mediators, and moderators of ADHD outcome with special attention to the emergence of SUDs (see Molina & Pelham, 2014, for review of pathways to SUD in ADHD). Given the wide age range of the sample at initial follow-up (as young as age 11) and the upper age range of the sample currently (age 40), our measures have been selected to accommodate the changing demography of our participants. For example, although the quality of the parent–son/daughter relationship has been continually assessed with one measure, the questionnaire assessing parental monitoring of the adolescent's daily whereabouts and activities was stopped after age 18. Our multiple reporter strategy also shifted with developmental stage. In childhood, we emphasized parent and teacher report, observation and performance of the children during their participation in the STP, and counselor/clinician ratings. During adolescence, we collected parent, teacher, and self-report as well as academic performance and discipline ratings directly from the school and medication treatment records from physicians. In adulthood, we ended collection of teacher and school reports, preferring instead to ask the young adults to report their academic outcomes; parent report has been continued but adjusted as the participants age. Beginning at age 30, the parent report assessments are relatively brief, and additional informant reports were added in recent years (romantic partners and friends). Other guidelines that we have adopted reflect a merging of standard procedures used in longitudinal studies across developmental stages with methods that we deemed necessary to validly measure functioning among adults with ADHD histories.

Sample Retention

Small numbers of participants have either died or permanently declined further participation. As of March 2015, thirteen ADHD and three non-ADHD are deceased, and only twenty-three ADHD and ten non-ADHD have declined further participation. Thus, our retention rates remain high. Also since March 2015, the majority of our continuing participants (86% from the ADHD group and 95% from the non-ADHD group, excluding those newly recruited since 2012) have completed nine or more waves of data collection over the course of the study. Figures such as these are an important measure of retention in longitudinal studies where analyses make use of recurring assessments (Chassin et al., 2004; Muthen & Muthen, 2004). We have written about the efforts required to maintain a sample such as the PALS longitudinally (Faden et al., 2004).

RESULTS

Overview

We include our findings with respect to alcohol and other substance use outcomes (including predictors, mediators, and moderators), as well as our findings characterizing other health-related outcomes (e.g., driving and risky sex), course of delinquency and academic/vocational outcomes, persistence of ADHD into adolescence and adulthood, and several additional reports of interest (e.g., comorbid psychopathology in adulthood). Due to limited space, we include only selected findings and refer readers to our PALS publications (see papers including Molina and Pelham as authors). For example, readers interested in the outcomes for the females may read these publications (Babinski, Pelham, Molina, Gnagy et al., 2011; Babinski, Pelham, Molina, Waschbusch et al., 2011).

Magnitude and Age-specificity of Risk for Alcohol Outcomes

Our initial test of the hypothesis that childhood ADHD increases risk of alcoholism was conducted with the first adolescent follow-up study (Molina & Pelham, 2003). To our knowledge, this was the first study designed to measure alcohol use using a developmentally informed assessment. Follow-up recruitment of this sample began in 1994 and ended in 2000. Participants averaged 15.18 years of age in both groups (SD = 1.42 non-ADHD, 1.44 ADHD), and most were boys (95% non-ADHD, 93.7% ADHD) (see Molina & Pelham, 2003 for additional sample description). At the time, the sample was comparable in size to other well-known longitudinal studies of children diagnosed with ADHD (e.g., Barkley et al., 1990; Biederman et al., 1997; Gittelman et al., 1985).

Results indicated that approximately half of the sample, regardless of ADHD history, reported some use of alcohol in their lifetime (46% non-ADHD, 52% ADHD, ns), and there were no group differences in the age when alcohol was first consumed or led to drunkenness. Group differences emerged, however, for frequency of drunkenness and a dimensional measure of alcohol problems. For example, 23.2% of the ADHD group compared with only 12.0% of the non-ADHD group reported more than one episode of drunkenness in the prior six months. Effect sizes were in the range of .39 (frequency of drunkenness) to .43 (alcohol problems), indicating modest-sized group differences in these more sensitive indicators of emerging alcohol problems among teens. Given the young mean-age of the sample, with no ADHD group differences in pertinent demographic characteristics, these findings suggested that some concern was warranted regarding ADHD risk for later alcohol problems.

These findings were partially replicated with the first wave of annual interviews conducted for the ongoing PALS study (Molina et al., 2007). Similar to national survey data at the time (Substance Abuse and Mental Health Services Administration [SAMHSA], 2003), about 40% of the adolescents (41% non-ADHD, 37% ADHD, ns) reported having consumed alcohol at least once in their lifetimes (more than just a sip). The age range included 11- to 17-year-olds, with n = 120 non-ADHD and n = 163 ADHD. Group differences were not found for frequency and typical quantity of drinking, but age-specific findings resulted for other variables assessing heavier levels of use. Specifically, adolescents with ADHD histories reported more binge drinking (five or more drinks at a time), more frequent drunkenness, and more symptoms of alcohol use disorder (AUD), compared with the non-ADHD group, in the 15- to 17-year-old age range. Figure 5.1 displays the findings for these outcome variables, which also reveal the relative importance of assessing frequency/quantity indicators compared with alcohol use disorder diagnoses and symptoms.

In the same paper (Molina et al., 2007), we examined alcohol outcomes for the older participants at the first annual interview (for these analyses, n = 118 non-ADHD, n = 195 ADHD, all aged 18–25 years). Although the young adults reported frequent drinking, frequent binge drinking, and more AUD symptoms than the adolescents (as expected), no ADHD group differences were found for any of the alcohol outcome variables (frequency and quantity of drinking, frequency of binge drinking and drunkenness, and AUD symptoms). For example, the average number of times drunk in the past year was 25 for both groups. As discussed later, we

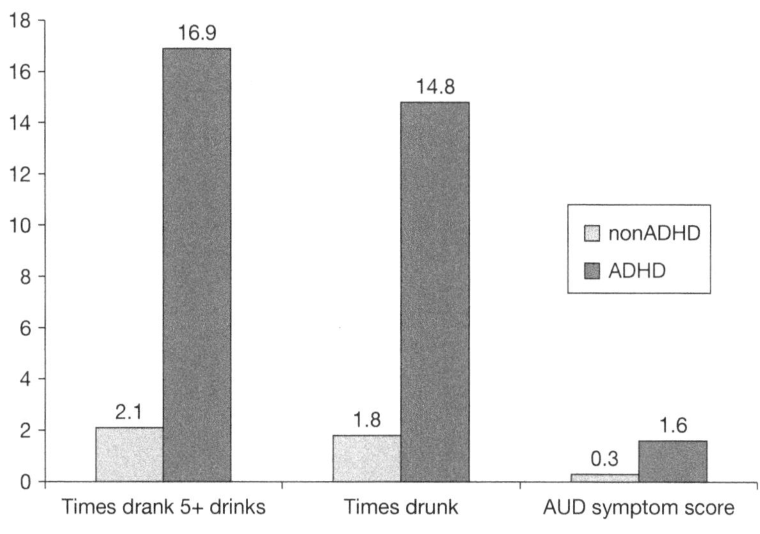

Figure 5.1 Alcohol consumption in the past year for 15- to 17-year-olds with and without childhood ADHD (Molina et al., 2007). Values are mean scores. See also color plate section.

found appreciably higher drinking scores among the probands with antisocial personality disorder (ASPD) comorbidity (e.g., 42.6% with ASPD had an AUD vs. 19.6% without ASPD had an AUD vs. 23% for the non-ADHD group). The ADHD group with ASPD also reported, on average, 43 episodes of drunkenness in the past year compared to 18 and 22 episodes for the ADHD without ASPD and non-ADHD groups, respectively. The relatively low percentage (27%) of the ADHD group (n = 54/197) who had ASPD may explain the failed overall ADHD group differences for the alcohol variables. In addition, heavy drinking is common in the 18- to 25-year-old age range, which we expect contributes to developmentally limited increased drinking in the non-ADHD group (SAMHSA, 2003). We will be able to test this hypothesis directly when all participants have completely passed the high-risk drinking period.

A recent report of age-20 heavy drinking for these participants examined hypothesized pathways from adolescence to heavy drinking in early adulthood (Molina et al., 2014). As expected, ADHD group differences were not found for age-20 heavy drinking (an average of binge drinking frequency and drunkenness frequency in the past 12 months), but childhood ADHD predicted adolescent delinquency, which, in turn, predicted age-20 delinquency, which, in turn, was associated with age-20 heavy drinking. Thus, analyzed in a slightly different way, the Molina et al. (2014) findings reaffirmed the contribution of involvement in conduct problem behaviors along the pathway to excessive drinking.

Taken together, our findings suggest a modest and variable association of childhood ADHD with important alcohol outcomes that are affected by developmental stage, type of alcohol measure, and conduct-problem comorbidity. Importantly, where previous research focused only on AUD or on any lifetime use of alcohol, a more nuanced measurement that captures variability in drinking characteristics and emerging problems, known to be prognostic of later AUD, is important for this type of research. We are continuing to follow our sample into their thirties to determine whether the developmental issues (especially group differences in adolescence that disappear in early adulthood) will lead to higher rates of heavy drinking and AUD once developmentally limited heavy drinking in early adulthood is complete.

Attention Deficit Hyperactivity Disorder Risk for Nonalcohol Substance Use

When examining nonalcohol substance use outcomes in adolescence with our first sample (Molina & Pelham, 2003), we again found group differences that depended on the measure. Lifetime use (any use ever) of marijuana did not differ between the groups (26% non-ADHD vs. 35% ADHD), but a medium effect size emerged in the comparison of marijuana use frequency (Cohen's d effect size of .48). The non-ADHD group averaged responses between "never" and "once" while the ADHD group averaged responses between "once" and "two-to-three times" in the past six months. The dimensional marijuana use problem score did not differ between groups. Analyses of our young adult data, at a mean age of 21, found no group differences in rates of having ever tried marijuana (64% non-ADHD vs. 68% ADHD), marijuana use frequency in the past year, or rates of marijuana use disorder (19.5% non-ADHD vs. 23% ADHD; Harty et al., 2015). An earlier age of first use was reported, however, for the ADHD group, M = 15.36, compared with the non-ADHD group, M = 16.05.

Use of other illicit drugs (e.g., hallucinogens, inhalants) was examined in our initial adolescent sample (Molina & Pelham, 2003). Adolescents in the ADHD group were more likely to report lifetime and past six months' use compared with the non-ADHD group. For example, 7% versus 20.4% of the non-ADHD and ADHD groups reported some illicit drug use in their lifetime, with an odds ratio of 3.41 and $p < .01$. Children with ADHD experienced their first illicit drug use at younger mean ages as well, at 16.92 years old versus 17.61 years old for those without ADHD, $p < .01$. For a young sample (mean age of 15), which usually corresponds to ninth and tenth grades in the United States, these are meaningful group differences that would have been missed had substance use *disorder* been the exclusive focus of assessment.

ADHD group differences for cigarette use have been robust and replicated within the PALS. In the first adolescent sample (Molina & Pelham, 2003), trying cigarettes was common for both groups (49% non-ADHD vs. 59.3% ADHD, ns), but probands smoked higher quantities of cigarettes (effect size of $d = .54$) and daily smoking was more common ($OR = 3.16$, $p < .01$). Age of first cigarette and age at which daily smoking began were also earlier by about a year for the ADHD group. Figure 5.2 illustrates the mean ages by which these behaviors emerged for each group.

From the first wave of annual interviews, adolescents with ADHD aged 11–17 were more likely to have tried cigarettes, and adolescents with ADHD aged 15-17 were more likely to be daily smokers, than same-aged adolescents without ADHD histories (Rhodes et al., in press). For example, among those 15–17 years old, 33% of the 15- to 17-year-olds reported daily smoking versus only 5% of the non-ADHD adolescents, $p < .001$, $OR = 8.7$. Group differences were also apparent among the adults, but only

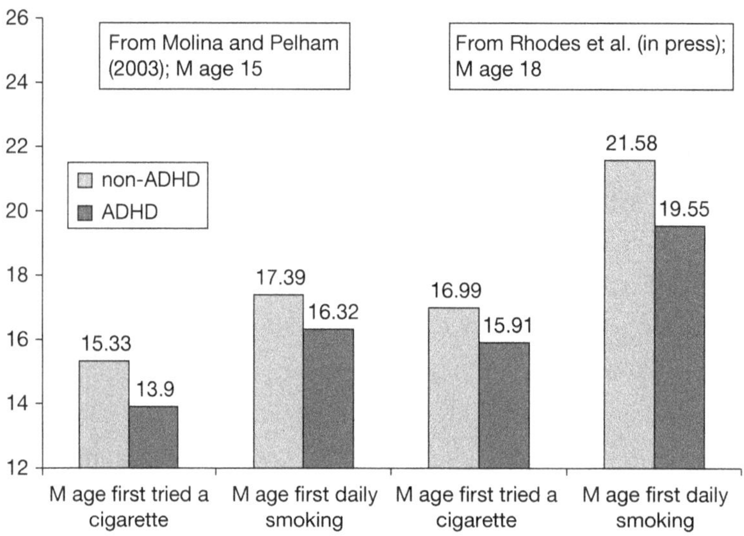

Figure 5.2 Mean ages of initiation, from Kaplan-Meier survival curves, for cigarette use behaviors, from Molina and Pelham (2003) and Rhodes et al. (in press). All group differences are statistically significant. See also color plate section.

for rates of daily smoking among the 21+ year olds because the majority of participants had tried cigarettes by adulthood. A sample finding is that among those 21–28 years old, 68% of the ADHD group (n = 73) reported daily smoking compared with 41% of the non-ADHD group (n = 34), $p < .01$. The large percentage of daily smokers in the non-ADHD group, compared with national norms for males aged 18–24 (20.1%; Centers for Disease Control [CDC], 2014), was surprising and we look forward to reanalyzing these data when all participants in the PALS are older. Our earlier finding of younger ages of initiation (Molina & Pelham, 2003) was replicated; age first tried cigarettes and age began daily smoking were significantly earlier for the ADHD than non-ADHD group Figure 5.2. Progression from initial to daily smoking was also more rapid in the ADHD than non-ADHD group (1 versus 2 years, respectively). Number of cigarettes smoked per day and standard measures of nicotine dependence did not differentiate the groups, with both groups demonstrating mild dependence, but more severe symptoms of craving and withdrawal (difficulty concentrating) during abstinence were reported by ADHD compared with the non-ADHD smokers.

These findings replicated and extended prior reports of more daily smoking in ADHD samples (e.g., Lambert, 2005; Milberger et al., 1997; Molina et al., 2013 from the Multimodal Treatment of ADHD study [MTA]) but, importantly, our rates were high. For example, in the age 17 follow-up of the children in the MTA study, 16.7% of the ADHD group versus 7.9% of the non-ADHD group were daily smokers (Molina et al., 2013) compared with 33% (ADHD) and 5% (non-ADHD) for the 15- to 17-year-olds in the PALS. One partial reason for the greater rates of smoking in the PALS may be the higher rate of conduct problems in the PALS versus MTA samples (see review by Molina, 2011). However, although conduct problems contribute to ADHD risk of smoking, this particular substance use outcome is the least dependent on conduct disorder comorbidity. For example, in Molina and Pelham (2003), comorbidity of CD was not crucial for elevated cigarette smoking risk. Our PALS findings by early adulthood are remarkably similar to Barkley's age-27 follow-up figures describing those who "currently smoke tobacco" (64% for ADHD vs. 30% non-ADHD, p. 301,

Barkley et al., 2008). Thus, given that cigarette smoking is the leading cause of preventable death in the United States (Rostron, 2013), and relatively few dependent smokers (< 10%) quit for six months or longer (Messer et al., 2008), more research is needed to understand precipitating factors and the efficacy of current evidence-based smoking treatments in this population.

Theoretical Model of Substance Use Disorder Risk in Attention Deficit Hyperactivity Disorder

We articulated theoretically derived pathways to SUD for children with ADHD in Molina and Pelham (2014). These include deviance-proneness and impairment pathways; cognition-mediated pathways that involve the anticipated, and experienced, effects of substances in this population; negative affect, stress, and coping pathways; and, finally, contextual variables that moderate the impact of these influences (e.g., parenting, treatment). These models are reproduced in Figures 5.3 and 5.4. The PALS data have been used to test elements of these models and we continue to turn to them in our ongoing data analyses.

The Contribution of ADHD Symptom Persistence, Delinquency, and Risky Behavior to ADHD-Related SUD Risk

ADHD symptom persistence should theoretically contribute to substance use for several reasons including indirect effects through impairments known to predict substance use (e.g., academic underperformance) and direct effects on substance use (e.g., impulsive decision-making). Persisting symptoms also may reflect the same traits tapped in adult studies of behavioral disinhibition that relate to differential response to alcohol.

In Molina and Pelham (2003), we found that persisting ADHD in adolescence was associated, even in the absence of adolescent conduct disorder, with frequency of drunkenness, alcohol problems, and cigarette use. In Molina et al. (2012), we found that persisting symptoms in adolescence were associated with more frequent alcohol use by age 17 and more

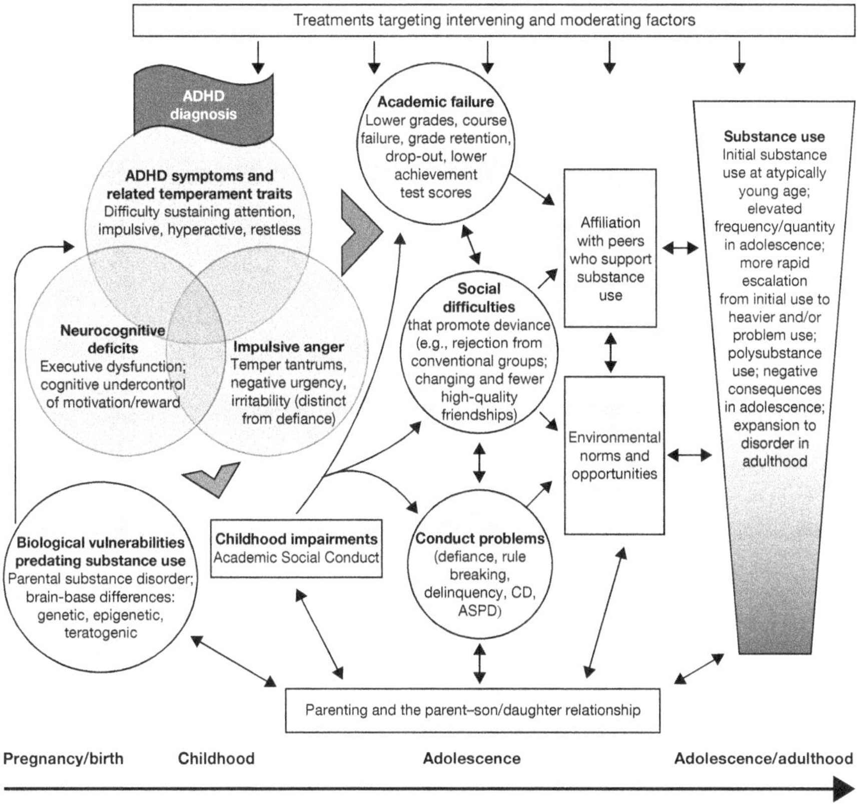

Figure 5.3 Attention deficit hyperactivity disorder (ADHD)-related impairment pathways to substance use disorder. Double-headed arrows indicate bidirectional associations. Abbreviations: ASPD, antisocial personality disorder; CD, conduct disorder. (Molina and Pelham, 2014) See also color plate section.

rapid increases in drinking frequency through adolescence; these effects included a control for delinquency in the models.

In both reports, delinquency was clearly contributory; for example, the highest rates of use for all substances and for alcohol problems were seen among the teens who had CD—which always included persisting ADHD (Molina & Pelham, 2003). Thus, our findings suggest that ADHD symptom persistence is an important contributor to SUD vulnerability in adolescence, often through its combination with conduct problems. A similar finding was recently reported by the MTA group (Howard et al., 2015), where binge drinking and marijuana use in early adulthood were associated with worse ADHD symptom and delinquency trajectories through

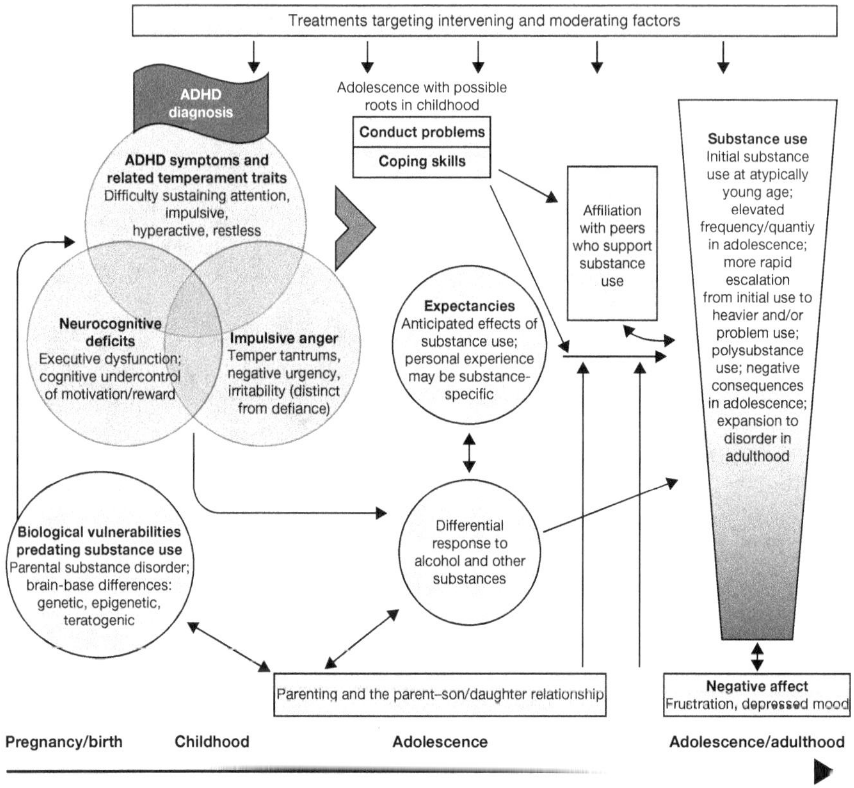

Figure 5.4 Negative affect, expectancies, and coping pathways to substance use disorder. Double-headed arrows indicate bidirectional associations. Abbreviation: ADHD, attention deficit hyperactivity disorder. (Molina and Pelham, 2014) See also color plate section.

adolescence. Our most recent report of heavy drinking in early adulthood, at age 20, found support for a mediational pathway from childhood ADHD to adolescent delinquency to age-20 delinquency, which, in turn, was associated with age-20 heavy drinking. Although ADHD symptom persistence was not included, it is easy to speculate that those young adults who drank most heavily and reported delinquent activity probably were also ADHD symptom persistent. Barkley and colleagues (2008) and Knop et al. (2009) also have reported the contribution of symptom persistence for substance use outcomes. An interesting speculation is whether direct treatment of ADHD symptoms (implying medication treatment) should dampen SUD vulnerability. The data from other studies have not strongly supported this possibility; however, there are also no data yet to suggest that medication treatment directly increases SUD risk. An alternative (additional) approach to SUD prevention and treatment is to target both the symptoms and impairments that are common in ADHD because, as we show below from the PALS data, some of the impairments are clear contributors and could be addressed in treatment (Molina and Pelham, 2014).

The Contribution of Social Impairment and Peer Choice to ADHD-Related SUD Risk

It is well-established that children with ADHD often have problems in the domain of social functioning. They are less liked by their classmates (Hoza et al., 2005), and their social problems extend into adolescence and adulthood (Bagwell et al., 2001; Barkley, Fischer, Smallish, & Fletcher, 2006; Molina et al., 2009; 2014). These social difficulties have potentially significant and diverse implications for substance use vulnerability; we have investigated some of this in the PALS.

Affiliation with peers who use substances and who approve of substance use in adolescence is among the strongest proximal predictors of adolescent alcohol and drug use (e.g., Barnes et al., 2006). Marshal and colleagues (2003) examined, in our first adolescent follow-up sample, the association between this variable and adolescent self-reported use of various substances. Probands reported more friendships with peers who used and approved of substance use, and the cross-sectional association between perceived peer use/tolerance and substance use was stronger for the ADHD than for the non-ADHD group. This finding applied to heavy alcohol use, to alcohol problems, and to illicit drug use (excluding marijuana), but not to cigarette and marijuana use. Recently, Belendiuk et al. (2016) replicated these associations longitudinally with the annual PALS interview data for adolescent alcohol use. These findings need to be examined in adulthood, but together they provide strong support for the hypothesis that the peer context is part and parcel of the vulnerability to adolescent substance use and particularly for alcohol consumption.

An interesting complication related to study of the social processes involved in substance use vulnerability for this population stems from the heterogeneity of their interpersonal difficulties, which include aggression and being actively rejected, as well as social isolation and shyness. These difficulties have potentially very different implications for substance use vulnerability (Molina & Pelham, 2014). Some of this complexity was discovered within the PALS data collected across four years in adolescence (from ages 14 to 17) when parent-rated social impairment was found to have a dual relationship with alcohol use (Molina et al., 2012; 2014). First, children with ADHD were rated as more socially impaired by their parents (usually mothers) as adolescents compared with the non-ADHD group. Specifically, their relationships with same-aged people were rated as more problematic and in need of treatment, counseling, or extra help, compared with the non-ADHD group. Second, higher social impairment was related to alcohol use frequency by age 17, but via two opposing mediational pathways. In one, social impairment was correlated with adolescent delinquency, which, in turn, predicted alcohol use frequency by age 17; in the other, social impairment was directly and inversely associated with alcohol use frequency by age 17 (Molina et al., 2012). Thus, social difficulties when coupled with conduct problems appear to increase alcohol use consumption. This finding dovetails quite sensibly with our finding in Marshal and Molina (2006; first adolescent sample) where we found that a mediational pathway from childhood ADHD to substance use through affiliation with substance using and tolerant peers was significant only in the presence of co-occurring conduct problems. The finding that social impairment, independent of delinquency, was negatively related to alcohol frequency suggests that another opposing process may be occurring. Specifically, some probands with social deficits may be shielded from the social contexts that increase alcohol exposure. Interestingly, this effect may extend into early adulthood for some, as we demonstrated in our age-20 follow-up (Molina et al., 2014).

The heterogeneous nature of the social impairments associated with ADHD may partly explain the modest and inconsistent prediction of elevated substance use and SUD from childhood ADHD: children whose social impairments lead them to a deviant peer culture may have increased risk while social inhibition or isolation may be protective, at least in adolescence. Whether these same processes apply in adulthood, when substance use opportunities and motives for substance use broaden, remains a question for future analyses.

The Contribution of Parenting Practices and the Parent– Teen Relationship to ADHD-Related SUD Risk

Parenting variables, such as developmentally appropriate limit setting with enforcement, and the parent–child relationship (e.g., warmth and support) are well-established predictors of substance use both in adolescence and even into early adulthood (Guo et al., 2001; Raudino et al., 2013). The parenting domain is also a target of intervention in evidence-based psychosocial treatment for ADHD (Pelham & Fabiano, 2008). In the PALS, three studies have directly addressed the role of these variables on substance use vulnerability in adolescence.

In Molina et al. (2005), parental social support was assessed with adolescent report of items such as "How much can you count on your mother to be there when you need her, no matter what?" Group differences were found, such that probands reported less support from their parents compared with the non-ADHD group. Moreover, parent support mediated the association between childhood ADHD and adolescent cigarette smoking, such that children with ADHD reported less support, and less support was associated with more smoking. Another paper with this same subsample of adolescents from our first study examined three other parenting variables: parental knowledge of the adolescents' whereabouts and activities, consistency of parenting (e.g., parents remembering, or not, about the rules they made), and conflict between the parent and teen (Walther et al., 2012). All of these variables were different between the groups, with effect sizes ranging from .29 (consistency) to .56 (support). However, when examined for their relations to heavy alcohol use, cigarette use, marijuana use, and delinquency, parental knowledge stood out as the most robust correlate of these outcomes. Moreover, it was more strongly associated with heavy alcohol use for the ADHD compared with the non-ADHD group. Another study from the PALS longitudinal data revealed that this same variable moderated the association between childhood ADHD and adolescent alcohol use over time, such that childhood ADHD predicted age-17 alcohol use frequency when parental knowledge was below median levels for the sample. Thus, when teens reported that their parents knew "most of the time" what they were doing and with whom, risk was significantly dampened. These findings, although subject to multiple interpretations, provide some support for the idea that normative age-related reductions in parental monitoring may be ill-advised for this population.

Substance use Cognitions and ADHD

Substance use expectancies, widely studied predictors of alcohol and drug use (e.g., Del Boca, Darkes, Goldman, & Smith, 2002; Goldman, 2002; Malmberg et al., 2012), are cognitions related to the positive (e.g., alcohol makes people outgoing) or negative (e.g., alcohol makes people have difficulty concentrating) anticipated outcome(s) of consuming a drug. Despite differences in rates of substance use for individuals with and without ADHD, limited research has examined whether there are mean level differences in substance use expectancies between these groups or how expectancies relate to drinking/drug use behavior for the ADHD population. To address the gap in the literature on how substance use expectancies function for individuals with a history of diagnostic ADHD, we examined alcohol and marijuana expectancies in PALS.

To further our understanding of how expectancies relate to alcohol use for the ADHD population, we (Pedersen et al., 2014) examined self-reported alcohol expectancies and alcohol use for 286 adolescents ages 11–17 (ADHD n = 165; non-ADHD n = 121) over a one-year period. Results showed that adolescents with a history of ADHD had lower mean levels of alcohol expectancies compared with adolescents without ADHD. Specifically, at Time 1, childhood ADHD predicted lower levels of sociability, cognitive and behavioral impairment, and liquid courage expectancies. Further, the association between negative alcohol expectancies at Time 1 and alcohol use a year later differed for individuals with and without a history of ADHD. Negative alcohol expectancies were not related to later alcohol use for individuals with a history of ADHD.

Building off of the alcohol expectancies findings, Harty and colleagues (2015) examined the marijuana expectancies of the young adults in the PALS ($N = 306$; 190 ADHD and 116 non-ADHD; $M\ age = 20.06$, $SD = 2.03$). Mean level differences were largely consistent with our alcohol expectancy findings. Individuals in the ADHD group reported lower levels of social enhancement, tension reduction, and cognitive and behavioral impairment expectancies compared with individuals in the non-ADHD group. Further paralleling the alcohol expectancy findings, a specific domain of negative expectancies, cognitive and behavioral impairment, was also less related to marijuana use for individuals with ADHD compared with those without. We also found, however, that sexual enhancement expectancies were more strongly associated with marijuana use among individuals with ADHD histories compared with those without ADHD histories.

These findings highlight that an important predictor of substance use may function differently for individuals with ADHD. Specifically, negative substance use expectancies may be less effective in deterring use for this population. Research based on the dual process model of alcohol cognition (Stacy & Wiers, 2010; Wiers & Stacy, 2006) has found that individuals in nonclinical populations with reduced executive control may rely less on a rationale or "cool" cognitive processing system (explicit expectancies) and more on an automatic, reflexive, or "hot" processing system (implicit associations) when making decisions to use drugs or alcohol. Our results are in line with this model. Research on implicit substance-related cognitions, assessed indirectly typically outside of one's awareness, could provide important insight into why individuals with ADHD use drugs and alcohol.

Susceptibility to Stressful Life Events: Parental Alcoholism, Coping, and Substance Use

Negative life events and stress across various domains have been associated with greater alcohol and drug use in adolescence (Cerbone & Larison, 2000; Hawkins, Catalano, & Miller, 1992) (Wills, Sandy, & Yaeger, 2002). Studying the association between stress and alcohol use for adolescents with ADHD may be particularly important. Individuals with ADHD are likely to experience more "controllable" stressful life events, that is, those directly related to the adolescents' own behavior (e.g., earning poor grades, fighting with peers) (Barkley, Anastopoulos, Guevremont, & Fletcher, 1992) as well as "uncontrollable" stressful life events, such as exposure to marital conflict, divorce, general family adversity, and parental alcoholism (Counts, Nigg, Stawicki, Rappley, & Von Eye, 2005; Knopik et al., 2006; Wymbs et al., 2008). Additionally, cross-sectional analyses with our first adolescent sample (Marshal, Molina, Pelham, & Cheong, 2007) found a stronger association between academic stress and alcohol use for adolescents with versus without ADHD. These results highlight that individuals with ADHD may be more susceptible to the effects of stress, but we needed to test this hypothesis longitudinally.

Recently, we (King et al., under review) extended these findings to a longitudinal framework examining multiple domains of stress in association with alcohol use from ages 14 to 17 (N = 259; 146 ADHD, 113 non-ADHD) in the PALS. Utilizing state-trait modeling we found that individuals with ADHD reported higher average levels and a more negative perception of stressful events from age 14 to 17 compared with individuals without a history of ADHD. Specifically, adolescents with ADHD perceived family and school stressors to be more negative, on average, across adolescence. We also found some indication that the associations between stressors and alcohol use were stronger for individuals with a history of ADHD than for individuals without ADHD.

These findings dovetail nicely with prior work from the PALS examining the interplay among ADHD, parental alcoholism, and stress. Parental alcoholism has been shown to increase the likelihood of alcohol use disorder in offspring (e.g., Sher, 1991). One pathway through which this may occur is by increasing the amount of stress experienced in the environment. Marshal and colleagues (2007) found, in our first adolescent sample, that parental alcoholism was related to elevated family and peer stress, which, in turn, was related to heavier alcohol use. Importantly, this pathway was only significant for individuals with a history of ADHD. Taken together, individuals with ADHD may experience more stress in their environments as a result of their continued impairments but also because of more distal risk factors, such as parental alcoholism.

Individuals with ADHD also may be more vulnerable to these stressors, ultimately increasing alcohol- and substance-use risk. For example, Molina and colleagues (2005) found that adolescents had lower cognitive (e.g., my child reminds himself that it could be worse) and behavioral (e.g., my child gets information that is necessary to deal with the problem) coping skills than adolescents without ADHD. These lower coping skills, in turn, were related to higher levels of cigarette use. These reduced coping skills may be one explanation for why King and colleagues (under review) found that stressful life events were more strongly related to alcohol use for adolescents with ADHD. In light of this growing body of work, it may be particularly important to target the coping skills of individuals with ADHD, given that they are likely to experience a disproportionate amount of stress, which, in turn, contributes to substance use.

Psychological Functioning: Attention Deficit Hyperactivity Disorder Persistence, Internalizing and Externalizing Problems

Beginning with the first annual follow-up of the PALS participants, psychological functioning was carefully assessed through a combination of semistructured interviews and informant- and self-ratings. As PALS participants entered adolescence and adulthood, collection of complete and accurate symptom reports met the usual challenges of assessing ADHD in older individuals. For one, perceptual biases among adolescents and adults with ADHD make it challenging for them to report on subjective (and sometimes objective) symptoms and behaviors (Molina & Sibley, 2014). Second, valid informant reports of adolescent and young adult functioning may be challenging to obtain. In adolescence, teachers may spend less than an hour a day with students (Eccles, 2004) and youth may participate in a range of unsupervised activities (i.e., social activities, independent work completion), limiting teacher and parent awareness of daily functioning. By young adulthood, many individuals do not attend school full-time and may not live at home, creating further challenges to the assessment of ADHD and comorbid disorders. As such, an early task in the PALS was to determine the optimal method of assessing psychological symptom severity in the sample.

With respect to ADHD symptoms, Sibley et al., (2012a/b) found that for adolescents with ADHD histories, self-reports of symptoms did not offer additional diagnostic information above the reports of parents and teachers, due to vast symptom under-reporting by these youth. Young adults with ADHD demonstrated levels of under-reporting similar to adolescents; however, there was slight benefit (in about 7% of cases) to integrating self and parent reports in young adulthood, when teacher reports were no longer available. As such, we made the decision to combine parent and teacher symptom reports for adolescents and parent and self symptom reports for young adults in subsequent analyses. We conducted similar analyses for self and informant reports of delinquent externalizing behaviors (Sibley et al., 2010)—a domain in which self-report is the gold standard due to the covert nature of many delinquent acts (Loeber, 1988). Results indicated that for participants with ADHD, there was benefit to integrating parent and self-reports of delinquency due to a tendency of youth with ADHD to deny delinquent acts reported by the parent or recant acts they previously reported.

In adolescence, symptomatic ADHD persistence in the PALS was approximately 70% using strict DSM-IV-TR guidelines (American Psychological Association [APA], 2000). Notably, an additional 10% displayed clinically significant impairment and subthreshold ADHD symptom severity. Analyses using norm-referenced ADHD symptom data from the non-ADHD comparison group indicated that relaxing the DSM threshold based on developmental norms increased persistence rate to approximately 75%, including more individuals with a childhood history of ADHD, elevated symptoms, and current impairment. This method did not appear to create clinically significant false positive diagnoses in the non-ADHD group. In the PALS young adults, symptomatic persistence was 19.7% using strict DSM-IV-TR guidelines; however, using a norm-referenced diagnostic cutoff, the persistence rate increased nearly fourfold to 75.6%. Nearly all individuals with elevated symptoms also possessed clinically significant impairment, suggesting that the higher percentage captured individuals continuing to experience meaningful difficulties in their daily lives. The PALS adolescent and young adult ADHD symptom papers (Sibley et al., 2012a/b) indicated potential value to reforming the DSM diagnostic threshold for older individuals, based on the finding that norm-based thresholds are more inclusive of impaired individuals with a childhood diagnosis. In Sibley et al. (2012b), we also evaluated the utility of recently posited adult-specific ADHD symptoms (e.g., Barkley et al., 2008). We replicated the previous finding that some of these symptoms are endorsed at higher rates than DSM symptoms among adults with ADHD—however, endorsement of many adult-specific ADHD symptoms also was elevated in the non-ADHD group, indicating poor specificity.

Comorbid externalizing and internalizing problems in adolescence also were examined in the larger PALS sample. With respect to delinquency (Sibley et al., 2011), males with ADHD histories were more likely than those without ADHD to commit severe delinquent acts (32% vs. 12%), initiate delinquent offending earlier (age 11 vs. age 12), and commit a greater variety of delinquent acts (seven vs. five types of acts). Estimates were particularly elevated for those with comorbid childhood CD (45% of those with childhood CD committed a severe delinquent act vs. 23% of probands with ADHD only). This finding is not surprising given the overlap between these constructs. Delinquency, however, encompasses a wider variety of criminal and violent behaviors than does CD, with an emphasis on offending outside of the home and classroom (Loeber, 1988). Problems with behavioral self-regulation including impulse control are core features of ADHD and often serve as an impetus for the development of childhood conduct problems (Patterson et al., 2000), which may eventually escalate into antisocial behaviors that culminate with delinquent offending. Thus, many PALS participants with CD at baseline likely had initiated a deviancy pathway leading to non-normative delinquency in adolescence (Moffitt & Caspi, 2001). It is important, however, to note that adolescent delinquency is not present in all individuals with childhood CD, many of whom see a remittance of symptoms prior to adolescence

(Lahey, McBurnett, & Loeber, 2000). In addition, some children with ADHD but without CD develop enough conduct problems to warrant the diagnosis later, as shown in Figure 5.5 (Molina, Pelham, Marshal, Curran et al., 2007). Thus, discontinuity, as well as stability, in serious conduct problems is evident in this population, which suggests the presence of (1) remission for some, (2) risk of later emergence of behavior problems for some children with ADHD, and (3) chronic antisocial behaviors for approximately one half to two thirds of the children with both ADHD and CD (amounting to 15%–27% of the PALS children with ADHD).

Generally, mood and anxiety disorders (Bagwell et al., 2006) in adolescence were found to occur at similar rates among the participants with and without ADHD in the initial adolescent follow-up (e.g., 5% vs. 8.8% with any depressive disorder in the non-ADHD and ADHD groups, respectively). However, childhood externalizing disorder symptoms and social problems (e.g., "doesn't get along with other kids," "not liked by other kids") predicted adolescent anxiety and mood disorders, suggesting that a subgroup of children with ADHD appear to be at increased risk of internalizing disorder. By young adulthood in the larger PALS study, there were

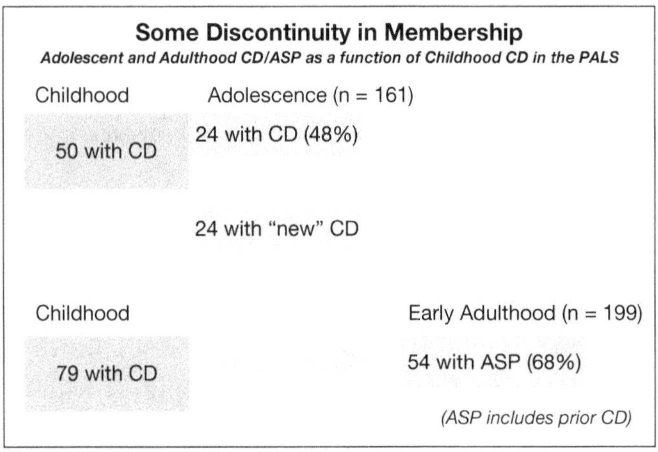

Figure 5.5 Conduct Disorder (CD) and Antisocial Personality (ASP) outcomes of childhood CD in the PALS (Molina, Pelham, Marshal, Curran et al., 2007). 24/161 = 15% of PALS children followed into adolescence who continued to have CD; 54/199 = 27% of the PALS children followed into early adulthood in Wave One of the PALS who had ASPD including childhood CD.

clear elevations in depressive symptoms for the ADHD group compared with the non-ADHD group (Meinzer et al., 2015), which appeared closely tied to daily life functioning. Thus, the relationship between ADHD and internalizing symptoms may be age-specific—perhaps young adulthood is a critical period for the development of internalizing problems in individuals with ADHD.

Overall, the findings of the PALS suggest that ADHD in childhood is an important precursor to additional psychological disorders in adolescence and adulthood. It appears that ADHD may impart direct risk for comorbid disorders through the persistence of its symptoms into adulthood (e.g., impulsive behaviors leading to higher levels of delinquency) and through maladjustment that develops as a consequence of mounting psychosocial impairments (e.g., depressive symptoms that relate to overall problem severity in young adulthood). Thus, both remediation of current ADHD symptoms (e.g., medication in adulthood) and prevention efforts to reduce later maladjustment (e.g., targeting impairments through psychosocial treatments in childhood and adolescence) may be equally necessary to mitigate risk for ADHD persistence and comorbidity.

Risky Behavior Outcomes in Attention Deficit Hyperactivity Disorder

Models of adolescent risky behavior point to predictors that overlap with, or are the same as, the core features of ADHD (i.e., behavioral impulsivity, inattention); these predictors are suggested to have direct and indirect influences on risky behavior in adolescence and adulthood (i.e., substance abuse, delinquency; Sher et al., 2005; Zucker, 2006). Direct effects of ADHD on risky outcomes may occur due to a tendency toward risky decision-making (Toplak et al., 2005) that primes individuals with ADHD to prefer more immediate rewards (e.g., fun, physical sensations) over larger delayed rewards (e.g., evading prison, long-term physical health). Indirect effects of ADHD on risky outcomes may occur due to slowly escalating disruptive behavior and functional impairments that make conventional environments aversive (e.g., school failure and peer rejection), driving individuals with ADHD to seek reinforcement from deviant or atypical sources.

It is highly likely that the risky or otherwise health-endangering behavior of adolescents and young adults with ADHD is pervasive—influencing the lives of these individuals in ways that have yet to be measured or detected. Three PALS papers sought to broaden the range of risky outcomes associated with childhood ADHD beyond substance use and criminality.

In the first (Flory et al., 2006), we examined risky sexual behavior among the young adult males in the PALS. Findings indicated that participants with ADHD reported more frequent instances of casual sex in the past year, as well as more lifetime sexual partners, more frequent unprotected sex, and more pregnancies in their partners. Overall, the ADHD group reported earlier initiation of sexual intercourse, but also more individuals who completely refrained from sexual intercourse. The latter finding was interesting and could represent under-reporting by individuals in the ADHD group (Sibley et al., 2010) or a tendency for social impairments among some individuals with ADHD (Bagwell et al., 2001; Molina et al., 2014) to prevent sexual interactions during the adolescent and young adult years. Overall, risky sexual behavior was associated with childhood ADHD, above and beyond childhood conduct problems. This finding suggests that there may be a unique influence of ADHD symptoms (e.g., impulsivity) on the sexual behavior of individuals with ADHD.

In the second paper (Thompson et al., 2007), we examined risky driving outcomes among the adolescents and young adults of the PALS from the first annual interview. Results indicated that by an average age of 17 years, the ADHD group reported more traffic tickets and accidents, were less likely to have obtained a driver's license, and reported higher levels of driving without a license. Risky driving behavior was associated with concurrent conduct problems. The results indicated that individuals with ADHD began driving at later ages—which may reflect difficulties passing a driving test, poor motivation to begin driving, or parental beliefs that teens or young adults with ADHD are not responsible enough to earn driving privileges. On the other hand, among those who were licensed, the same individuals who often displayed rule-breaking behaviors also reported frequent driving infractions. Additional analyses on PALS driving outcomes are planned as the sample ages—particularly past the age of 25, which marks a documented transition to safer driving practices by adults (Jessor et al., 1997).

Finally, Wymbs et al. (2013) investigated participation in recreational motorsports among the adolescents and young adults of the PALS and found that the ADHD group was more likely to engage in car racing, ATV/four-wheeler use, and/or motorcycle trail biking. Individuals who were rated by parents as being more impulsive and antisocial, as well as those who self-identified as heavy drinkers, were at highest risk for participation in recreational motorsports activities. This paper offered preliminary evidence that individuals with ADHD may self-select into recreational activities that offer specific perceived benefits, which may include sensation seeking. Further work is needed to investigate additional activities that may be particularly appealing to individuals with ADHD. Overall, full characterization of impulsive and risky behavior patterns among adolescents and adults with ADHD is an interesting area that warrants additional research.

In line with this, recent research has shown that disaggregating the broad construct of "impulsivity" provides a more specific understanding of who is at risk for engagement in various risky behaviors. To increase our understanding of various aspects of impulsivity for individuals with ADHD, a measurement of five facets of impulsivity was added to the PALS ongoing study starting in 2009. In recent analyses ($N = 302$; $n = 179$ ADHD; $n = 123$ non-ADHD) in adulthood ($M = 28.75$, $SD = 3.38$), we found evidence for an emotional impulsivity pathway whereby individuals with childhood ADHD have elevated levels of emotional impulsivity in adulthood, which, in turn, is related to more alcohol problems (Pedersen et al., 2016). The ADHD and non-ADHD groups did not differ on one of the specific facets, sensation-seeking, which is an interesting finding given speculation about its possible importance for this population (such as our risky motorsports finding). An important next step is to examine sensation seeking in interaction with other facets of impulsivity; specifically, although sensation-seeking per se may not be higher in ADHD, its presence may have important risk behavior implications in the presence of poor inhibitory control (i.e., impulsivity), which is typically higher in ADHD.

Academic and Vocational Outcomes

It is well established that across development, individuals with ADHD display higher levels of academic impairment than typically developing peers and that this risk is highly implicated in the onset of serious adult outcomes (Barbaresi et al., 2007; Loe & Feldman, 2007). PALS educational analyses aimed to examine lesser-known facets of academic functioning among individuals with ADHD (see Table 5.2).

Robb et al. (2011) monetized the K–12 educational experience of the PALS ADHD and non-ADHD groups. Direct costs of major and minor disciplinary incidents, special education services, grade retention, and transfer to alternative educational settings were considered as well as indirect costs of lost instructional time to classmates and lost teacher and administrator time dealing with disciplinary infractions. Educational history was obtained from a combination of prospective and retrospective parent reports obtained at Wave 1 and each subsequent wave that the participant was enrolled in K–12 education. Cost estimates were derived from publicly available statistics from the U.S. Department of Labor, Census Bureau, and Department of Education. Due to the occurrence of elevated disciplinary and academic problems across grade levels, an individual with ADHD was estimated to cost the educational system an additional $5,007 (2010 dollars) per year when compared with individuals without ADHD. Extrapolated, this cost amounts to $13.4 billion per year to the U.S. education system. The PALS estimate, which included indirect costs, was significantly greater than previous educational costs of ADHD estimated by the Fast Track sample (Jones et al., 2009) and others (Forness & Kavale, 2002).

Though the academic experience of elementary school age children with ADHD is well characterized (DuPaul & Eckert, 1998), there are very few

TABLE 5.2

ACADEMIC AND VOCATIONAL OUTCOMES OF THE PITTSBURGH ADHD LONGITUDINAL STUDY (PALS) PARTICIPANTS

	ADHD	Comparison
Annual Cost of K–12 Education	$5,007	$381
HIGH SCHOOL (AGE 14–18)		
9th Grade GPA (0–100)	73.24 (18.18)	82.11 (16.08)
12th Grade GPA (0–100)	76.86 (19.13)	80.39 (16.48)
Days Absent from School per Year	17.0 (14.1)	10.1 (14.6)
Days Tardy for School	8.0 (11.3)	4.2 (11.9)
Working up to Potential (%)	30.0	61.0
Percentage of Work Turned In	64.0	83.0
Remedial Class Placement (%)	39.8	9.3
Course Failure (%)	30.9	9.9
Dropout (%)	13.1	1.4
COLLEGE YEARS (AGE 18–22)		
No Postsecondary Education (%)	26.9	4.9
Community College or Vocational Training	43.6	18.3
Bachelor's Degree	29.5	76.8
POST COLLEGE YEARS (AGE 23–32)		
Unemployed and Not Enrolled in School	16.6	2.4
Unskilled/Labor Job	72.5	36.0
Clerical Job	21.8	44.0
Professional Job	5.6	20.0

available details about how students with ADHD function in high school (for exceptions, see Barkley et al., 2002, 2006; Molina et al., 2009). Using a combination of official school records and teacher and parent reports of academic functioning, Kent et al. (2011) provided a close look at the PALS participants in high school in the larger PALS sample. Compared with the non-ADHD group, the ADHD group exhibited poorer attendance records, greater difficulty arriving at class on time, lower levels of work completion, and poorer academic effort. High school students with ADHD also were more likely to be placed in remedial classes, to fail courses regardless of class placement, and to eventually drop out of high school. With respect to grade point average (GPA), significant group differences persisted across all four years of high school. On average, the ADHD group displayed lower average grades in academic classes (C– average) than the non-ADHD group (B– average). This outcome is particularly concerning because GPA is an ecologically valid index of cumulative academic functioning that is used to determine selection into advanced classes, eligibility for extracurricular activities, college admission, and financial assistance in postsecondary education (Zimmerman, Caldwell, & Bernat, 2002).

Academic trajectory across the high school years also differed for ADHD and non-ADHD participants. While non-ADHD participants tended to display slightly poorer academic performance as high school progressed, the ADHD group displayed notable academic impairment in 9th grade that improved and stabilized beginning in 10th grade. These data may indicate that the transition to high school is particularly difficult for students with ADHD such that they experience a large performance drop between middle and high school followed by nominal (non-normalizing) improvement. In this study, there was slight evidence that conduct problems, low IQ, and poor parent education in childhood may relate to academic performance in high school. Thus, it appears that malleable factors in childhood (e.g., behavior problems) and adolescence (e.g., attendance, work completion, academic effort) may be appropriate prevention strategies for high school failure among individuals with ADHD.

Intervening to prevent high school dropout may have important implications for adult outcomes. Kuriyan et al. (2013) extended the PALS educational analyses to the post-high school period, additionally evaluating vocational outcomes of the sample. Overall, the ADHD group participants were less likely than the non-ADHD group participants to pursue education after high school, with only 29.5% pursuing a bachelor's degree (76.8% of the non-ADHD group did so). Within the ADHD group, enrollment in university was significantly below national averages during the same time period: 39%–42% of all 18- to 24-year-olds in the United States enrolled in four-year institutions between 1999 and 2009 (e.g., National

Center for Education Statistics, Digest of Education Statistics, 2010). The most common post-high school educational option for the ADHD group was vocational school or community college (43.6% of those pursuing postsecondary education). During the post-college years (ages 23–32), the ADHD group was about seven times more likely to be neither employed nor in school (16.6% vs. 2.4%). Those in the ADHD group who were employed were twice as likely to hold unskilled or labor jobs in their mid-twenties to early thirties (72.5% vs. 36%). Cumulative academic and disciplinary problems over the course of K–12 education were the strongest predictors of postsecondary education and vocational outcomes.

Our findings indicate that the academic difficulties of children and adolescents with ADHD are pervasive and forge a path for educational and vocational underperformance as individuals move from the teen years into their twenties. As participants age into their thirties, continued examination of the PALS educational and vocational outcomes is planned. In the Kuriyan et al. analyses, many participants were still enrolled in school; thus, the ultimate educational attainment of the sample is not yet known. Similarly, vocational trajectories are often not clear until education is completed.

Social Functioning

The social deficits and impairments of children with ADHD are well established; however, less is known about the social functioning of adolescents and adults with ADHD. In the initial PALS adolescent sample, Bagwell et al. (2001) reported that teens with ADHD had fewer close friendships (2.96 vs. 3.4, $p < .001$) and greater overall peer rejection than the non-ADHD group. For example, 11% of the ADHD group versus only 1% of the non-ADHD group had no close friends based on parent report. Compared with the ADHD group, the non-ADHD group reported that their friends were more likely to be involved in extracurricular activities. Meanwhile, parents in the ADHD group were more likely to report that their son/daughters' friends were a bad influence. Thus, adolescents with

ADHD had fewer friends and tended to choose peers who were unconventional or less prosocial.

Additional research in the PALS sought to untangle the causes and consequences of ADHD-related social impairment in adolescence. Bagwell et al. (2001) additionally reported that within the ADHD group, those who fared best (i.e., avoided social rejection, possessed more close friends) were those whose ADHD symptoms partially desisted by adolescence. Thus, ongoing symptoms of ADHD (i.e., inattention, impulsivity) may play a direct role in the social behavior of teens with ADHD (i.e., difficulties engaging in developmentally appropriate conversation, aversive interactions that annoy peers).

With respect to deviant peer affiliations, Bagwell et al. (2001) indicated that children with ADHD who have a history of conduct problems are those most likely to gravitate toward rule-breaking peers in adolescence. One serious consequence of these deviant friendships is synergistic escalation of risk behaviors, such as substance use and delinquency (Patterson et al., 1985). Marshal et al. (2003) reported that the PALS children with ADHD reported more friends who used and approved of substance use in adolescence than the comparison peers. Moreover, an ADHD history tightened the connection between having these types of friendships and reporting substance use and conduct problems themselves. Thus, a critical point of intervention to prevent substance use in teens with ADHD may be preventing unsupervised activities with deviant peers—potentially through increased parental monitoring of social activities (Molina et al., 2012; Walther et al., 2012).

Unexpectedly, PALS findings also indicated that adolescents with ADHD who display the highest levels of social impairment may be protected against problematic substance use—at least during the teen and young adult years (Molina et al., 2012; 2014). It may be the case that adolescents with fewer friends display low social access to alcohol prior to the legal age of consumption. This protective effect is striking, given the critical role of early substance use in the development of serious outcomes that include high school dropout, juvenile incarceration, and addiction (Sher et al., 2005). It is likely, however, that the best strategy to improve the social functioning and long-term behavioral health of adolescents with ADHD is a combination of treatment for ADHD symptoms and increased parental monitoring of and limit setting for teen social activities. Further work is needed to understand the specific mechanisms through which ADHD symptoms produce social rejection and friendship problems in teens, in order to promote prosocial interactions in adolescence.

In the Molina et al. 2014 paper we found that childhood ADHD predicted adolescent social impairment, which also predicted adult social impairment. Although the measurement of social impairment was limited to parental ratings, the findings provide some evidence of life course stability in social impairment among individuals with ADHD, which may create new problems in adulthood. Formation of healthy intimate relationships is an important developmental milestone in young adulthood (Collins & Sroufe, 1999). Other findings from the PALS (Wymbs et al., 2012) suggest that adults with ADHD struggled to maintain mutually respectful intimate relationships. Young adults with ADHD reported more aggression, both verbal and physical, in their relationships with their romantic partners, indicating difficulties with conflict management (Wymbs et al., 2012). Moreover, heavy drinking and relationship aggression were associated in the ADHD, but not in the non-ADHD, group (Wymbs et al., 2014). Given the higher rates of divorce among the parents of children with ADHD (Wymbs et al., 2008), together these findings suggest a strong familial theme of interpersonal difficulties in households affected by ADHD. These findings concur with other longitudinal studies revealing high conflict between individuals with ADHD and their parents (Edwards et al., 2001) and highlight the importance of attending to social deficits in this population throughout the life course.

OVERALL SUMMARY AND CONCLUSIONS

In this chapter we described the program of research conducted as the Pittsburgh ADHD Longitudinal Study (PALS). Initiated in 1994 as a one-time adolescent follow-up study (e.g., Molina & Pelham, 2003) and now ongoing as age-specific interviews through adolescence into the fourth decade of life, the PALS has published findings testing our model-driven hypotheses about alcohol and substance use (Molina & Pelham, 2014), as well as multiple papers on ADHD symptom persistence, conduct problems and delinquency, social functioning, stress and coping, risky behaviors such as unprotected sex, depression and anxiety, academic and vocational outcomes, and cost. A diversity of outcomes is apparent, with findings depending upon the variable of interest.

Alcohol

Although a meta-analysis concluded that childhood ADHD increases risk of alcohol use disorder (abuse or dependence) by adulthood (Lee et al., 2011), the pathways to that outcome as well as long-term adulthood risk for heavy drinking and its associated consequences have needed investigation. PALS findings have shown that childhood ADHD does not increase the likelihood of alcohol initiation by adolescence, but it does predict elevated drinking and drinking problems. Teenagers with childhood ADHD report more heavy drinking and more problems stemming from their drinking than do teenagers without childhood ADHD. For example, 23% report being drunk in the past six months compared with only 12% of those without ADHD histories. By early adulthood, heavy drinking is common independent of ADHD (e.g., 25 episodes of drunkenness in the past year), but serious conduct problems dramatically increase the risk of heavy and problem drinking. To the extent that childhood ADHD increases risk for delinquency and antisocial behavior, childhood ADHD also increases the risk for negative alcohol outcomes in adolescence and early adulthood. Future analyses will continue to investigate the course to these outcomes as well as the factors that serve to maintain them beyond early adulthood.

Other Drug Use

Our findings on drug use, somewhat similar to our findings on alcohol use, show a moderately increased risk for certain marijuana use outcomes but not others; these include more frequent use in adolescence and an earlier age of first use, but no difference in marijuana problems or disorder but high rates of disorder in early adulthood for all participants (about 20% with a marijuana use disorder by early adulthood). Use of other illicit drugs (e.g., heroin, cocaine, inhalants) is infrequent and group differences in adolescence were only detected by summing across these drugs. Cigarette smoking, as shown in other studies, is dramatically increased in the PALS participants and includes starting younger, progressing to daily use more quickly, and a dramatically increased risk of daily smoking once initiation has occurred. These findings, particularly in the context of rapidly changing access to marijuana nationally, and in light of new access to alternative forms of nicotine (e.g., e-cigarettes), warrant ongoing investigation of ADHD-related risk.

Contributing Factors

Given the PALS' focus on alcohol and other drug use outcomes in ADHD, multiple factors have been investigated for the contribution to elevated risk for alcohol and drug use in ADHD. We found,

- Both ADHD symptom persistence and conduct problems (measured as CD symptoms, delinquency, or antisocial personality disorder) contribute to elevated risk, even when accounting for other impairments including academic and social. The implications of this finding are that interventions should target symptom relief and management as well as deflection from delinquency trajectories (both pharmacologic as well as psychologic interventions).
- Adolescents with ADHD histories are more likely than their non-ADHD peers to have friendships with peers who use, and support the use of, drugs and alcohol. These affiliations are more strongly associated in the ADHD versus the non-ADHD group, indicating that social milieu, which likely

includes both selection of risky friendships as well as influence by risky friendships, is a key component of drug and alcohol risk in ADHD. Some teens with ADHD histories appear to be "protected" from these relationships by aspects of social impairment, which may partly explain the complicated and inconsistent risk of adverse alcohol outcomes for children with ADHD.

- Parenting practices and parent–teen relationships are, on average, of lower quality in the presence of teen ADHD histories. Better functioning in these domains, however, is associated with less cigarette and alcohol use.
- Cognitive factors known to predict alcohol and marijuana use in typical populations do not appear to operate similarly in the face of an ADHD history. For example, beliefs about the anticipated negative effects of alcohol and marijuana use do not protect individuals with ADHD histories from future use as much as they do those without ADHD histories. This finding has unfortunate implications about the likelihood of decreasing substance use risk by increasing awareness of its associated negative outcomes.
- Children with ADHD have an increased likelihood of negative and potentially stressful life events associated with their ADHD and with their membership in families affected by alcohol problems. Moreover, their vulnerability to these stressors, be they impairments caused by ADHD or events usually perceived as uncontrollable stressors (e.g., parental job loss), heightens their risk of alcohol use. In addition, adolescents with ADHD histories have fewer adaptive coping skills, which is associated with increased rates of cigarette use. Together, these vulnerabilities suggest that family-level vulnerabilities and psychological resilience through skill-building may need to be considered in the future development of interventions for this population.

Attention Deficit Hyperactivity Disorder Persistence, Internalizing, and Externalizing Outcomes

Perhaps one of our most important findings is that ADHD symptom persistence into adolescence and particularly into adulthood is underestimated by reliance on self-report. Although we acknowledge the difficulty of continuing to rely on parent report into later adulthood, our findings into early adulthood (and more recently, continuing analyses to age 25 for other variables [Molina et al., 2015]), indicates that individuals with ADHD histories report less symptomatology and impairment than what is reported by their parents.

As reflected earlier in our summary, a substantial minority (about a quarter to one third) of the PALS sample, like other clinic-based samples of children with ADHD followed longitudinally (for review, see Molina, 2011), has serious conduct problems sufficient to be diagnosed with CD in childhood, serious delinquency in adolescence, or antisocial personality disorder in early adulthood. This comorbidity is strongly connected to, though not necessary for, the presence of other functioning difficulties throughout life.

In early adulthood, internalizing (depression) symptoms become elevated for the PALS participants compared with the non-ADHD group, and they are tied to ADHD-related impairment, suggesting the possibility that interventions targeting impairments may assuage low mood. This finding is important given our failure to find internalizing disorder group differences in adolescence.

Additional Risky Behaviors

Children with ADHD have increased risk of additional risky behaviors including unprotected sex, more sexual partners, and more pregnancies at a younger age. They have more vehicular moving violations and accidents, but they do not perceive themselves as more risky drivers overall—consistent with their general pattern of under-reporting symptoms and impairment. They also engage in more motorsports, which is correlated with impulsivity, antisocial behavior, and alcohol use.

Academic and Vocational Outcomes

There are clear and robust group differences in academic outcomes for the PALS children with ADHD compared with the non-ADHD group. Moreover, these group differences provide clear targets for improvements from interventions; they include lower attendance at school, less work completion, lower grade point average, and decreased likelihood of enrollment in secondary education. Moreover, the cost to educate a child with ADHD is about $5,000 more than that to educate a child without ADHD. The ADHD group is also more likely to be employed in unskilled labor jobs after the college age range, although we await the results of our 30-year-old follow-up to determine a more stable estimate of vocational disposition in adulthood.

Social Functioning

Although social deficits have long been documented for children with ADHD, this common impairment has only recently been studied at older ages. In the PALS, we found that teens with ADHD histories have fewer friends and their friends are less prosocial, on average. The long-term effects of ADHD on social functioning in adolescence were more pronounced for probands with persistent ADHD or conduct disorder in adolescence. Social impairment, as rated by parents, exhibited significant stability from adolescence into early adulthood, and young adults with ADHD histories also reported more verbal and physical aggression in their intimate relationships in early adulthood. These negative outcomes, however, characterize only portions of children with ADHD (e.g., no more than 15% of the ADHD group reported physical violence compared with 6% of the non-ADHD group), but the social features of children with ADHD are highly variable, with diverse implications for outcomes in other domains (e.g., alcohol). More work is needed to understand the specific behaviors that produce these variable social profiles, their associated consequences in adolescence and adulthood, and their malleability given the challenges associated with improving social skills in this population.

REFERENCES

American Psychiatric Association. (2000). *Diagnostic and Statistical Manual of Mental Disorders* (4th ed.). Washington, DC: Author.

Bagwell, C. L., Molina, B. S. G., Kashdan, T. B., Pelham, W. E., & Hoza, B. (2006). Anxiety and mood disorders in adolescents with childhood attention-deficit hyperactivity disorder. *Journal of Emotional and Behavioral Disorders, 14*(3), 178–187. doi:10.1177/10634266060140030501

Bagwell, C. L., Molina, B. S., Pelham, W. E., Jr., & Hoza, B. (2001). Attention-deficit hyperactivity disorder and problems in peer relations: predictions from childhood to adolescence. *Journal of the American Academy of Child and Adolescent Psychiatry, 40*(11), 1285–1292. doi: 10.1097/00004583-200111000-00008

Barbaresi, W. J., Katusic, S. K., Colligan, R. C., Weaver, A. L., & Jacobsen, S. J. (2007). Long-term school outcomes for children with attention-deficit/hyperactivity disorder: a population-based perspective. *Journal of Developmental and Behavioral Pediatrics, 28*(4), 265–273. doi: 10.1097/DBP.0b013e31811ff87d

Barkley, R. A., Anastopoulos, A. D., Guevremont, D. C., & Fletcher, K. E. (1992). Adolescents with attention deficit hyperactivity disorder: mother–adolescent interactions, family beliefs and conflicts, and maternal psychopathology. *Journal of Abnormal Child Psychology, 20*(3), 263–288.

Barkley, R. A., Fischer, M., Edelbrock, C. S., & Smallish, L. (1990). The adolescent outcome of hyperactive children diagnosed by research criteria: I. An 8-year prospective follow-up study. *Journal of the American Academy of Child and Adolescent Psychiatry, 29*(4), 546–557. doi: 10.1097/00004583-199007000-00007

Barkley, R. A., Fischer, M., Smallish, L., & Fletcher, K. (2002). The persistence of attention-deficit/hyperactivity disorder into young adulthood as a function of reporting source and definition of disorder. *Journal of Abnormal Psychology, 111*(2), 279–289. doi:10.1037//0021-843x.111.2.279

Barkley, R. A., Fischer, M., Smallish, L., & Fletcher, K. (2006). Young adult outcome of hyperactive children: adaptive functioning in major life activities. *Journal of the American Academy of Child and Adolescent Psychiatry, 45*(2), 192–202. doi: 10.1097/01.chi.0000189134.97436.e2

Barkley, R. A., Murphy, K. R., & Fischer, M. (2008). *ADHD in Adults: What the Science Says.* New York: Guilford.

Babinski, D. E., Pelham, W. E., Jr., Molina, B. S., Gnagy, E. M., Waschbusch, D. A., Yu, J., . . . Karch, K. M. (2011). Late adolescent and young adult outcomes of girls diagnosed with ADHD in childhood: an exploratory investigation. *Journal of Attention Disorders, 15*(3), 204–214. doi: 10.1177/1087054710361586

Babinski, D. E., Pelham, W. E., Jr., Molina, B. S., Waschbusch, D. A., Gnagy, E. M., Yu, J., . . . Biswas, A. (2011). Women with childhood ADHD: comparisons by diagnostic group and gender. *Journal of Psychopathology and Behavioral Assessment, 33*(4), 420–429. doi: 10.1007/s10862-011-9247-4

Barnes, G. M., Hoffman, J. H., Welte, J. W., Farrell, M. P., & Dintcheff, B. A. (2006). Effects of parental monitoring and peer deviance on substance use and delinquency. *Journal of Marriage and Family*, *68*(4), 1084–1104. doi: DOI 10.1111/j.1741-3737.2006.00315.x

Belendiuk, K. A., Pedersen, S.P., King, K.M., Pelham, W.E. & Molina, B. S.G. (2016). Change over time in adolescent and friend alcohol use: Differential associations for youth with and without childhood Attention-Deficit/Hyperactivity Disorder (ADHD). *Psychology of Addictive Behaviors*, 30(1), 29–38. *PMCID: PMC4752397*

Biederman, J., Wilens, T., Mick, E., Faraone, S. V., Weber, W., Curtis, S., Thornell, A., Pfister, K., Garcia Jetton, J., & Soriano, J. (1997). Is ADHD a risk factor for psychoactive substance use disorders? Findings from a four-year prospective follow-up study. *Archives of General Psychiatry, 36*(1), 21–29.

Centers for Disease Control and Prevention. (2014). Current cigarette smoking among adults—United States, 2005–2012. *Morbidity and Mortality Weekly Report, 63*(02),29–34.

Cerbone, F. G., & Larison, C. L. (2000). A bibliographic essay: the relationship between stress and substance use. *Substance Use & Misuse*, 35(5), 757–786.

Chassin, L., Hussong, A., Barrera, Jr., M., Molina, B. S. G., Trim, R., & Ritter, J. (2004). Adolescent substance use. In R. M. Lerner & L. Steinberg (Eds.), *Handbook of Adolescent Psychology* (2nd. ed.) (pp. 665–696). Hoboken, NJ: John Wiley & Sons, Inc.

Collins, W. A., & Sroufe, L. A. (1999). Capacity for intimate relationships: A developmental construction. In W. Furman, C. Feiring, & B. B. Brown (Eds.), *The Development of Romantic Relationships in Adolescence* (pp. 123–147). New York: Cambridge University Press.

Counts, C. A., Nigg, J. T., Stawicki, J. A., Rappley, M. D., & von Eye, A. (2005). Family adversity in DSM-IV ADHD combined and inattentive subtypes and associated disruptive behavior problems. *Journal of the American Academy of Child and Adolescent Psychiatry, 44*(7), 690–698. doi: 10.1097/01.chi.0000162582.87710.66

Del Boca, F. K., Darkes, J., Goldman, M. S., & Smith, G. T. (2002). Advancing the expectancy concept via the interplay between theory and research. *Alcoholism, Clinical and Experimental Research, 26*(6), 926–935.

DuPaul, G. J., & Eckert, T. L. (1998). Academic interventions for students with attention-deficit/hyperactivity disorder: A review of the literature. *Reading & Writing Quarterly Overcoming Learning Difficulties, 14*, 59–82.

Eccles, J. (2004). Schools, academic motivation, and stage-environment fit. In R. M. Lerner, & L. Steinberg (Eds.), *Handbook of Adolescent Psychology* (2nd ed.) (pp. 125–153). Hoboken, NJ: John Wiley.

Edwards, G., Barkley, R.A., Laneri, M., Fletcher, K., & Metevia, L. (2001). Parent-adolescent conflict in teenagers with ADHD and ODD. *Journal of Abnormal Child Psychology*, *29*(6), 557–572.

Faden, V. B., Day, N. L., Windle, M., Windle, R., Grube, J. W., Molina, B. S., . . . Sher, K. J. (2004). Collecting longitudinal data through childhood, adolescence, and young adulthood: methodological challenges. *Alcoholism, Clinical and Experimental Research*, *28*(2), 330–340.

Flory, K., Molina, B. S., Pelham, W. E., Jr., Gnagy, E., & Smith, B. (2006). Childhood ADHD predicts risky sexual behavior in young adulthood. *Journal of Clinical Child and Adolescent Psychology*, *35*(4), 571–577. doi: 10.1207/s15374424jccp3504_8

Forness, S. R., & Kavale, K. A. (2002). Impact of ADHD on school systems. In: P. S. Jensen & J. R. Cooper (Eds.), *Attention Deficit Hyperactivity Disorder.* Kingston, NJ: Civic Research Institute, 24–31

Gittelman, R., Mannuzza, S., Shenker, R., & Bonagura, N. (1985). Hyperactive boys almost grown up. I. Psychiatric status. *Archives of General Psychiatry*, *42*(10), 937–947.

Goldman, M. S. (2002). Expectancy and risk for alcoholism: the unfortunate exploitation of a fundamental characteristic of neurobehavioral adaptation. *Alcoholism, Clinical and Experimental Research*, *26*(5), 737–746.

Guo, J., Hawkins, J. D., Hill, K. G., & Abbott, R. D. (2001). Childhood and adolescent predictors of alcohol abuse and dependence in young adulthood. *Journal of Studies on Alcohol*, *62*(6), 754–762.

Hartsough, C. S., & Lambert, N. M. (1987). Pattern and progression of drug use among hyperactives and controls: A prospective short-term longitudinal study. *Journal of Child Psychology and Psychiatry*, *28*(4), 543–553.

Harty, S. C., Pedersen, S. L., Gnagy, E. M., Pelham, W. E., & Molina, B. S. G. (2015). ADHD and marijuana use expectancies in young adulthood. *Substance Use and Misuse*. *50*(11), 1470–1478.

Hawkins, J. D., Catalano, R. F., & Miller, J. Y. (1992). Risk and protective factors for alcohol and other drug problems in adolescence and early adulthood: implications for substance abuse prevention. *Psychology Bulletin*, *112*(1), 64–105.

Howard, A. L., Molina, B. S. G., Swanson, J. M., Hinshaw, S. P., Belendiuk, K. A., Harty, S. C.,. . .Wigal, T. (in press). Developmental progression to early adult binge drinking and marijuana use from worsening versus stable trajectories of adolescent ADHD and delinquency. *Addiction*, *110*(5), 784–795. PMCID: PMC4398637

Hoza, B., Mrug, S., Gerdes, A. C., Hinshaw, S. P., Bukowski, W. M., Gold, J. A., . . . Arnold, L. E. (2005). What aspects of peer relationships are impaired in children with attention-deficit/hyperactivity disorder? *Journal of Consulting and Clinical Psychology*, *73*(3), 411–423. doi: 10.1037/0022-006X.73.3.411

Jessor, R., Turbin, M. S., & Costa, F. M. (1997). Predicting developmental change in risky driving: The transition to young adulthood. *Applied Developmental Science*, *1*(1), 4–16.

Jones, D. E., Foster, E. M., & Conduct Problems Prevention Research Group. (2009). Service use patterns for adolescents with ADHD and comorbid conduct disorder. *Journal of Behavioral Health Services Research*, *36*(4), 436–449. doi: 10.1007/s11414-008-9133-3

Kent, K. M., Pelham, W. E., Jr., Molina, B. S., Sibley, M. H., Waschbusch, D. A., Yu, J., . . . Karch, K. M. (2011). The academic experience of male high school students with ADHD. *Journal of Abnormal Child Psychology, 39*(3), 451–462. doi: 10.1007/s10802-010-9472-4

King, K. M., Pedersen, S. L., Louie, K., Pelham, W. E., & Molina, B. S. G. (under review). ADHD, negative life events and alcohol use in adolescence: A state trait perspective.

Knop, J., Penick, E. C., Nickel, E. J., Mortensen, E. L., Sullivan, M. A., Murtaza, S., . . . Gabrielli, W. F. (2009). Childhood ADHD and Conduct Disorder as independent predictors of male alcohol dependence at age 40. *Journal of Studies on Alcohol and Drugs, 70*(2), 169–177.

Knopik, V. S., Heath, A. C., Jacob, T., Slutske, W. S., Bucholz, K. K., Madden, P. A., . . . Martin, N. G. (2006). Maternal alcohol use disorder and offspring ADHD: disentangling genetic and environmental effects using a children-of-twins design. *Psychological Medicine, 36*(10), 1461–1471. doi: 10.1017/S0033291706007884

Kuriyan, A. B., Pelham, W. E., Jr., Molina, B. S., Waschbusch, D. A., Gnagy, E. M., Sibley, M. H., . . . Kent, K. M. (2013). Young adult educational and vocational outcomes of children diagnosed with ADHD. *Journal of Abnormal Child Psychology, 41*(1), 27–41. doi: 10.1007/s10802-012-9658-z

Kuriyan, A. B., Pelham, W. E., Jr., Molina, B. S., Waschbusch, D. A., Sibley, M. H., & Gnagy, E. M. (2014). Concordance between parent and physician medication histories for children and adolescents with attention-deficit/hyperactivity disorder. *Journal of Child and Adolescent Psychopharmacology, 24*(5), 269–274. doi: 10.1089/cap.2013.0081

Lahey, B. B., McBurnett, K., & Loeber, R. (2000). Are attention-deficit/hyperactivity disorder and oppositional defiant disorder developmental precursors to conduct disorder? In A. J. Sameroff, M. Lewis & S. M. Miller (Eds.), *Handbook of Developmental Psychopathology* (pp. 431–446). Springer US.

Lambert, N. M. (2005). The contribution of childhood ADHD, conduct problems, and stimulant treatment to adolescent and adult tobacco and psychoactive substance abuse. *Ethical Human Psychology and Psychiatry, 7*(3), 197–221.

Lee, S. S., Humphreys, K. L., Flory, K., Liu, R., & Glass, K. (2011). Prospective association of childhood attention-deficit/hyperactivity disorder (ADHD) and substance use and abuse/dependence: A meta-analytic review. *Clinical Psychology Review, 31*, 328–341.

Loe, I. M., & Feldman, H. M. (2007). Academic and educational outcomes of children with ADHD. *Journal of Pediatric Psychology, 32*(6), 643–654. doi: 10.1093/jpepsy/jsl054

Loeber R. (1988). Natural histories of conduct problems, delinquency, and associated substance use: Evidence for developmental progressions. In B. B. Lahey & A. E. Kazdin (Eds.), *Advances in Clinical Child Psychology,* Vol. 11 (pp. 73–123). New York: Plenum Press

Loney, J. (1993). Alcohol outcomes in an ADHD longitudinal study. Paper presented at the Society for Research in Child and Adolescent Psychopathology, February 1993, Santa Fe, New Mexico.

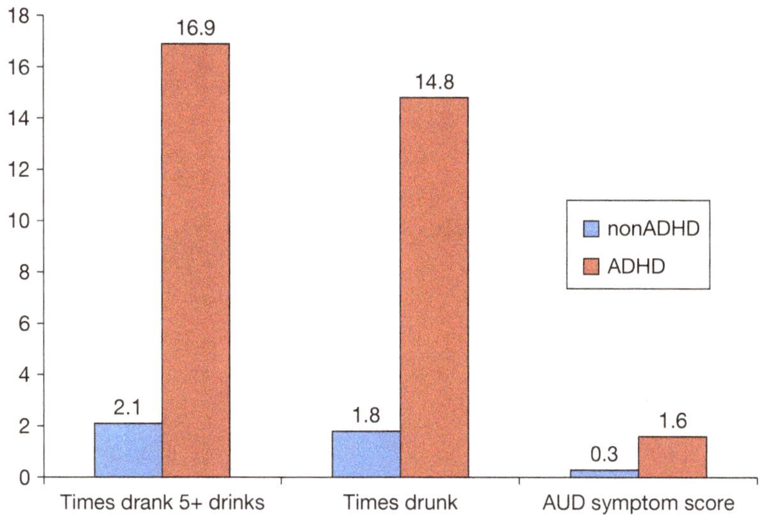

Figure 5.1

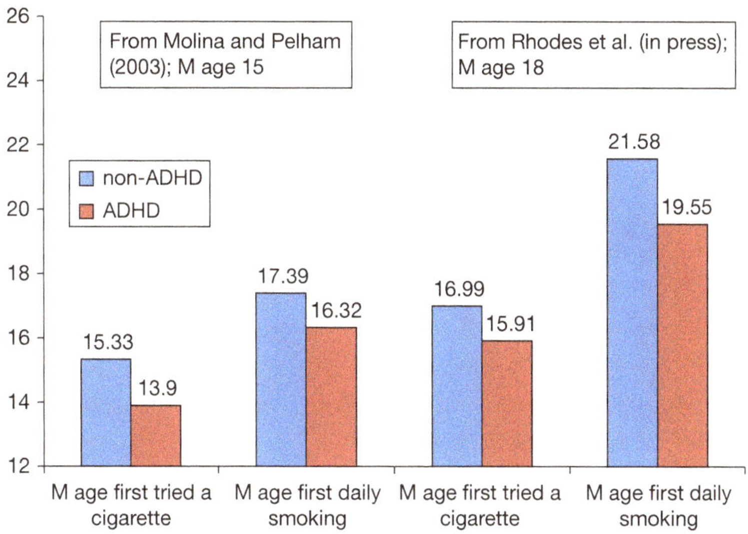

Figure 5.2

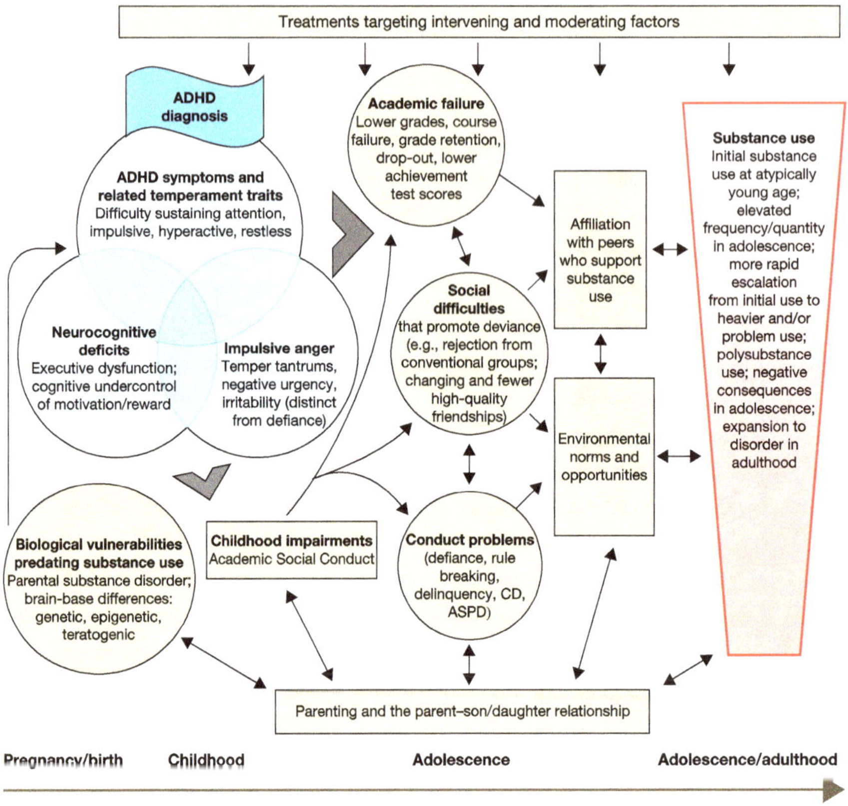
Treatments targeting intervening and moderating factors
ADHD diagnosis
ADHD symptoms and related temperament traits
Difficulty sustaining attention, impulsive, hyperactive, restless
Neurocognitive deficits
Executive dysfunction; cognitive undercontrol of motivation/reward
Impulsive anger
Temper tantrums, negative urgency, irritability (distinct from defiance)
Academic failure
Lower grades, course failure, grade retention, drop-out, lower achievement test scores
Social difficulties
that promote deviance (e.g., rejection from conventional groups; changing and fewer high-quality friendships)
Conduct problems
(defiance, rule breaking, delinquency, CD, ASPD)
Affiliation with peers who support substance use
Environmental norms and opportunities
Substance use
Initial substance use at atypically young age; elevated frequency/quantity in adolescence; more rapid escalation from initial use to heavier and/or problem use; polysubstance use; negative consequences in adolescence; expansion to disorder in adulthood
Biological vulnerabilities predating substance use
Parental substance disorder; brain-base differences: genetic, epigenetic, teratogenic
Childhood impairments
Academic Social Conduct
Parenting and the parent–son/daughter relationship
Pregnancy/birth
Childhood
Adolescence
Adolescence/adulthood

Figure 5.3

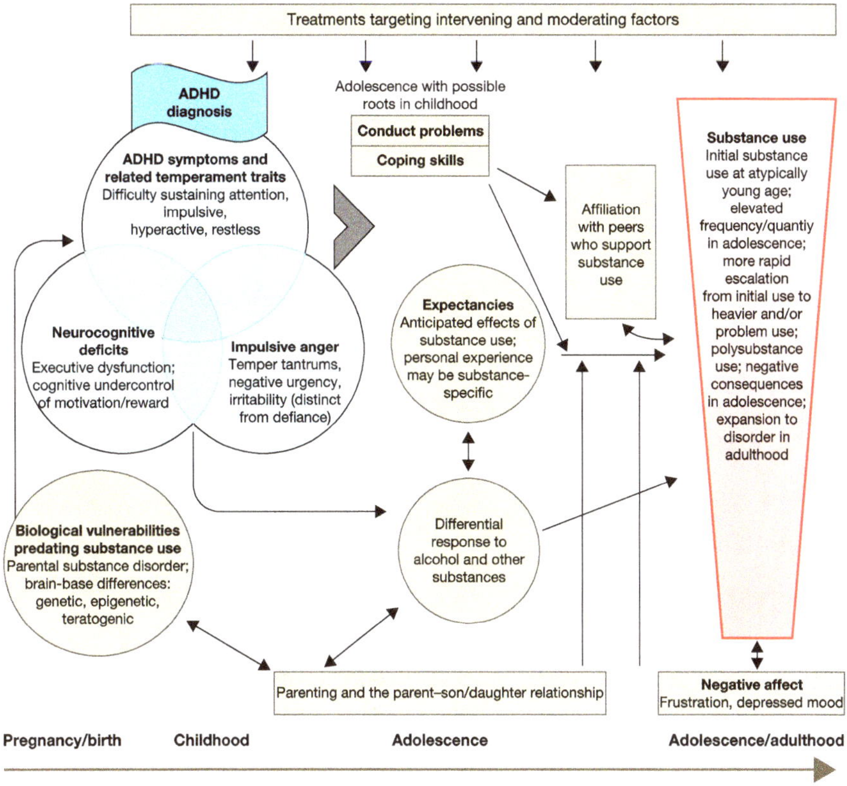

Figure 5.4

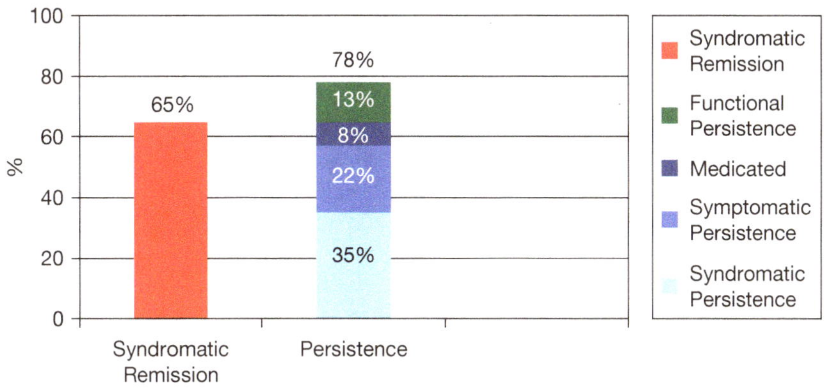

Figure 6.1

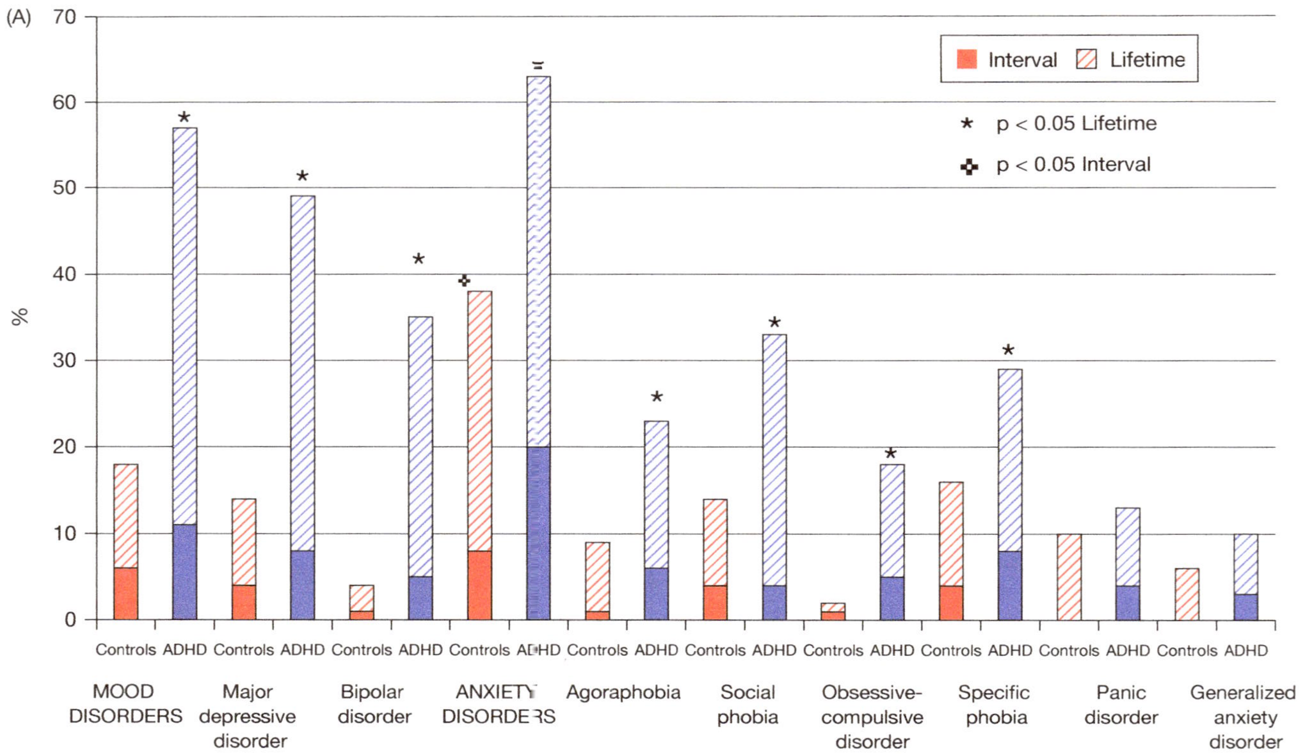
(A)
%
70
60
50
40
30
20
10
0
Interval
Lifetime
p < 0.05 Lifetime
p < 0.05 Interval
Controls
ADHD
MOOD DISORDERS
Major depressive disorder
Bipolar disorder
ANXIETY DISORDERS
Agoraphobia
Social phobia
Obsessive-compulsive disorder
Specific phobia
Panic disorder
Generalized anxiety disorder

Figure 6.2a

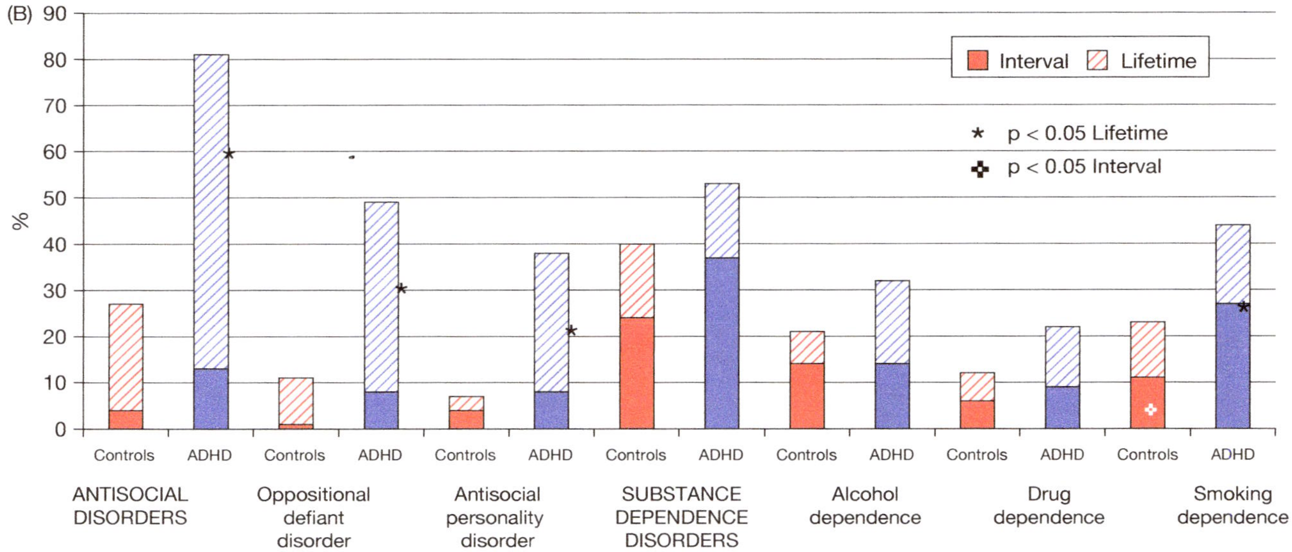
(B)
%
Interval
Lifetime
* p < 0.05 Lifetime
p < 0.05 Interval
Controls
ADHD
ANTISOCIAL DISORDERS
Oppositional defiant disorder
Antisocial personality disorder
SUBSTANCE DEPENDENCE DISORDERS
Alcohol dependence
Drug dependence
Smoking dependence

Figure 6.2b

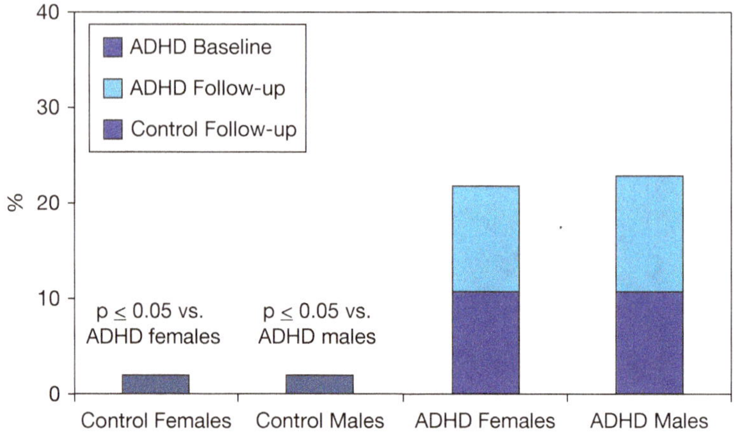

Figure 6.3

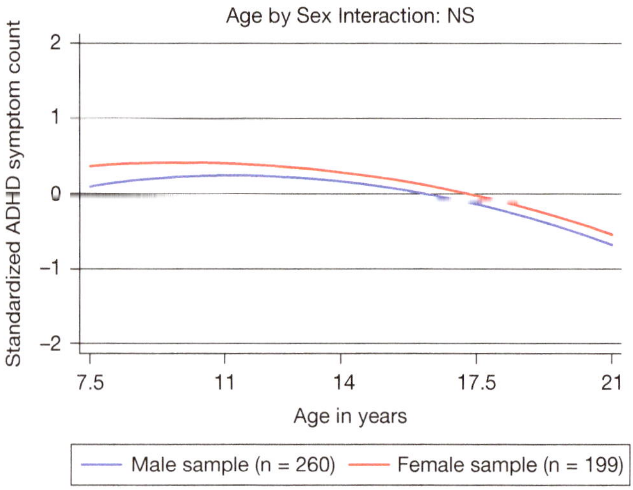

Figure 6.4

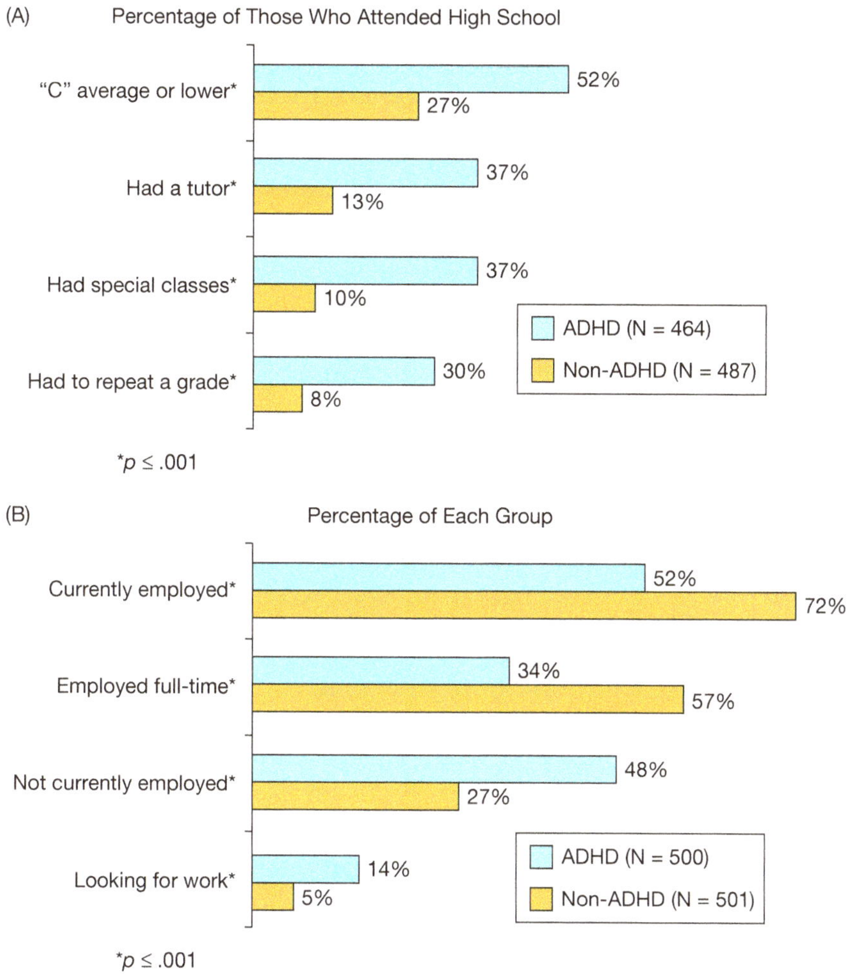

(A)
Percentage of Those Who Attended High School
"C" average or lower*
52%
27%
Had a tutor*
37%
13%
Had special classes*
37%
10%
Had to repeat a grade*
30%
8%
ADHD (N = 464)
Non-ADHD (N = 487)
*p ≤ .001
(B)
Percentage of Each Group
Currently employed*
52%
72%
Employed full-time*
34%
57%
Not currently employed*
48%
27%
Looking for work*
14%
5%
ADHD (N = 500)
Non-ADHD (N = 501)
*p ≤ .001

Figure 6.5ab

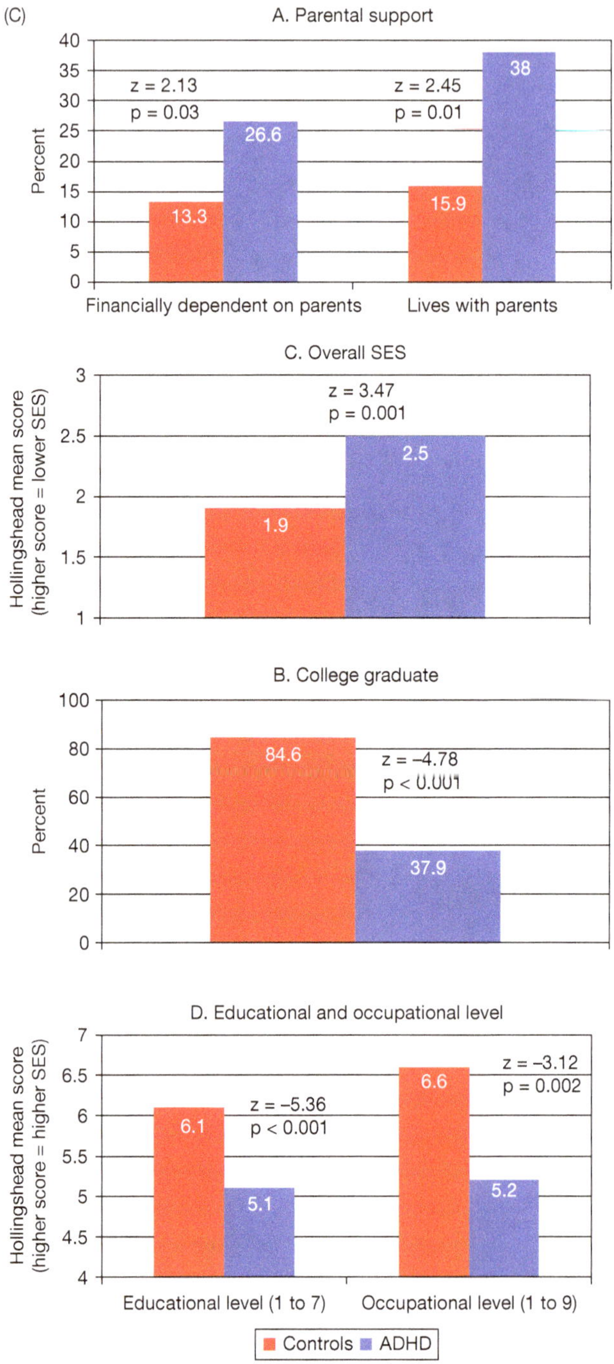
(C)
A. Parental support
Percent
z = 2.13
p = 0.03
z = 2.45
p = 0.01
13.3
26.6
15.9
38
Financially dependent on parents
Lives with parents
C. Overall SES
Hollingshead mean score (higher score = lower SES)
z = 3.47
p = 0.001
1.9
2.5
B. College graduate
Percent
84.6
37.9
z = –4.78
p < 0.001
D. Educational and occupational level
Hollingshead mean score (higher score = higher SES)
6.1
5.1
z = –5.36
p < 0.001
6.6
5.2
z = –3.12
p = 0.002
Educational level (1 to 7)
Occupational level (1 to 9)
Controls
ADHD

Figure 6.5c

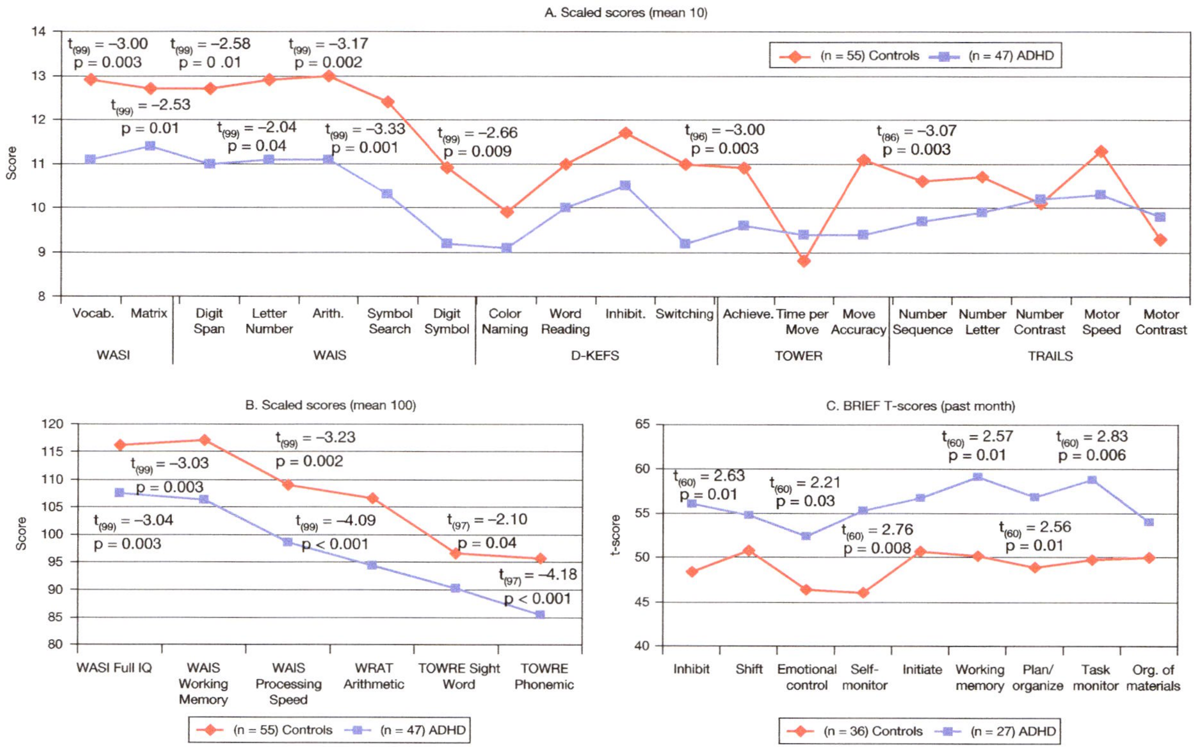
A. Scaled scores (mean 10)
(n = 55) Controls
(n = 47) ADHD
Score
$t_{(99)} = -3.00$ p = 0.003
$t_{(99)} = -2.58$ p = 0 .01
$t_{(99)} = -3.17$ p = 0.002
$t_{(99)} = -2.53$ p = 0.01
$t_{(99)} = -2.04$ p = 0.04
$t_{(99)} = -3.33$ p = 0.001
$t_{(99)} = -2.66$ p = 0.009
$t_{(96)} = -3.00$ p = 0.003
$t_{(86)} = -3.07$ p = 0.003
Vocab. Matrix
WASI
Digit Span
Letter Number
Arith.
Symbol Search
Digit Symbol
WAIS
Color Naming
Word Reading
Inhibit.
Switching
D-KEFS
Achieve.
Time per Move
Move Accuracy
TOWER
Number Sequence
Number Letter
Number Contrast
Motor Speed
Motor Contrast
TRAILS
B. Scaled scores (mean 100)
Score
$t_{(99)} = -3.23$ p = 0.002
$t_{(99)} = -3.03$ p = 0.003
$t_{(99)} = -3.04$ p = 0.003
$t_{(99)} = -4.09$ p < 0.001
$t_{(97)} = -2.10$ p = 0.04
$t_{(97)} = -4.18$ p < 0.001
WASI Full IQ
WAIS Working Memory
WAIS Processing Speed
WRAT Arithmetic
TOWRE Sight Word
TOWRE Phonemic
(n = 55) Controls
(n = 47) ADHD
C. BRIEF T-scores (past month)
t-score
$t_{(60)} = 2.57$ p = 0.01
$t_{(60)} = 2.83$ p = 0.006
$t_{(60)} = 2.63$ p = 0.01
$t_{(60)} = 2.21$ p = 0.03
$t_{(60)} = 2.76$ p = 0.008
$t_{(60)} = 2.56$ p = 0.01
Inhibit
Shift
Emotional control
Self-monitor
Initiate
Working memory
Plan/ organize
Task monitor
Org. of materials
(n = 36) Controls
(n = 27) ADHD

Figure 6.6

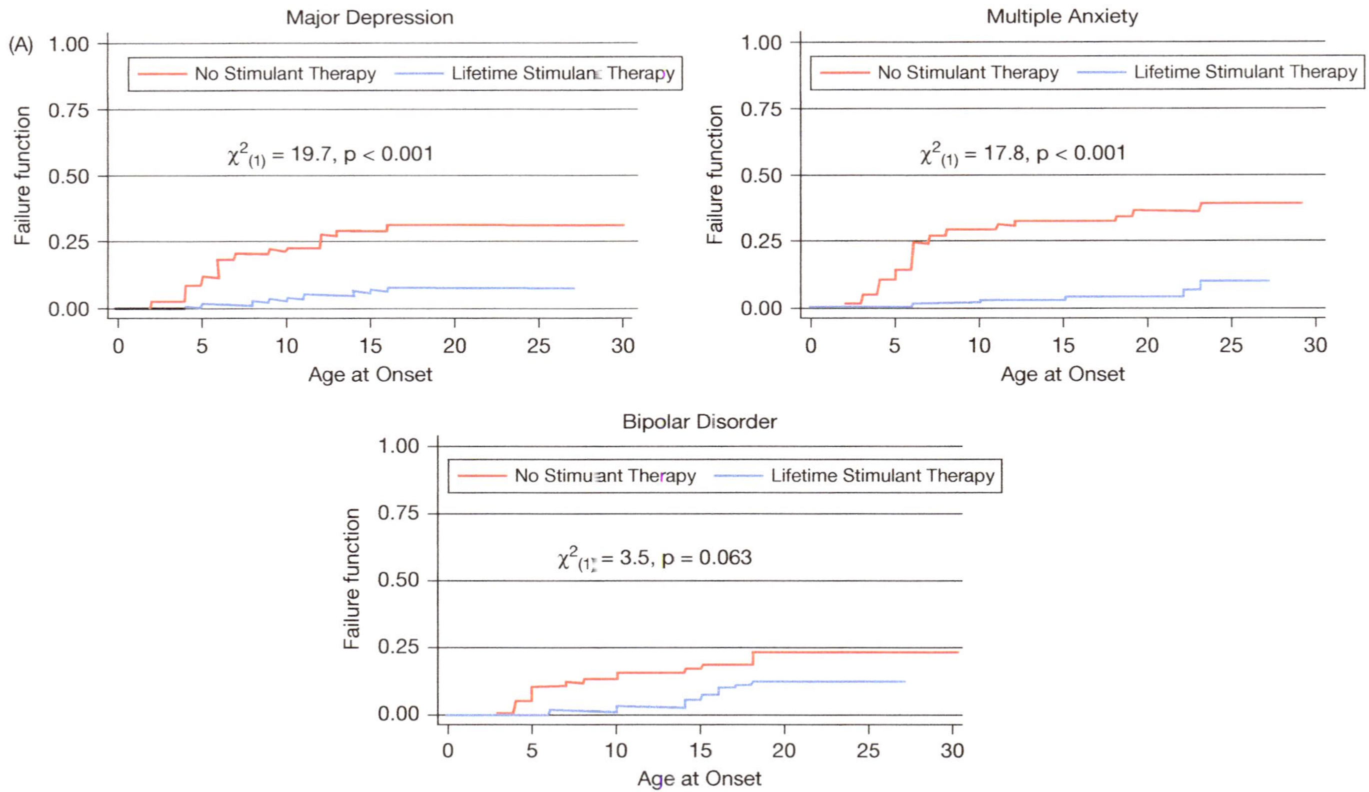

(A)
Major Depression
No Stimulant Therapy
Lifetime Stimulant Therapy
χ2(1) = 19.7, p < 0.001
Failure function
1.00
0.75
0.50
0.25
0.00
0
5
10
15
20
25
30
Age at Onset
Multiple Anxiety
No Stimulant Therapy
Lifetime Stimulant Therapy
χ2(1) = 17.8, p < 0.001
Failure function
Age at Onset
Bipolar Disorder
No Stimulant Therapy
Lifetime Stimulant Therapy
χ2(1) = 3.5, p = 0.063
Failure function
Age at Onset

Figure 6.7a

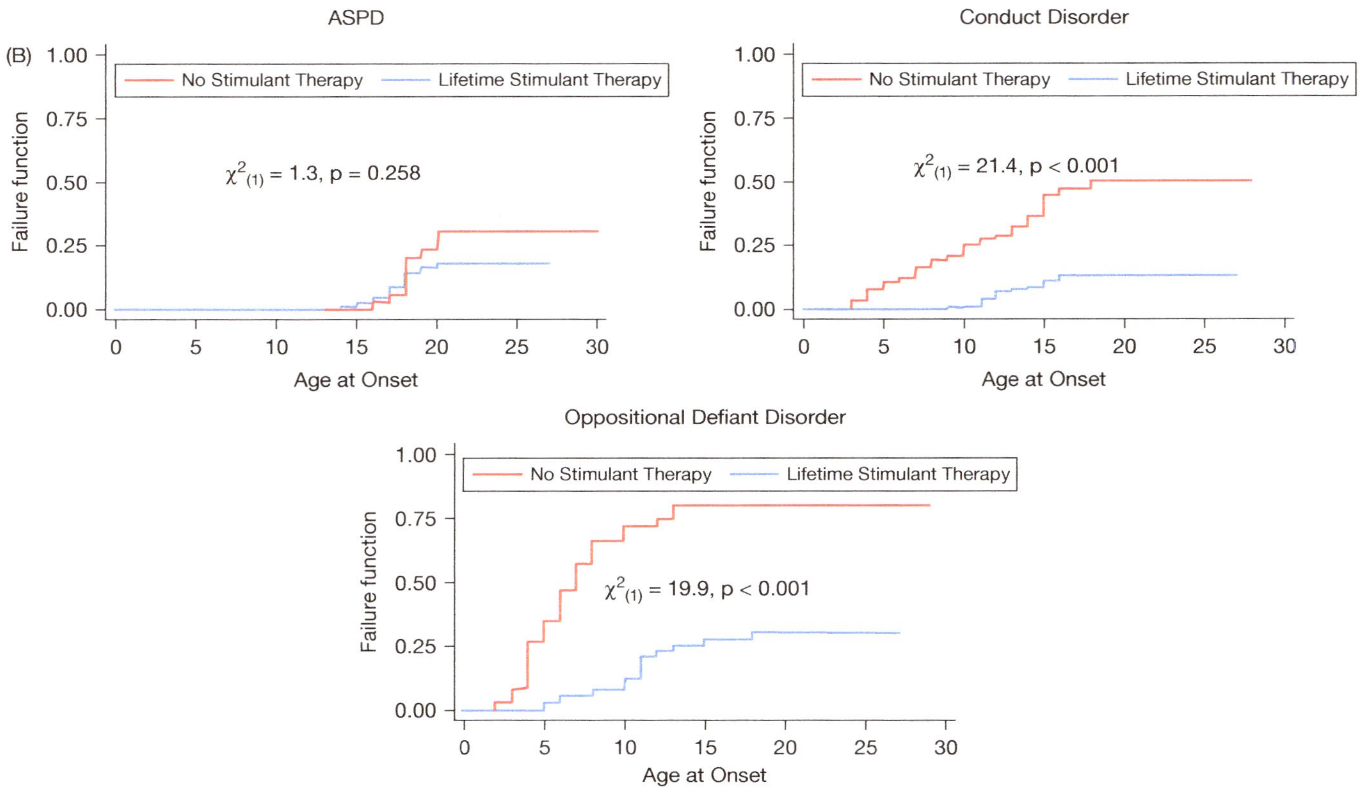
ASPD
(B)
Failure function
No Stimulant Therapy
Lifetime Stimulant Therapy
χ2(1) = 1.3, p = 0.258
Age at Onset
Conduct Disorder
Failure function
No Stimulant Therapy
Lifetime Stimulant Therapy
χ2(1) = 21.4, p < 0.001
Age at Onset
Oppositional Defiant Disorder
Failure function
No Stimulant Therapy
Lifetime Stimulant Therapy
χ2(1) = 19.9, p < 0.001
Age at Onset

Figure 6.7b

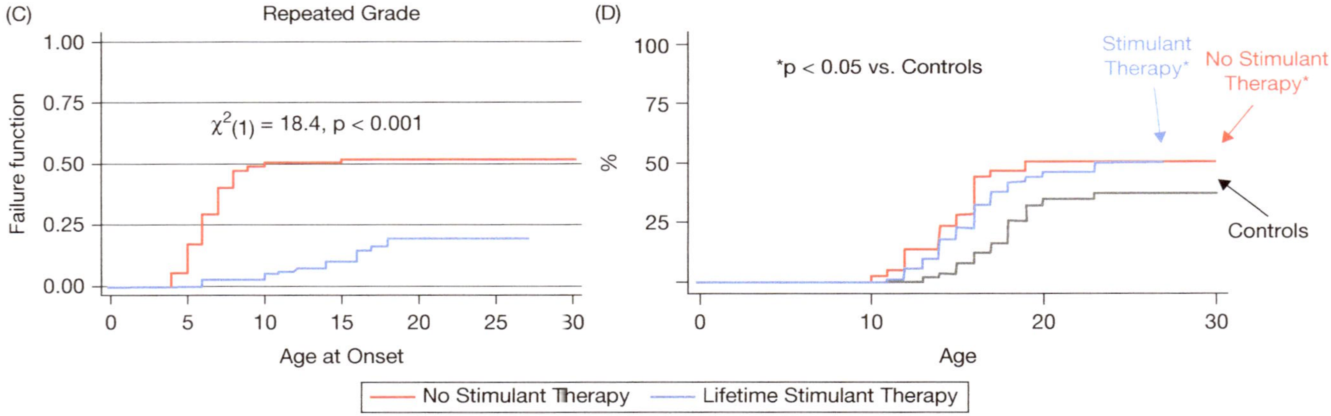
(C)
Repeated Grade
Failure function
1.00
0.75
0.50
0.25
0.00
$\chi^2(1) = 18.4, p < 0.001$
0
5
10
15
20
25
30
Age at Onset
(D)
%
100
75
50
25
*p < 0.05 vs. Controls
Stimulant Therapy*
No Stimulant Therapy*
Controls
0
10
20
30
Age
No Stimulant Therapy
Lifetime Stimulant Therapy

Figure 6.7cd

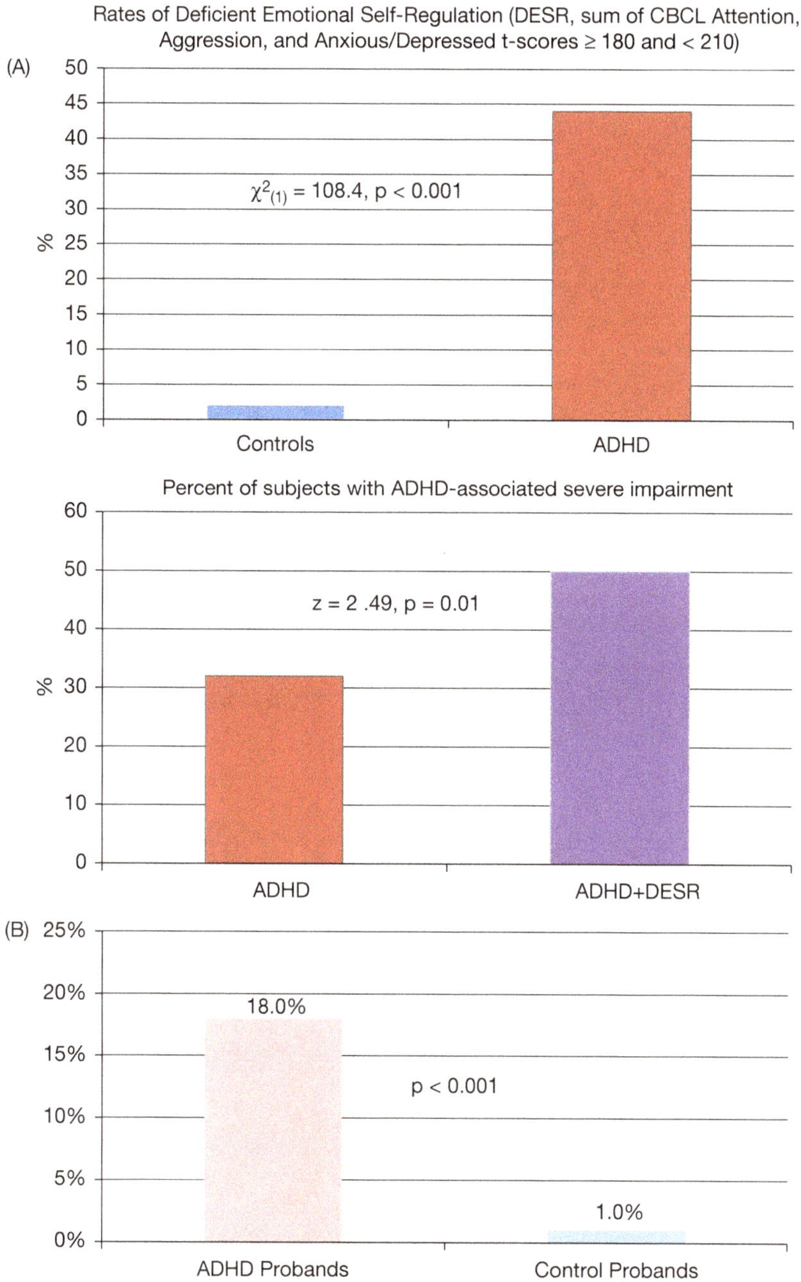

Rates of Deficient Emotional Self-Regulation (DESR, sum of CBCL Attention, Aggression, and Anxious/Depressed t-scores ≥ 180 and < 210)
(A)
%
50
45
40
35
30
25
20
15
10
5
0
$\chi^2_{(1)} = 108.4$, $p < 0.001$
Controls
ADHD
Percent of subjects with ADHD-associated severe impairment
%
60
50
40
30
20
10
0
z = 2 .49, p = 0.01
ADHD
ADHD+DESR
(B)
25%
20%
15%
10%
5%
0%
18.0%
p < 0.001
1.0%
ADHD Probands
Control Probands

Figure 6.8

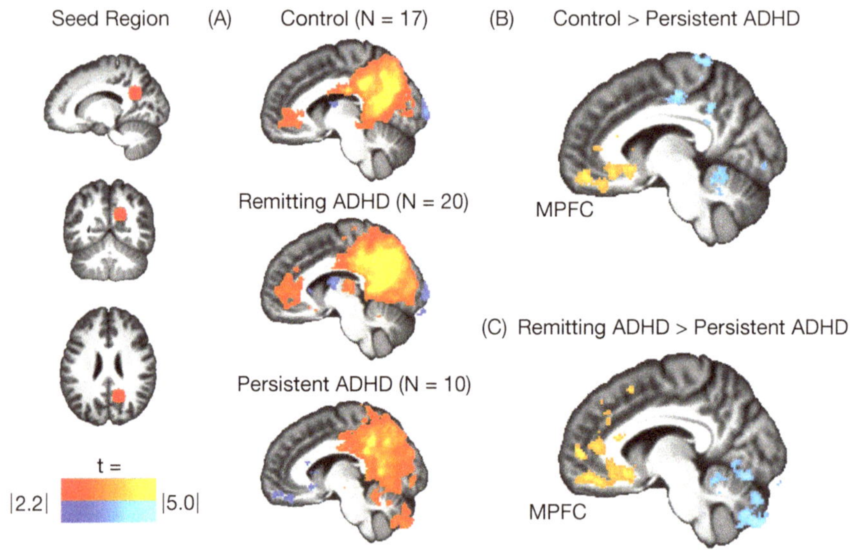

Figure 6.9

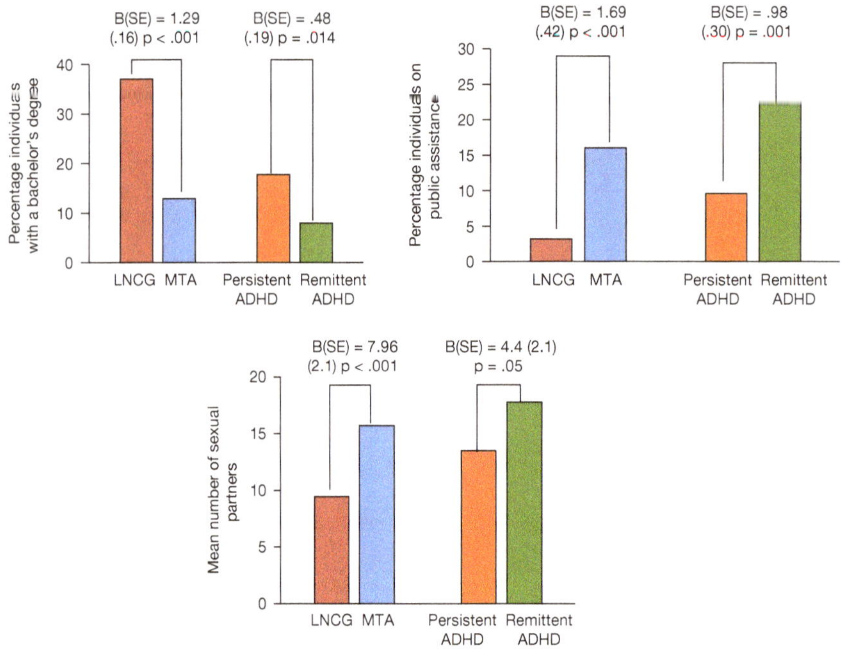

Figure 8.2

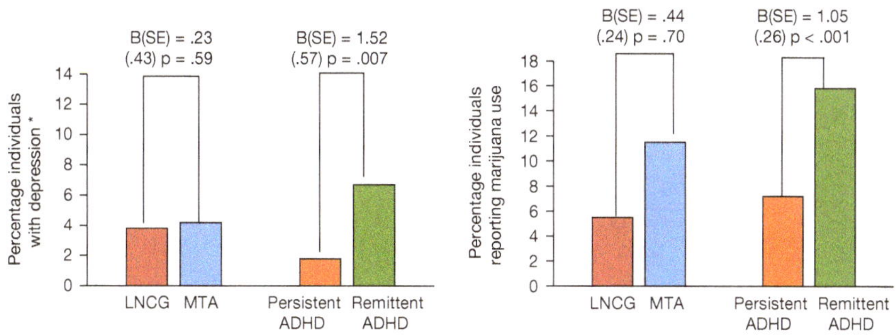

Figure 8.3

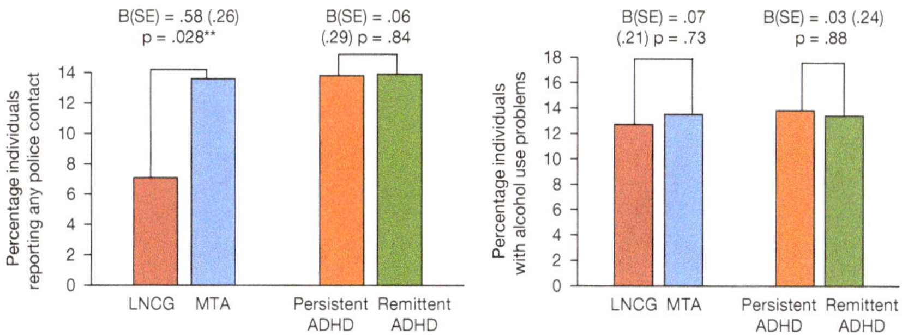

Figure 8.4

Malmberg, M., Kleinjan, M., Vermulst, A. A., Overbeek, G., Monshouwer, K., Lammers, J., & Engels, R. C. (2012). Do substance use risk personality dimensions predict the onset of substance use in early adolescence? A variable- and person-centered approach. *Journal of Youth and Adolescence, 41*(11), 1512–1525. doi: 10.1007/s10964-012-9775-6

Mannuzza, S., Klein, R. G., Bonagura, N., Malloy, P., Giampino, T. L., & Addalli, K. A. (1991). Hyperactive boys almost grown up. V. Replication of psychiatric status. *Archives of General Psychiatry, 48*(1), 77–83.

Marshal, M. P., Molina, B. S., & Pelham, W. E., Jr. (2003). Childhood ADHD and adolescent substance use: an examination of deviant peer group affiliation as a risk factor. *Psychology of Addictive Behaviors, 17*(4), 293–302. doi: 10.1037/0893-164X.17.4.293

Marshal, M. P., & Molina, B. S. G. (2006). Antisocial behaviors moderate the deviant peer pathway to substance use in children with ADHD. *Journal of Clinical Child and Adolescent Psychology, 35*(2), 216–226. doi: 10.1207/s15374424jccp3502_5

Marshal, M. P., Molina, B. S., Pelham, W. E., & Cheong, J. (2007). Attention-deficit hyperactivity disorder moderates the life stress pathway to alcohol problems in children of alcoholics. *Alcoholism, Clinical and Experimental Research, 31*(4), 564–574. doi: 10.1111/j.1530-0277.2007.00340.x

Meinzer, M.C., Pettit, J.W., Waxmonsky, J.G., Gnagy, E., Molina, B.S.G., & Pelham, W.E. (2016). Does childhood attention-deficit/hyperactivity disorder (ADHD) predict levels of depressive symptoms during emerging adulthood? *Journal of Abnormal Child Psychology, 44*(4), 787–797.

Messer, K., Trinidad, D. R., Al-Delaimy, W. K., & Pierce, J. P. (2008). Smoking cessation rates in the United States: A comparison of young adult and older smokers. *American Journal of Public Health, 98*(2), 317–322.

Milberger, S., Biederman, J., Faraone, S. V., Chen, L., & Jones, J. (1997). ADHD is associated with early initiation of cigarette smoking in children and adolescents. *Journal of the American Academy of Child and Adolescent Psychiatry, 36*(1), 37–44.

Moffitt, T. E., & Caspi, A. (2001). Childhood predictors differentiate life-course persistent and adolescence-limited antisocial pathways among males and females. *Development and Psychopathology, 13*(2), 355–375. doi: 10.1017/S0954579401002097

Molina, B. S. G. (2011). Delinquency and substance use in Attention Deficit Hyperactivity Disorder: Adolescent and young adult outcomes in developmental context. In S. W. Evans & B. Hoza (Eds.), *Treating Attention Deficit Hyperactivity Disorder: Assessment and Intervention in Developmental Context* (19:1–52). Kingston, NJ: Civic Research Institute: Kingston.

Molina, B. S., Hinshaw, S. P., Eugene Arnold, L., Swanson, J. M., Pelham, W. E., Hechtman, L., . . . MTA Cooperative Group. (2013). Adolescent substance use in the multimodal treatment study of attention-deficit/hyperactivity disorder (ADHD) (MTA) as a function of childhood ADHD, random assignment to childhood treatments, and subsequent medication. *Journal of the American Academy of Child and Adolescent Psychiatry, 52*(3), 250–263. doi: 10.1016/j.jaac.2012.12.014

Molina, B. S., Hinshaw, S. P., Swanson, J. M., Arnold, L. E., Vitiello, B., Jensen, P. S., . . . MTA Cooperative Group. (2009). The MTA at 8 years: prospective follow-up of children treated for combined-type ADHD in a multisite study. *Journal of the*

American Academy of Child and Adolescent Psychiatry, *48*(5), 484–500. doi: 10.1097/CHI.0b013e31819c23d0

Molina, B. S., Marshal, M. P., Pelham, W. E., Jr., & Wirth, R. J. (2005). Coping skills and parent support mediate the association between childhood attention-deficit/hyperactivity disorder and adolescent cigarette use. *Journal of Pediatric Psychology*, *30*(4), 345–357. doi: 10.1093/jpepsy/jsi029

Molina, B. S. G., & Pelham, W. E. (2003). Childhood predictors of adolescent substance use in a longitudinal study of children with ADHD. *Journal of Abnormal Psychology*, *112*(3), 497–507. doi: 10.1037/0021-843x.112.3.497

Molina, B. S. G., Pelham, W. E., Marshal, M. P., Curran, P. J., Gnagy, E. M., Thompson, A. L., Cheong, J. W. (2007, July). *Developmental influences on the associations among childhood ADHD, antisocial behaviors, and alcohol use*. In B.S.G. Molina (Chair), *Disinhibition and use of alcohol and drugs among youth in high risk longitudinal samples: A developmental perspective*. Symposium at the annual meeting of the Research Society on Alcoholism, Chicago, IL.

Molina, B. S., & Pelham, W. E., Jr. (2014). Attention-deficit/hyperactivity disorder and risk of substance use disorder: developmental considerations, potential pathways, and opportunities for research. *Annual Review of Clinical Psychology*, *10*, 607–639. doi: 10.1146/annurev-clinpsy-032813-153722

Molina, B. S., Pelham, W. E., Cheong, J., Marshal, M. P., Gnagy, E. M., & Curran, P. J. (2012). Childhood attention-deficit/hyperactivity disorder (ADHD) and growth in adolescent alcohol use: the roles of functional impairments, ADHD symptom persistence, and parental knowledge. *Journal of Abnormal Psychology*, *121*(4), 922–935. doi: 10.1037/a0028260

Molina, B. S., Pelham, W. E., Gnagy, E. M., Thompson, A. L., & Marshal, M. P. (2007). Attention-deficit/hyperactivity disorder risk for heavy drinking and alcohol use disorder is age specific. *Alcoholism, Clinical and Experimental Research*, *31*(4), 643–654. doi: 10.1111/j.1530-0277.2007.00349.x

Molina, B. S. G., & Sibley, M. H. (2014). The case for including informant reports in the assessment of adulthood ADHD. *The ADHD Report*, *22*(8), 1–7. doi: 10.1521/adhd.2014.22.8.1

Molina, B. S., Walther, C. A., Cheong, J., Pedersen, S. L., Gnagy, E. M., & Pelham, W. E. (2014). Heavy alcohol use in early adulthood as a function of childhood ADHD: developmentally specific mediation by social impairment and delinquency. *Experimental and Clinical Psychopharmacology*, *22*(2), 110–121. doi: 10.1037/a0035656

Molina, B. S. G., Walther, C. A., Pedersen, S. L., Gnagy, E. M., & Pelham, W. E. (2015, June). Parent- versus self-reported alcohol problems for young adults with childhood ADHD. Poster presented at the Annual Meeting of the Society for Research on Alcoholism, Austin, TX.

Muthén, B. O., & Muthén, L. K. (2004). *Mplus User's Guide* (3rd ed.). Los Angeles, CA: Muthen & Muthen.

Owens, J. S., Goldfine, M. E., Evangelista, N. M., Hoza, B., Kaiser, N. M. A critical review of self-perceptions and the positive illusory bias in children with ADHD. (2007). *Clinical Child and Family Psychology Review*, *10*(4), 335–351.

Patterson, G. R., & Dishion, T. J. (1985). Contributions of families and peers to delinquency. *Criminology, 23*(1), 63–79.

Pedersen, S.L., Walther, C.A.P., Harty, S.C., Gnagy, E.M., Pelham, W.E., Molina, B.S.G. (2016). The indirect effects of childhood ADHD on alcohol problems in adulthood through unique facets of impulsivity. *Addiction*. PMCID: PMC Journal - In Process NIHMS#770862

Pedersen, S. L., Harty, S. C., Pelham, W. E., Gnagy, E. M., & Molina, B. S. (2014). Differential associations between alcohol expectancies and adolescent alcohol use as a function of childhood ADHD. *Journal of Studies on Alcohol and Drugs, 75*(1), 145–152.

Pelham, W. E., Evans, S. W., Gnagy, E. M., & Greenslade, K. E. (1992). Teacher ratings of DSM-III-R symptoms for the disruptive behavior disorders: Prevalence, factor analyses, and conditional probabilities in a special education sample. *School Psychology Review, 21*(2), 285–299.

Pelham, W. E., Jr., & Fabiano, G. A. (2008). Evidence-based psychosocial treatments for attention-deficit/hyperactivity disorder. *Journal of Clinical Child and Adolescent Psychology, 37*(1), 184–214. doi: 10.1080/15374410701818681

Pelham, W. E., Gnagy, E. M., Greiner, A. R., Waschbusch, D. A., Fabiano, G. A., & Burrows-MacLean, L. (2010). Summer treatment programs for attention deficit/hyperactivity disorder. In A. E. Kazdin & J. R. Weisz (Eds.), *Evidence-Based Psychotherapies for Children and Adolescents* (2nd ed.) (pp. 277–292). New York: The Guilford Press.

Pelham, W. E., & Hoza, B. (1996). Intensive treatment: A summer treatment program for children with ADHD. In E. D. Hibbs & P. S. Jensen (Eds.), *Psychosocial Treatments for Child and Adolescent Disorders: Empirically Based Strategies for Clinical Practice* (pp. 311–340). New York: American Psychological Association Press.

Raudino, A., Fergusson, D. M., & Horwood, L. J. (2013). The quality of parent/child relationships in adolescence is associated with poor adult psychosocial adjustment. *Journal of Adolescence, 36*(2), 331–340. doi: 10.1016/j.adolescence.2012.12.002

Rhodes, J. D., Derefinko, K. J., Gnagy, E. M., Shiffman, S., Pelham, W. E., & Molina, B. S. G. (in press). Cigarette smoking and ADHD: An examination of prognostically-relevant smoking behaviors among adolescents and young adults. *Psychology of Addictive Behaviors*.

Robb, J. A., Sibley, M. H., Pelham, W. E., Jr., Foster, E. M., Molina, B. S., Gnagy, E. M., & Kuriyan, A. B. (2011). The estimated annual cost of ADHD to the U.S. education system. *School Mental Health, 3*(3), 169–177. doi: 10.1007/s12310-011-9057-6

Rostron, B. (2013). Smoking-attributable mortality by cause in the United States: revising the CDC's data and estimates. *Nicotine & Tobacco Research, 15*(1), 238–246. doi: 10.1093/ntr/nts120

Sher, K. J. (1991). Psychological characteristics of children of alcoholics. Overview of research methods and findings. *Recent Developments in Alcoholism, 9*, 301–326.

Sher, K. J., Grekin, E. R., & Williams, N. A. (2005). The development of alcohol use disorders. *Annual Review of Clinical Psychology, 1*, 493–523. doi: 10.1146/annurev.clinpsy.1.102803.144107

Sibley, M. H., Pelham, W. E., Molina, B. S. G., Gnagy, E. M., Waschbusch, D. A., Biswas, A., . . . Karch, K. M. (2011). The delinquency outcomes of boys with ADHD with and without comorbidity. *Journal of Abnormal Child Psychology, 39*(1), 21–32. doi: DOI 10.1007/s10802-010-9443-9

Sibley, M. H., Pelham, W. E., Jr., Molina, B. S., Gnagy, E. M., Waschbusch, D. A., Garefino, A. C., . . . Karch, K. M. (2012a). Diagnosing ADHD in adolescence. *Journal of Consulting and Clinical Psychology, 80*(1), 139–150. doi: 10.1037/a0026577

Sibley, M. H., Pelham, W. E., Molina, B. S., Gnagy, E. M., Waxmonsky, J. G., Waschbusch, D. A., . . . Kuriyan, A. B. (2012b). When diagnosing ADHD in young adults emphasize informant reports, DSM items, and impairment. *Journal of Consulting and Clinical Psychology, 80*(6), 1052–1061. doi: 10.1037/a0029098

Sibley, M. H., Pelham, W. E., Molina, B. S., Waschbusch, D. A., Gnagy, E. M., Babinski, D. E., & Biswas, A. (2010). Inconsistent self-report of delinquency by adolescents and young adults with ADHD. *Journal of Abnormal Child Psychology, 38*(5), 645–656. doi: 10.1007/s10802-010-9404-3

Stacy, A. W., & Wiers, R. W. (2010). Implicit cognition and addiction: a tool for explaining paradoxical behavior. *Annual Review of Clinical Psychology, 6*, 551–575. doi: 10.1146/annurev.clinpsy.121208.131444

Thompson, A. L., Molina, B. S., Pelham, W., Jr., & Gnagy, E. M. (2007). Risky driving in adolescents and young adults with childhood ADHD. *Journal of Pediatric Psychology, 32*(7), 745–759. doi: 10.1093/jpepsy/jsm002

Toplak, M. E., Jain, U., & Tannock, R. (2005). Executive and motivational processes in adolescents with Attention-Deficit-Hyperactivity Disorder (ADHD). *Behavioral and Brain Functions, 1*(1), 8.

U.S. Department of Education, National Center for Education Statistics. (2011). *Digest of Education Statistics 2010.* (Table 212). http://nces.ed.gov/programs/digest/d10/tables/dt10_212.asp

Walther, C. A., Cheong, J., Molina, B. S., Pelham, W. E., Jr., Wymbs, B. T., Belendiuk, K. A., & Pedersen, S. L. (2012). Substance use and delinquency among adolescents with childhood ADHD: the protective role of parenting. *Psychology of Addictive Behaviors, 26*(3), 585–598.

Weiss, G., & Hechtman, L. T. (1993). *Hyperactive Children Grown Up. ADHD in Children, Adolescents, and Adults* (2nd ed.). New York: The Guilford Press.

Wiers, R. W., & Stacy, A. W. (2006). Implicit cognition and addiction. *Current Directions in Psychological Science, 15*(6), 292–296. doi: 10.1111/j.1467-8721.2006.00455.x

Wills, T. A., Sandy, J. M., & Yaeger, A. M. (2002). Moderators of the relation between substance use level and problems: test of a self-regulation model in middle adolescence. *Journal of Abnormal Psychology, 111*(1), 3.

Wymbs, B. T., Molina, B. S. G., Belendiuk, K. A., Pedersen, S. L., Walther, C. A. P., Cheong, J.,. . .Pelham, W. E. (2013). Motorsports involvement among adolescents and young adults with childhood ADHD. *Journal of Clinical and Child Adolescence and Psychology, 42*(2), 220–231. doi: 10.1080/15374416.2012.759227

Wymbs, B., Molina, B., Pelham, W., Cheong, J., Gnagy, E., Belendiuk, K., . . . Waschbusch, D. (2012). Risk of intimate partner violence among young adult males with childhood ADHD. *Journal of Attention Disorders, 16*(5), 373–383. doi: 10.1177/1087054710389987

Wymbs, B. T., Pelham, W. E., Jr., Gnagy, E. M., & Molina, B. S. (2008). Mother and adolescent reports of interparental discord among parents of adolescents with and without attention-deficit hyperactivity disorder. *Journal of Emotional and Behavioral Disorders 16*(1), 29–41.

Wymbs, B. T., Pelham, W. E., Molina, B. S. G., Gnagy, E. M., Wilson, T. K., & Greenhouse, J. B. (2008). Rate and predictors of divorce among parents of youths with ADHD. *Journal of Consulting and Clinical Psychology, 76*(5), 735–744. doi: 10.1037/A0012719

Wymbs, B. T., Walther, C. A. P., Cheong, J., Belendiuk, K. A., Pedersen, S. L., Gnagy, E. M., Pelham, W. E., & Molina, B. S. G. (2014). Childhood ADHD potentiates the association between problematic drinking and intimate partner violence. *Journal of Attention Disorders.* Advance online publication. doi: 10.1177/1087054714557358.

Zimmerman, M. A., Caldwell, C. H., & Bernat, D. H. (2002). Discrepancy between self-report and school-record grade point average: correlates with psychosocial outcomes among African American adolescents. *Journal of Applied Social Psychology, 32*(1), 86–109. doi: 10.1111/j.1559-1816.2002.tb01421.x

Zucker, R. A. (2006). The developmental behavior genetics of drug involvement: overview and comments. *Behavior Genetics, 36*(4), 616–625. doi: 10.1007/s10519-006-9070-y

6

Young Adult Outcome of Attention Deficit Hyperactivity Disorder

Results from the Longitudinal Massachusetts General Hospital Sample of Pediatrically and Psychiatrically Referred Youth with and without ADHD of Both Sexes

MAI UCHIDA AND JOSEPH BIEDERMAN

INTRODUCTION

Long-term outcome studies of attention deficit hyperactivity disorder (ADHD) are critical for evaluating the course of a disorder from childhood into adulthood, for documenting its stability over time, and for helping link the pediatric and adult literature on the subject. Unique strengths of the Massachusetts General Hospital (MGH) Longitudinal Study of ADHD are its large sample size; its accelerated design; the inclusion of an equal number of boys and girls; its family–genetic design; the large scope of nonoverlapping outcome domains including a comprehensive assessment of comorbid psychiatric disorders beyond the disruptive behavior disorders such as mood and anxiety disorders; comprehensive functional assessments such as cognition, school, family, and interpersonal functioning; blindness of assessments; and ascertainment from pediatric and psychiatric sources.

SUBJECTS

Probands were predominantly Caucasian youth 6–17 years of age of both sexes with and without ADHD ascertained from pediatric and psychiatric sources. At baseline, we ascertained 140 boys and 140 girls with ADHD, and 120 boys and 122 girls without ADHD and their first-degree relatives. Diagnoses were made based on DSM-III-R criteria. Subjects were followed for an average of 11 years. Of the original subjects, 208 subjects with ADHD (112 boys and 96 girls) and 196 controls (105 boys and 91 girls) returned for the 10-year follow-up assessment. The ages at follow-up ranged from 15 to 31 years (mean = 22 years).

COURSE OF ATTENTION DEFICIT HYPERACTIVITY DISORDER

High Levels of Persistence of ADHD

At follow-up in young adult years (Figure 6.1), 77% of boys and girls with ADHD continued to display full or subsyndromic ADHD, clearly documenting that ADHD is a highly persistent disorder [1]. Predictors of persistence in both sexes were: (1) psychiatric comorbidity with disruptive mood and anxiety disorders, (2) familiality with ADHD, and (3) psychosocial adversity. By stressing that persistence of ADHD needs to consider not only the full syndromatic picture of ADHD but also subsyndromic forms of the disorder as well as impaired functioning, our work expanded

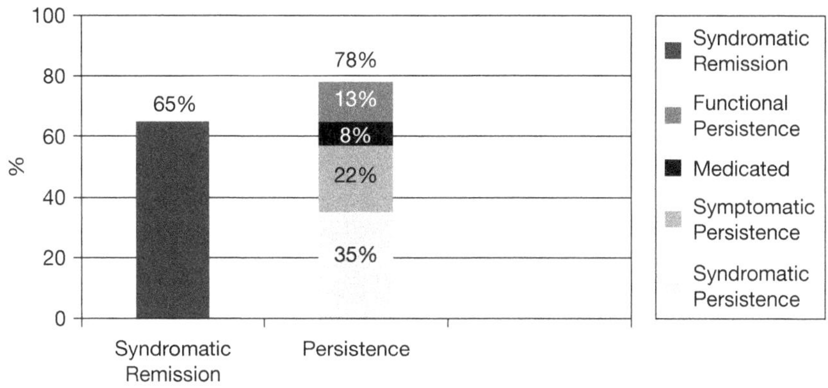

Figure 6.1 Persistence of attention deficit hyperactivity disorder at 10-year follow-up. See also color plate section.

the literature on the persistence of ADHD. For example, while only 35% of our ADHD children met the full DSM-IV criteria for ADHD in their adult years, an additional 43% continued to struggle with subthreshold symptoms of ADHD or associated functional impairments, had functional impairments associated with ADHD, or had medication induced remission of their ADHD symptoms [1]. Our work also showed that symptom decline was heterogeneous with symptoms of hyperactivity and impulsivity declining early on while symptoms of inattention, the most covert component of the clinical picture, remained highly persistent. Our work also documented that symptom decline was very similar in both sexes, as it was in psychiatrically and pediatrically referred children, expanding the generalizability of our findings to pediatrically referred children.

PATTERNS OF PSYCHIATRIC COMORBIDITY

Our studies confirmed that ADHD is highly associated with a much wider range of comorbid psychiatric disorders than previously thought (Figure 6.2). These included not only disruptive behavior disorders but also mood and anxiety disorders [2]. Our work also documented a wide discrepancy between very high lifetime rates of comorbid psychiatric disorders and low concurrent rates. In fact, in our longest reported 16-year

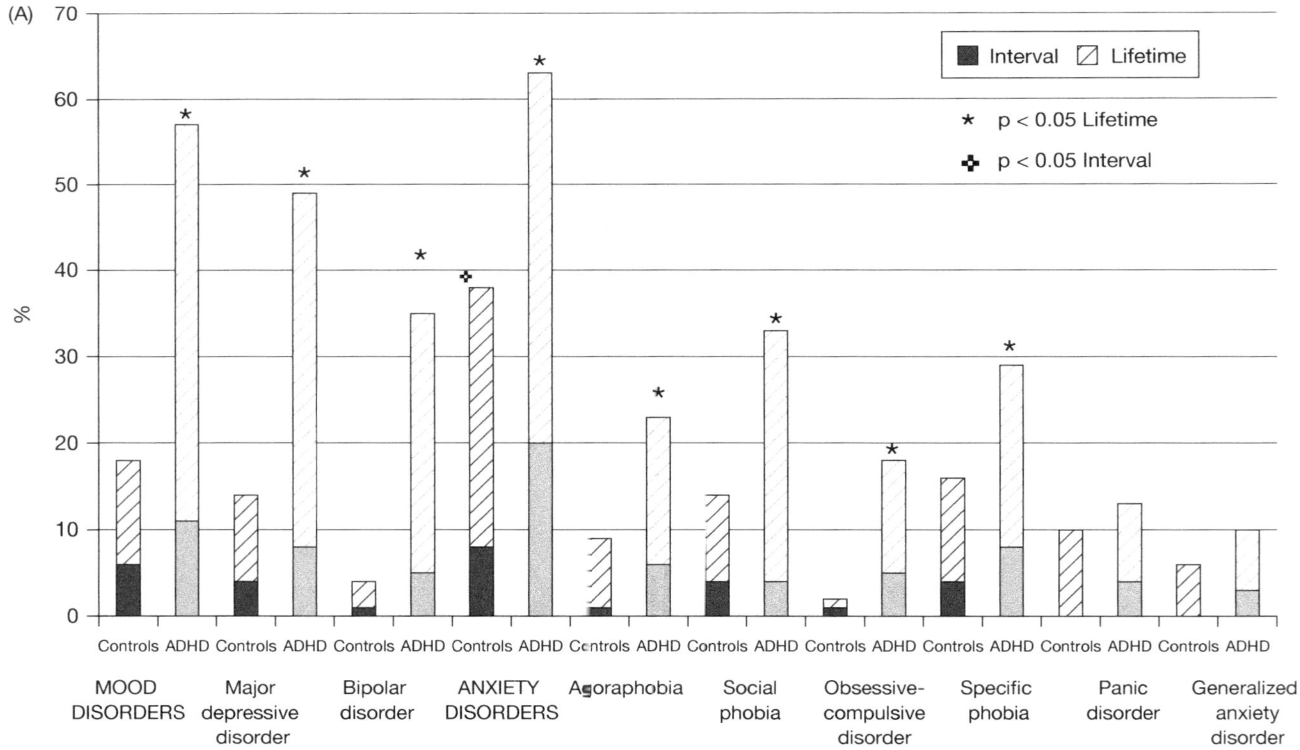

Figure 6.2 (a) Rates of lifetime versus interval disorders in ADHD subjects versus controls at the 16-year follow-up; (b) Rates of lifetime and interval disorders in ADHD subjects versus controls at the 16-year follow-up. See also color plate section.

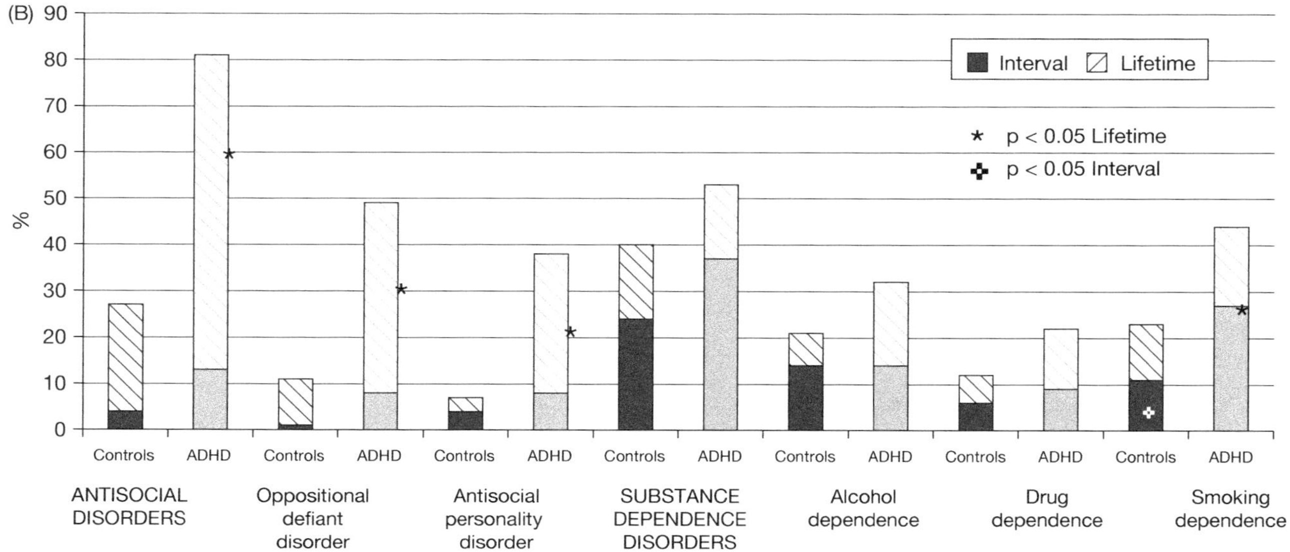

Figure 6.2 Continued

follow-up study, we documented that the only contemporaneous psychiatric disorders that separated subjects with ADHD from controls were anxiety disorders and nicotine addiction [3]. These findings are important in that they support the conclusion that the well-documented psychosocial and psychoeducational dysfunction associated with ADHD children in their adult years is due to ADHD proper and not to its comorbid disorders. Another key contribution of our work is that it provides clear documentation of the early onset of comorbid psychiatric disorders in the preadolescent years.

Comorbidity with Smoking, Alcohol and Drug Abuse and Dependence

Our work confirmed and expanded results from previous studies that documented that ADHD significantly increases the risk for all substances of abuse (Figure 6.2B). Our work also identified a developmental trajectory for substance use disorders that starts with cigarette smoking and continues with alcohol and drug use disorders. Furthermore, we were able to document that cigarette smoking is a gateway drug in that ADHD children who smoke are at a very significant risk to progress onto alcohol and drug use disorders in subsequent years [4].

Comorbidity with Bipolar-I Disorder

Our work clearly documented high rates of comorbid bipolar-I (BP-I) disorder in our ADHD children (Figure 6.3). BP-I disorder was diagnosed in 11% of our ADHD children versus 0% of our controls (selected only by the absence of ADHD) at the baseline assessment in childhood, with an additional 12% of ADHD children developing this disorder at the four-year follow-up (lifetime rate 23% by adolescence) [2, 5]. ADHD children with comorbid BP-I disorder at the baseline or follow-up assessment had significantly higher rates of additional psychopathology, psychiatric

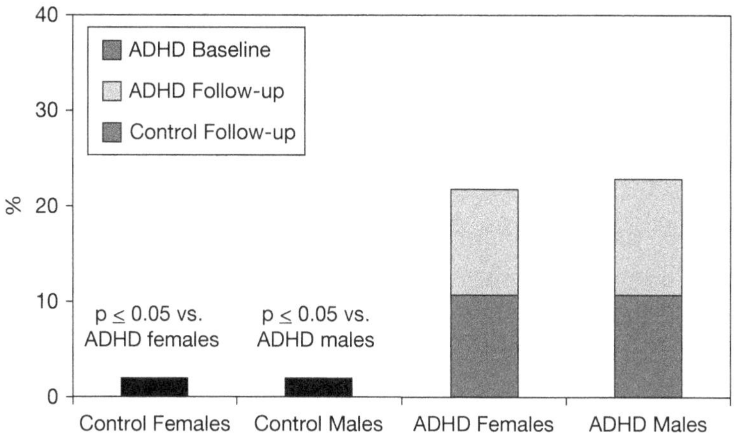

Figure 6.3 Bipolar disorder in girls and boys with and without ADHD. See also color plate section.

hospitalization, and severely impaired psychosocial functioning when compared with other ADHD children. The clinical picture of bipolarity was mostly irritable and mixed. ADHD children with comorbid BP-I disorder also had a very severe symptomatic picture of ADHD as well as prototypical correlates of BP-I disorder. A greater family history of mood disorders also was found in children with BP-I disorder compared with non-BP-I ADHD children [6]. Our work also documented that the high comorbidity between ADHD and BP-I disorder was not due to symptom overlap between ADHD and BP-I disorder [6]. The majority of children with the combined condition continued to meet diagnostic criteria of both BP-I disorder and ADHD after removing overlapping symptoms such as distractibility, motoric hyperactivity, and talkativeness, which indicates that BP-I disorder and ADHD comorbidity is not a methodological artifact of shared diagnostic criteria.

Our familial aggregation findings documented that comorbid ADHD plus BP-I disorder was familially distinct from other forms of ADHD, supporting the conclusion that childhood-onset BP-I disorder may be a developmentally distinct form of BP-I disorder [7]. Our findings showed that although relatives of ADHD probands were at significantly greater risk for ADHD irrespective of the comorbidity with BP-I, a fivefold elevated risk for BP-I was observed only among relatives of ADHD probands with comorbid BP-I disorder. We also found evidence for co-segregation between ADHD and BP-I disorder in relatives, supporting the hypothesis that ADHD with comorbid BP-I disorder represents a genetically distinct subtype of ADHD. We also documented that the risk for manic switches from unipolar major depressive disorder to bipolar disorder was significantly higher in youth with ADHD (28%) when compared with the risk in youth without ADHD (6%) [8]. Furthermore, in subjects with ADHD, the risk of switching from unipolar to bipolar disorder was predicted by the presence of comorbid conduct disorder, school behavior problems, a positive family history of parental mood disorder, and subthreshold manic symptoms [9].

THE INFLUENCE OF SEX ON THE COURSE OF ILLNESS

A key contribution of our work was the documentation that sex does not moderate the clinical features of ADHD, including the defining symptoms of the disorder, age of onset, associated impairment, patterns of comorbidity, neuropsychological underpinnings, or patterns of symptom decline [10]. We did observe, however, a phase delay in the onset of comorbid disruptive behavior disorder that developed later in girls than in boys, a finding that may account for the differential patterns of referrals between boys and girls (Figure 6.4).

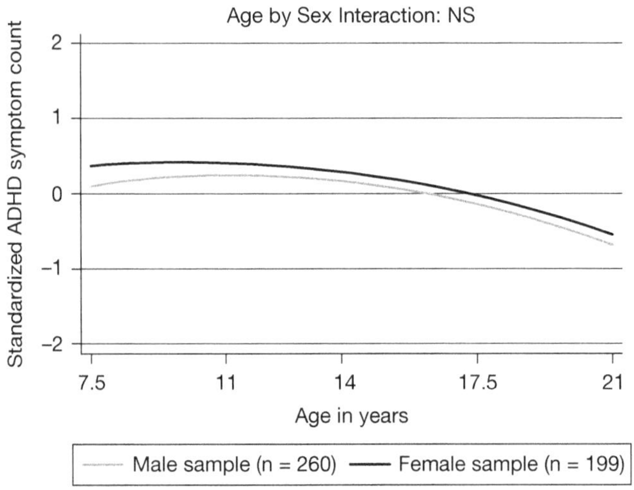

Figure 6.4 Course of ADHD symptoms over time by sex: A growth curve model. See also color plate section.

PATTERNS OF FAMILIALITY

Familial risk analysis confirmed the strong familial nature of ADHD. We observed an eightfold increase in the risk for ADHD in parents and siblings of ADHD children compared with controls [11]. Familial risk analysis provided evidence for the genetic heterogeneity of ADHD. Our familial risk studies also documented that (1) ADHD and major depression share common familial vulnerabilities [12, 13];

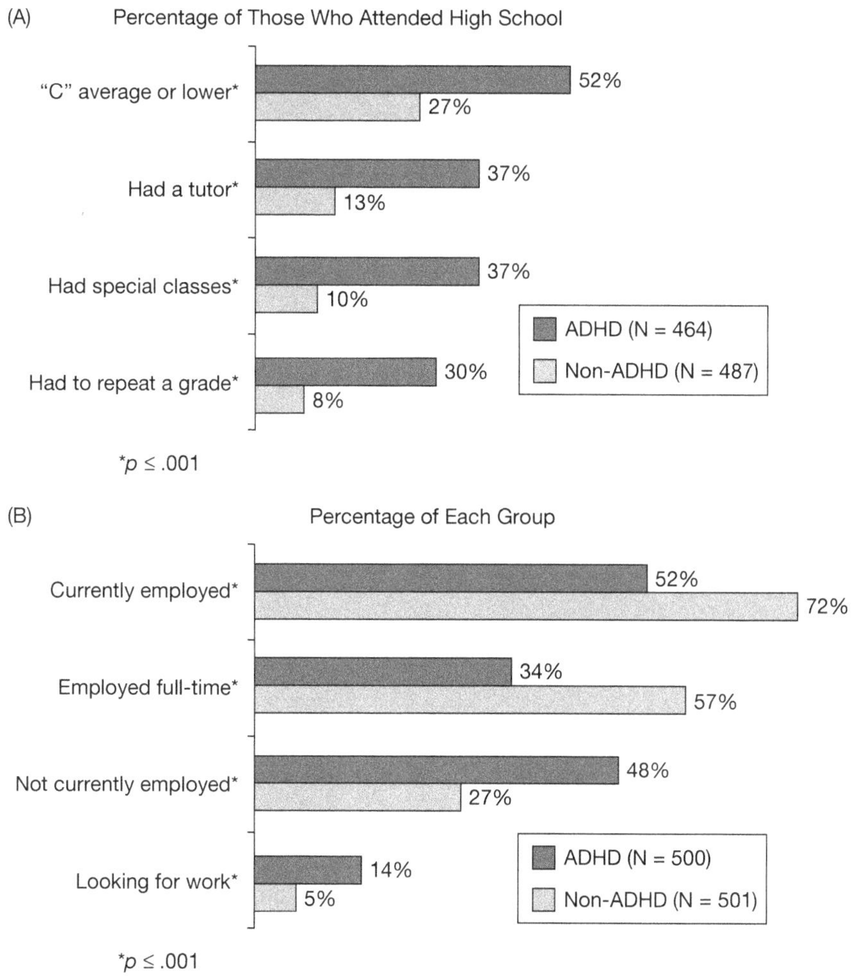

Figure 6.5 A: Educational Impairment in High School; B: Current Employment Status; C: Educational and occupational achievement in ADHD and control subjects at the year follow-up. See also color plate section.

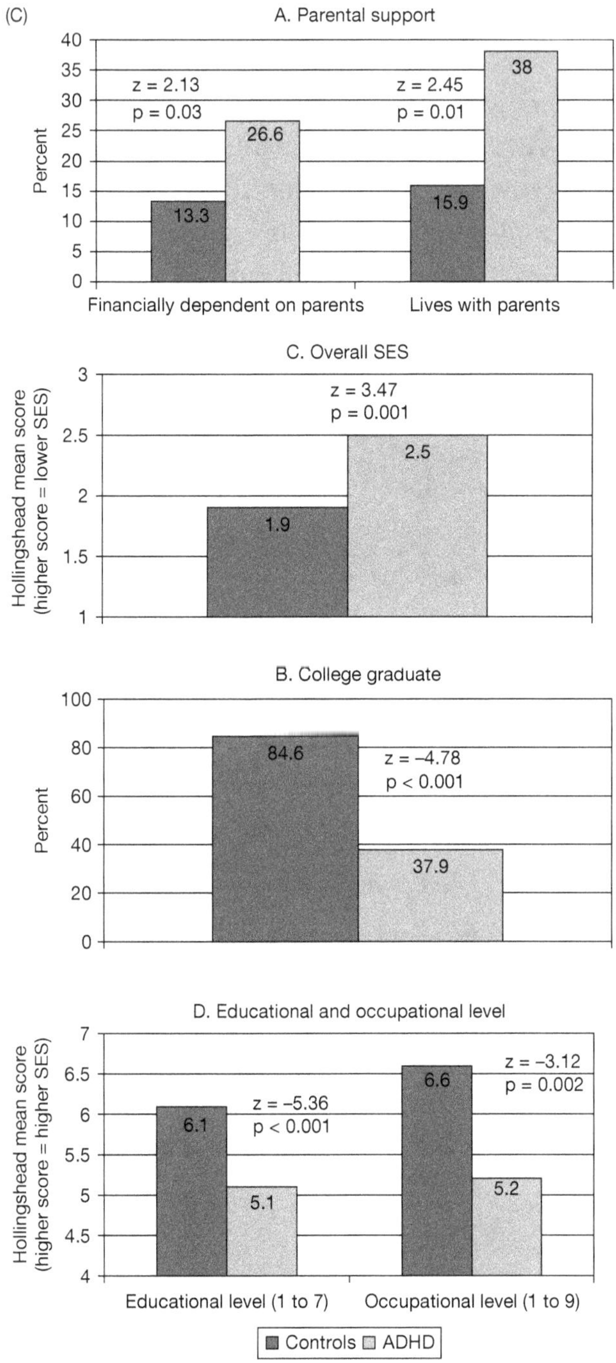

Figure 6.5 Continued

(2) ADHD children with conduct disorders and bipolar disorders represent a distinct familial subtype of ADHD [13, 14]; and (3) ADHD is familially independent from anxiety disorders [15] and learning disabilities [16].

EDUCATIONAL AND OCCUPATIONAL OUTCOMES

Our work documented that ADHD children had significantly more struggles in their school years than age and sex matched comparators without ADHD (Figure 6.5). Half of the ADHD children had an average grade lower than a "C." They also frequently required tutoring or placement in special classes, and a large percentage of them needed to repeat a grade in high school [17].

When compared with age and sex matched non-ADHD comparators, ADHD children in adulthood were significantly more likely to drop out of high school, not to complete college, to be jobless [17], to be financially dependent on their parents, and to attain a lower personal social class than their family of origin [3]. These outcomes remained significant after controlling for comorbid psychiatric disorders, indicating that they were due to ADHD itself.

COGNITIVE OUTCOMES

Our work documented that ADHD children were significantly more impaired than controls in all neuropsychological and academic achievement measures assessed and that they continued to be impaired in these domains in adulthood [3] (Figure 6.6). Considering the high level of persistence of neuropsychological deficits into adult years and the high level of morbidity associated with them, persistence of neuropsychological deficits needs to be considered in the conceptualization of persistence of ADHD.

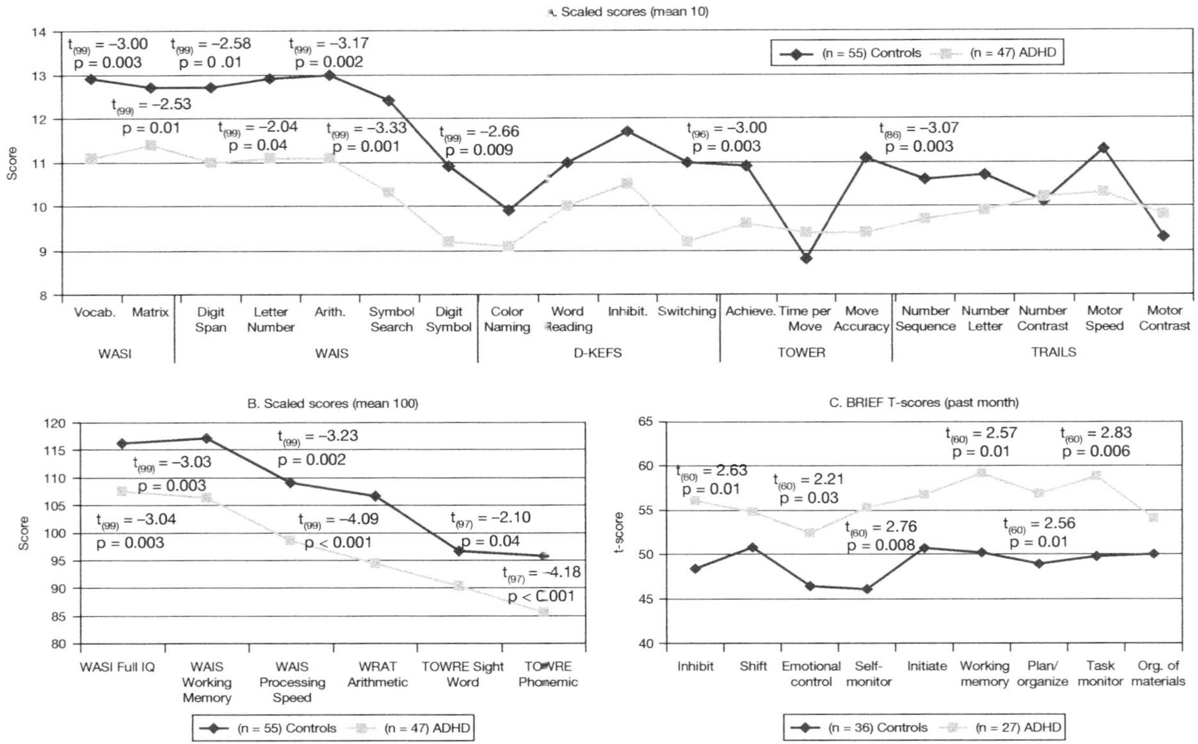

Figure 6.6 Cognitive outcomes in ADHD children grown up. See also color plate section.

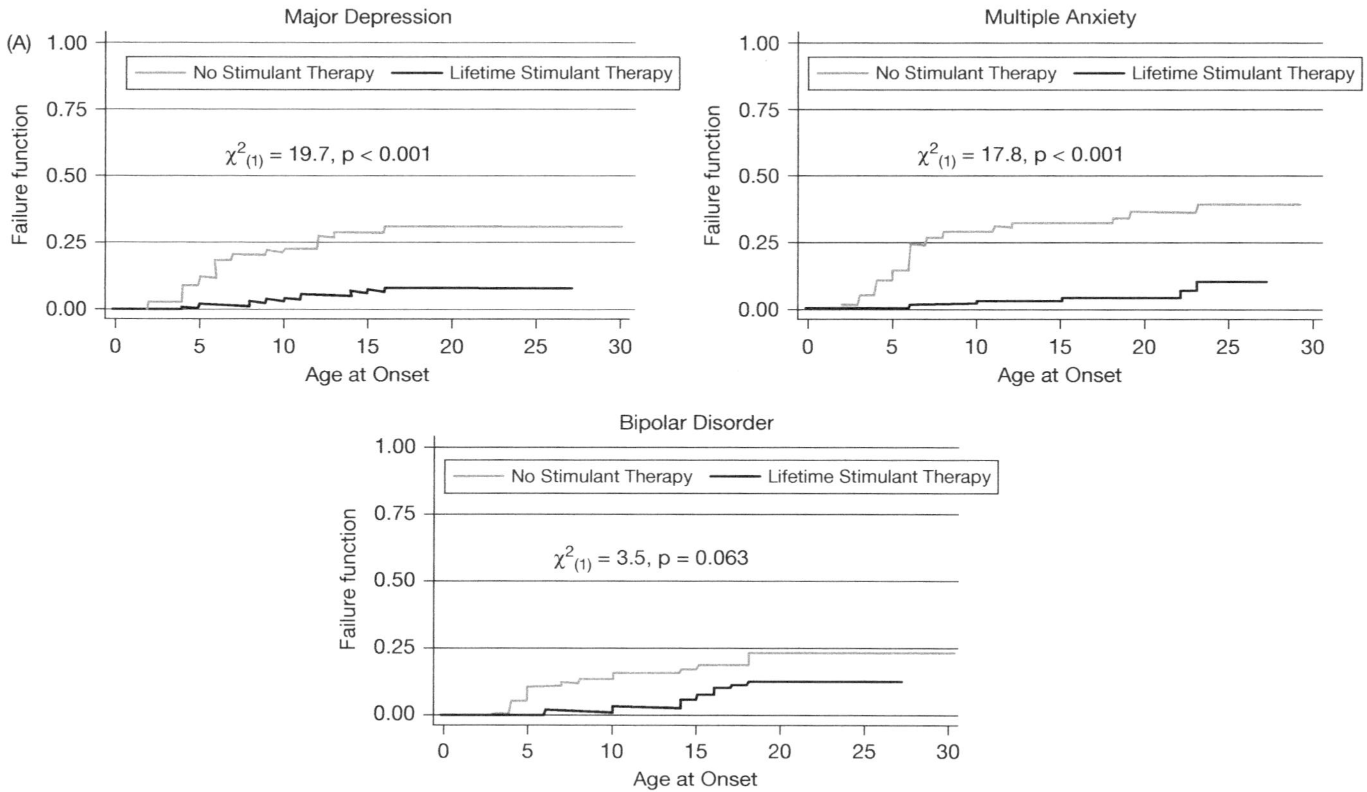

Figure 6.7 A: Protective effect of stimulants on comorbidity; B: Protective effect of stimulants on comorbidity; C: Protective effect of stimulants on grade retention; D: Stimulant therapy and subsequent risk for substance dependence disorders. See also color plate section.

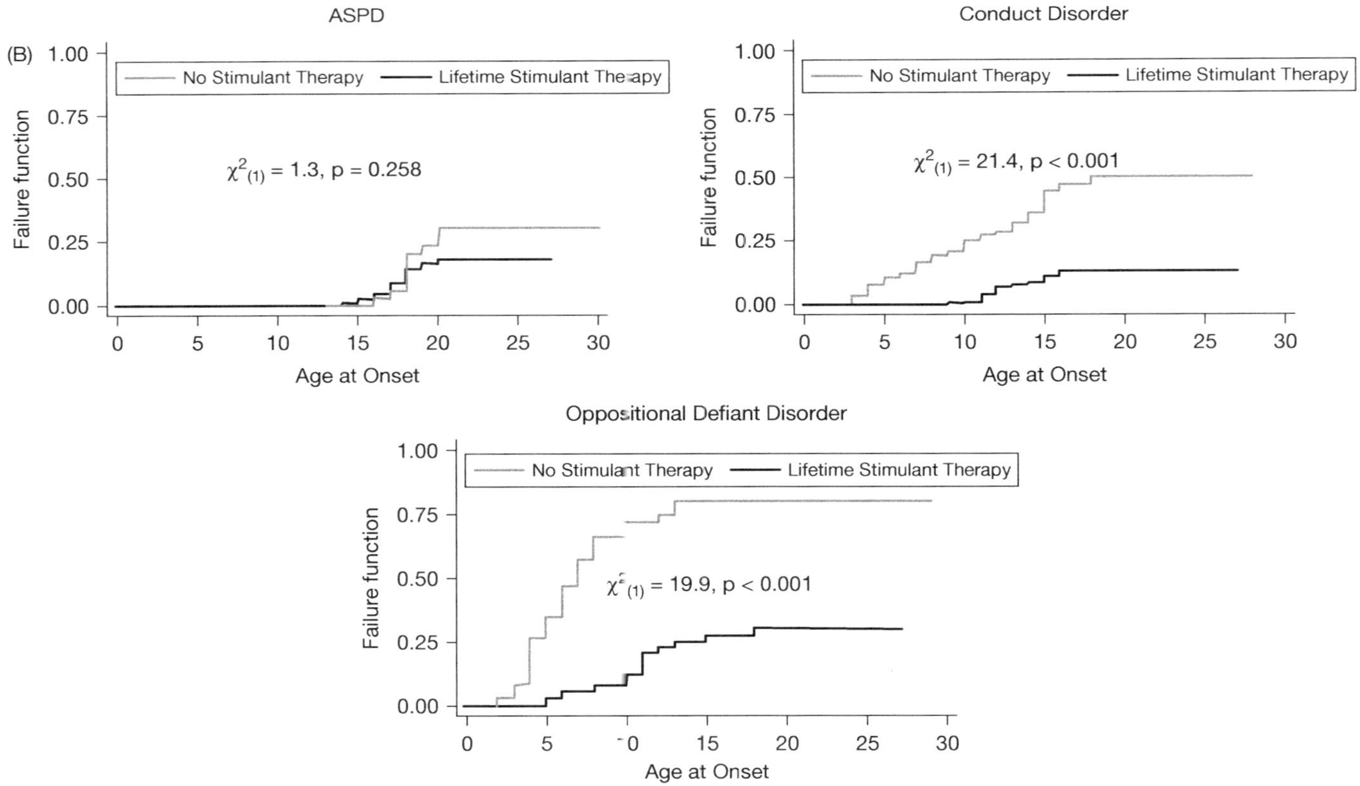

Figure 6.7 Continued

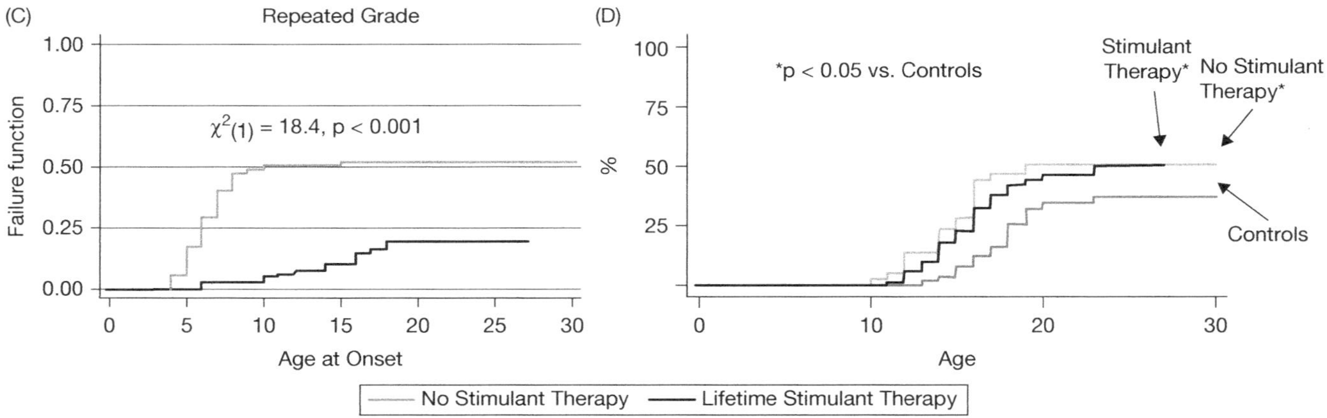

Figure 6.7 Continued

IMPACT OF STIMULANT TREATMENT

We were able to document that ADHD children treated with stimulants in childhood were significantly less likely to be held back in school, and to subsequently develop mood, anxiety, and disruptive behavior disorders [18], as well as addictive disorders [19] when compared with untreated ADHD children (Figure 6.7). These findings are consistent with findings from a separate study in which we were able to document that treatment with stimulants significantly decreased the risk for initiation of smoking [18]. Taken together, these findings provide strong support for the conclusion that treatment with stimulants in childhood has protective effects against the development of a wide range of ADHD-associated complications.

EFFECTS ON HEIGHT AND WEIGHT

Our work was the first to document that previous reports of stimulant-associated stunting of growth in height represent a temporary delay in the tempo of growth in height that was independent of stimulant treatment. Our work also was the first to find evidence that final adult height was NOT compromised in analysis that used parental height as a reference point [20].

NOVEL COMORBIDITIES

We documented that emotional dysregulation is highly prevalent in children with ADHD [21] (Figure 6.8). Emotional dysregulation refers to deficits in self-regulating the physiological arousal caused by strong emotions that is distinct from a mood disorder. Emotional dysregulation was associated at the follow-up assessment with higher rates of persistence of ADHD, more psychiatric comorbidity, and more social impairment problems. These findings suggest that the presence of emotional

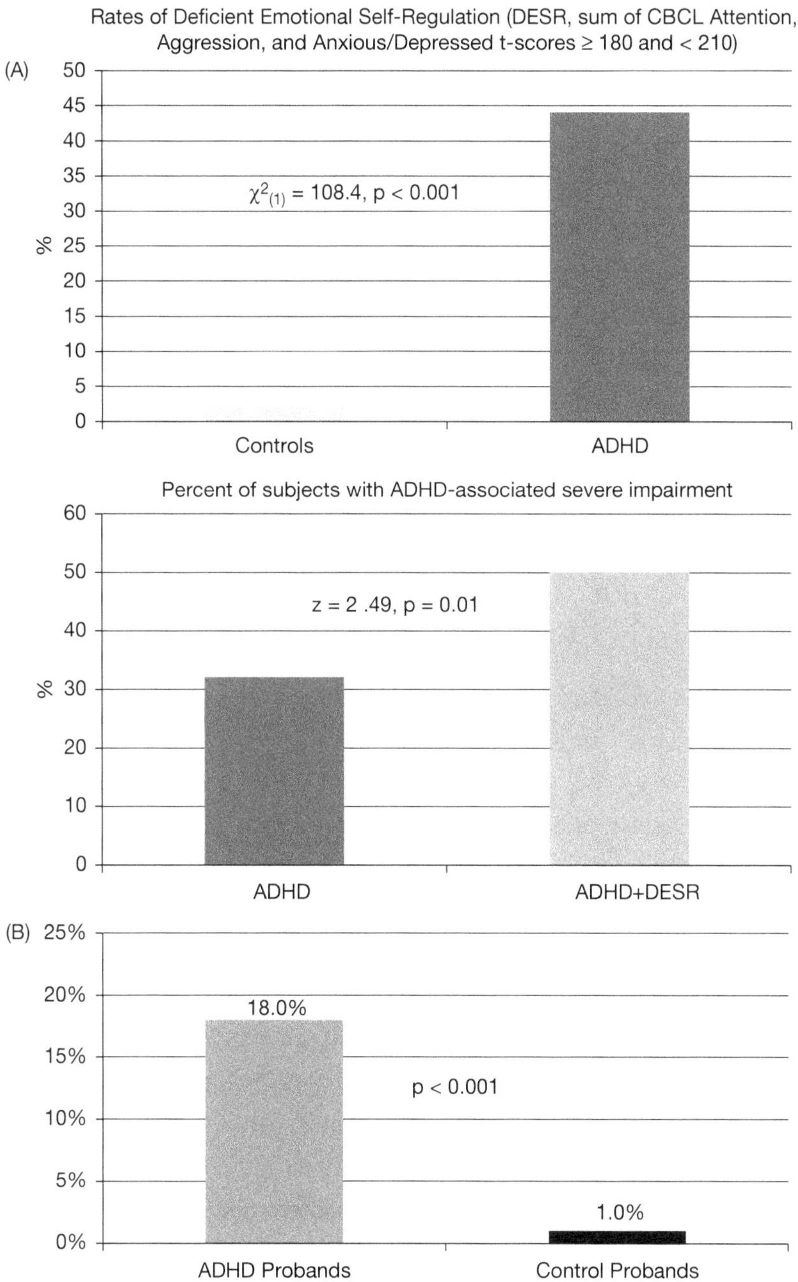

Figure 6.8 A: Emotional Dysregulation and ADHD; B: Autistic Traits in ADHD Children. See also color plate section.

dysregulation can help identify a clinically meaningful subgroup of children with ADHD with long-term compromised outcomes [21]. Our work also documented that a sizeable minority of children with ADHD manifest autistic traits even in the absence of a fully developed diagnosis of autism spectrum disorder and that its presence heralds more compromised social dysfunction [22]. Although some of the social impairments of children with ADHD are due to the core features of the disorder, including impulsivity, inattention, and hyperactivity, children with autistic traits struggle with a repertoire of interpersonal deficits that are reminiscent of more severe social interaction deficits seen in children with autism spectrum disorders (ASDs) [23, 24]. Recent work also has begun to document important associations among ADHD and post-traumatic stress disorder (PTSD), traumatic brain injury (TBI), and cardiovascular risk.

NEUROBIOLOGICAL UNDERPINNING OF PERSISTENT SYMPTOMS

Using resting-state functional magnetic resonance imaging (fMRI), we were able to document circuit-specific neural underpinnings in ADHD children grown up limited to those with a persistent course of the disorder [25] (Figure 6.9). Intrinsic functional brain organization was measured in patients who had a persistent diagnosis in childhood and adulthood, in patients who met diagnosis in childhood but not in adulthood, and in control participants who never had an ADHD diagnosis. Significant differences in intrinsic functional brain organization within the Default Mode Network (DMN) reflected the persistence of ADHD into adult years. The persistent ADHD group exhibited reduced positive posterior cingulate cortex (PCC)–medial prefrontal cortex (mPFC) functional connectivity relative to both the remitted ADHD and control groups, whereas the remitted ADHD and control groups did not differ from each other. In contrast, reduced medial–dorsolateral prefrontal cortex anticorrelation was related to childhood diagnosis of ADHD independent of adult diagnostic status. Both ADHD groups

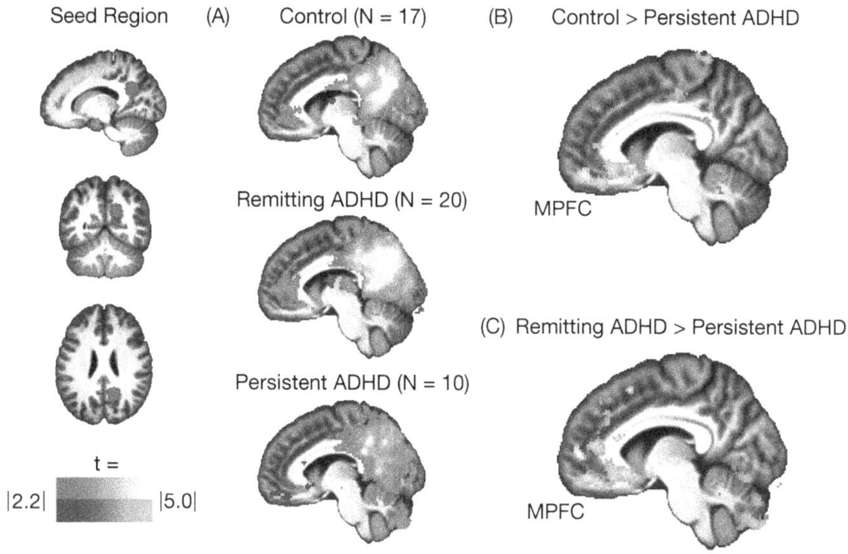

Figure 6.9 Reduced MPFC-PCC Coupling Reflects Current Diagnostic State of ADHD
See also color plate section.

exhibited reduced negative medial–dorsolateral prefrontal cortex connectivity relative to the control group, and the persistent and remitted ADHD groups did not differ from each other. This reduced posterior cingulate cortex–medial prefrontal cortex functional disconnectivity associated with the clinical state of ADHD may offer novel insight into brain mechanisms that are central to the diagnosis of ADHD itself. The neurobiological dissociation between the persistence and remittance of attention deficit hyperactivity disorder supports the idea that persistent ADHD diagnosis into adulthood reflects a biological abnormality in the brain.

SUMMARY

The Massachusetts General Hospital Longitudinal Study of ADHD evaluated and followed a large sample of both boys and girls with ADHD and controls without ADHD, along with their families, ascertained from psychiatric and pediatric sources. Our results confirmed that ADHD in both sexes is associated with high levels of persistence onto adulthood, high levels of familiality with ADHD and other psychiatric disorders, a wide range of comorbid psychiatric and cognitive comorbidities including mood, anxiety, and substance use disorders, learning disabilities with reading and math, executive function deficits, cardiovascular risk, TBI, PTSD, emotional dysregulation, and autistic traits, as well as educational, social, and occupational dysfunctions. Our studies also documented the protective effect of stimulants on the development of comorbid psychiatric disorders, substance use disorders, and functional outcomes. Our work also recently documented the neural basis of the persistence of ADHD using resting-state functional magnetic resonance imaging (fMRI).

REFERENCES

1. Biederman, J., Petty, C. R., Evans, M, Small, J., Faraone, S.V.. How persistent is ADHD? A controlled 10-year follow-up study of boys with ADHD. (2010). *Psychiatry Research*, *177*(3), 299–304.
2. Biederman, J., Monuteaux, M. C., Mick, E., Spencer, T., Wilens, T.E., Silva, J.M., . . .Faraone, S.V. Young adult outcome of attention deficit hyperactivity disorder: A controlled 10-year follow-up study. (2006). *Psychological Medicine*, *36*(2), 167–179.
3. Biederman, J., Petty, C. R., Woodworth, K. Y., Lomedico, A., Hyder, L.L., Faraone, S.V. (2012). Adult outcome of attention-deficit/hyperactivity disorder: A controlled 16-year follow-up study. *Journal of Clinical Psychiatry*, 73(7), 941–950.
4. Biederman, J., Petty, C. R., Hammerness, P., Batchelder, H., Faraone, S.V., (2012). Cigarette smoking as a risk factor for other substance misuse: 10-year study of individuals with and without attention-deficit hyperactivity disorder. *British Journal of Psychiatry*, *201*(3), 207–214.
5. Biederman, J., Monuteaux, M. Mick, E., et al., (2006). Psychopathology in females with attention-deficit/hyperactivity disorder: A controlled, five-year prospective study. *Biological Psychiatry*, *60*(10), 1098–1105.
6. Biederman, J., Faraone, S., Mick, E., Spencer, T., Wilens, T.E., Klein, K.L., Price, J.E., Faraone, S.V., (1996). Attention-deficit hyperactivity disorder and juvenile mania: An overlooked comorbidity? *Journal of the American Academy of Child and Adolescent Psychiatry*, *35*(8), 997–1008.
7. Faraone, S. V., Biederman, J., Mennin, D., Wozniak, J., Spencer, T. (1997). Attention-deficit hyperactivity disorder with bipolar disorder: A familial subtype? *Journal of the American Academy of Child and Adolescent Psychiatry*, *36*(10), 1378–1387; discussion 1387–1390.

8. Biederman, J., Petty, C. R., Byrne, D., Wong, P., Wozniak, J., Faraone, S.V., (2009). Risk for switch from unipolar to bipolar disorder in youth with ADHD: A long term prospective controlled study. *Journal of Affective Disorders, 119*(1-3), 16–21.
9. Uchida, M., Serra, G., Zayas, L., Kenworthy, T., Hughes, B., Faraone, S.V., Biederman, J., (2014). Can manic switches be predicted in pediatric major depression? A systematic literature review. *Journal of Affective Disorders, 172*(C), 300–306.
10. Monuteaux, M. C., Mick, E., Faraone, S. V., Biederman, J., (2010). The influence of sex on the course and psychiatric correlates of ADHD from childhood to adolescence: A longitudinal study. *Journal of Child Psychology and Psychiatry, 51*(3), 233–241.
11. Biederman, J., Faraone, S. V., Keenan, K., Knee, D., Tsuang, M.T.,(1990). Family-genetic and psychosocial risk factors in DSM-III attention deficit disorder. *Journal of the American Academy of Child and Adolescent Psychiatry, 29*(4), 526–533.
12. Biederman, J., Faraone, S. V., Keenan, K., Tsuang, M.T. (1991). Evidence of familial association between attention deficit disorder and major affective disorders. *Archives of General Psychiatry, 48*(7), 633–642.
13. Biederman, J., Faraone, S. V., Keenan, K., Benjamin, J., Krifcher, B., Moore, C.,. . . Tsuang, M.T., (1992). Further evidence for family-genetic risk factors in attention deficit hyperactivity disorder. Patterns of comorbidity in probands and relatives in psychiatrically and pediatrically referred samples. *Archives of General Psychiatry, 49*(9), 728–738.
14. Wozniak, J., Biederman, J., Mundy, E., Mennin, D., Faraone, S.V., (1995). A pilot family study of childhood-onset mania. *Journal of the American Academy of Child and Adolescent Psychiatry, 34*(12), 1577–1583.
15. Biederman, J., Faraone, S. V., Keenan, K., Steingard, R., Tsuang, M.T., (1991). Familial association between attention deficit disorder and anxiety disorders. *American Journal of Psychiatry, 148*(2), 251–256.
16. Faraone, S.V., Biederman, J. , Lehman, B. K., Keenan, K., Norman, D., Seidman, L.J.,. . .Chen, W.J., (1993). Evidence for the independent familial transmission of attention deficit hyperactivity disorder and learning disabilities: Results from a family genetic study. *American Journal of Psychiatry, 150*(6), 891–895.
17. Biederman, J., Faraone, S. V., Spencer, T. J., Mick, E., Monteaux, M.C., Aleardi, M., (2006). Functional impairments in adults with self-reports of diagnosed ADHD: A controlled study of 1001 adults in the community. *Journal of Clinical Psychiatry, 67*(4), 524–540.
18. Biederman, J., Monuteaux, M. C., Spencer, T., Wilens, T.E., Faraone, S.V., (2009). Do stimulants protect against psychiatric disorders in youth with ADHD? A 10-year follow-up study. *Pediatrics, 124*(1), 71–78.
19. Biederman, J., Monuteaux, M. C., Spencer, T., Wilens, T.E., Macpherson, H.A., Faraone, S.V., (2008). Stimulant therapy and risk for subsequent substance use disorders in male adults with ADHD: A naturalistic controlled 10-year follow-up study. *American Journal of Psychiatry, 165*(5), 597–603.
20. Biederman, J., Spencer, T. J., Monuteaux, M. C., Faraone, S.V., (2010). A naturalistic 10-year prospective study of height and weight in children with attention-deficit

hyperactivity disorder grown up: sex and treatment effects. *Journal of Pediatrics, 157*(4), 635–640, 640 e1.

21. Spencer, T.J., Faraone, S. V., Surman, C. B., Petty, C., Clarke, A., Batchelder, H., Wozniak, J., Biederman, J.,(2011). Toward defining deficient emotional self-regulation in children with attention-deficit/hyperactivity disorder using the Child Behavior Checklist: A controlled study. *Postgraduate Medicine, 123*(5), 50–59.
22. Kotte, A., Joshi, G., Fried, R., Uchida, M., Spencer, A., Woodworth, K.Y.,. . . Biederman, J., (2013). Autistic traits in children with and without ADHD. *Pediatrics, 132*(3), e612–e622.
23. Dalton, K. M., Nacewicz, B. M., Alexander, A. L., Davidson, R.J., (2007). Gaze-fixation, brain activation, and amygdala volume in unaffected siblings of individuals with autism. *Biological Psychiatry, 61*(4), 512–520.
24. Joseph, R. M., Ehrman, K., McNally, R., Keehn, B., (2008). Affective response to eye contact and face recognition ability in children with ASD. *Journal of the International Neuropsychological Society, 14*(6), 947–955.
25. Mattfeld, A. T., Gabrieli, J. D., Biederman, J., Spencer, T., Brown, A., Kotte, A.,. . . Whitfield-Gabrieli, S. (2014). Brain differences between persistent and remitted attention deficit hyperactivity disorder. Brain, 137(Pt 9), 2423–2428.

7

The Berkeley Girls with ADHD Longitudinal Study

ELIZABETH B. OWENS, CHRISTINE A. ZALECKI, AND STEPHEN P. HINSHAW

The Berkeley Girls with ADHD Longitudinal Study (BGALS) began in the mid-1990s as a cross-sectional investigation—with the hope of turning it into a prospective, longitudinal project—of impairment and competence in a severely understudied population: girls with attention deficit hyperactivity disorder (ADHD). The project was proposed against a backdrop of a long, uphill battle that had been fought (and, indeed, is still being fought) for clinical and research recognition of the presence and impact of ADHD in females. Believed to be a male disorder for much of the 20th century, only recently has recognition been given to the reality of ADHD in girls and women. Investigations across the past two decades have revealed mounting evidence for the substantial impairments incurred by females with this condition (meta-analyses: Gaub & Carlson, 1997; Gershon, 2002; long-term investigations: Biederman et al., 2010; Hinshaw et al., 2012). Previously, the official wisdom was that females could not really "have" ADHD. Along with a dearth of relevant research and services, this stance led to massive under-recognition of the presence of ADHD in this population, fostering the potential for these girls and women to experience internalized negative sequelae (see Nadeau, Littman, & Quinn, 1999).

At the time of the initial BGALS grant proposal, exceedingly few girls with ADHD had been investigated via multimethod and multi-informant research protocols, much less followed longitudinally for the purpose of understanding their developmental trajectories. One key reason was that most ADHD researchers typically recruited clinically referred participants. At that time, the ratio of boys-to-girls with ADHD presenting for services was between 5:1 and 10:1 (American Psychiatric Association, 1994), thus leading to the erroneous assumption that ADHD in girls is rare. Obtaining the number of female participants required for adequate statistical power to test sex differences seemed hardly feasible, and, therefore, efforts were usually abandoned. There was also growing recognition, however, that the prevalence of girls with ADHD in representative community samples might be much larger than initially estimated. Arnold (1996) estimated the boy-to-girl ratio for ADHD to be 2:1 to 3:1. Using the prevalence rates of ADHD at the time (American Psychiatric Association, 1994), the population of the United States in 1996 (http://www.census.gov/popest/data/intercensal/national/index.html), and this ratio, we estimate that there were almost one million girls (ages 4 to 18) with ADHD in the United States alone. Again, almost none of them had ever participated in a longitudinal study.

Nevertheless, some knowledge about sex differences had accumulated by this time. As noted, although it was clear that the disorder was (and is) more prevalent in boys than in girls, obtained sex ratios varied dramatically depending on how children were sampled (i.e., clinical vs. population-based samples). There was also evidence that among girls, ADHD-predominantly inattentive type (ADHD-I) was more likely to be diagnosed than it was among boys (Lahey et al., 1994). Girls appeared less likely than boys to show comorbid externalizing or disruptive comorbidity (Horn, Wagner, & Ialongo, 1989). It also appeared that girls and boys responded equally well to treatment (Pelham, Walker, Sturgis, & Hoza,

1989). Beyond these observations, all too little was known about whether and how risk factors, most co-occurring features, symptom presentation, neuropsychological performance, and developmental course and prognosis might be different for boys and girls. This gaping hole in our knowledge base constituted a primary rationale for the BGALS.

Another major impetus was to gain knowledge about ADHD-I, which was introduced as an ADHD subtype in the *Diagnostic and Statistical Manual of Mental Disorders-IV/DSM-IV* (American Psychiatric Association, 1994). As of the mid-1990s, no longitudinal studies had differentiated children with ADHD-I from children with ADHD-combined type (ADHD-C), and virtually all participants in longitudinal studies of ADHD prior to the mid-1990s had high levels of both inattention and hyperactivity/impulsivity. Furthermore, as noted earlier, there was reason to believe that the ADHD-I presentation was more prevalent among girls (Lahey et al., 1994). Thus, the BGALS was also intended to provide missing knowledge about ADHD-I, because the all-girl sample should include a critical mass diagnosed specifically with this subtype. Additional important features of the BGALS were its ethnic mix (most of the participants with ADHD up to that point had been Caucasian) and its nonreliance on exclusively clinically referred participants. Although the sample was not epidemiologically derived, it was representative of local community children with ADHD, given its mix of clinic-referred and school-referred participants, as well as those solicited by advertisement.

At our project's initiation, we had the goal of, but not yet the funds for, a prospective, longitudinal investigation. We had to ensure that our initial data collection was performed with a rigorously assessed sample—and that it produced valid findings—before we could even consider a well-thought-through prospective investigation. We did inform families, however, that our ultimate plans were to follow their daughters over time. Moreover, we did everything possible to facilitate recontacting families subsequent to the summer programs. In hindsight, planting this seed and making these preparations—along with providing an intensive program for their daughters with dedicated and caring staff—were crucial for our excellent retention rates.

Finally, during our grant preparation we made a crucial decision. That is, we debated for some time whether to sample boys and girls with ADHD or to constitute an all-female sample, in order to (a) maximize the number of female participants and (b) investigate the girls, via our summer-camp methodology, in the context of female peers. Taking the advice of prescient reviewer feedback, we became convinced of the wisdom of learning the maximum amount possible about an all-girl sample. Given what we have learned about our sample, we believe that this was a wise choice, even though making explicit sex comparisons is also a worthy goal.

OVERVIEW OF PROCEDURES

The BGALS has involved data collection from girls with ADHD (n = 140) and from girls without ADHD (n = 88), at one extended baseline assessment, which included many hours of initial evaluations plus an intensive summer research program, and two lengthy follow-ups. A third follow-up, 15 years after initial ascertainment, is being completed at the time of this writing. Wave 1 (W1) baseline data were collected prior to and during three 5-week summer camps held in 1997 (n = 79), 1998 (n = 77), and 1999 (n = 72). At W1, the girls were 6 to 12 years of age (mean = 9.6). Prior to the camp, data were collected from parents and teachers via interviews and questionnaires and from girls themselves in terms of achievement, IQ, and cognitive testing. Subsequently, the summer camps were intended to allow collection of naturalistic, ecologically valid data from observers and peers regarding the behavioral and social functioning of girls with and without ADHD, including peer sociometric appraisals, intensive daily behavior observations, ratings obtained from summer program teachers and counselors, and individualized neuropsychological testing. In nearly all activities, girls with ADHD and comparison girls participated alongside one another; staff were unaware of a participant's diagnostic group. Camps were *not* for the purposes of treatment, even though a token economy was used to assist with adherence to the program's structure. Daily activities included art, sports, outdoor play, peer group meetings, lunch, and academic time. Camps were free of charge, allowing the participation of a diverse sample.

Five years later, at Wave 2 (W2), girls and their parents were invited to participate in two half-day assessments. At W2, girls were 11- to 18-year-olds (mean = 14.2). Overall retention was 92%, reflecting the number of girls from whom at least some data were collected at W2. For the vast majority of these, data were complete. Five years later, at Wave 3 (W3), girls again were asked to participate in two half-day assessments with a parent participating in one half-day assessment. Young women ranged in age from 17 to 24 years (mean = 19.6) and overall retention was 95%, again with the vast majority providing complete data. As of this writing, a fourth wave of data collection (W4) is occurring and we expect that the young women will have an average age of about 25 years. At W4, the young women are invited to participate in one half-day assessment. Through the mail, we also collect questionnaire data from a parent, peer, and work supervisor.

PARTICIPANTS

Our aim was to recruit a socioeconomically and ethnically diverse sample of girls from local communities. It was not intended to comprise a representative sample, derived from epidemiologic methods, but it was not exclusively clinically referred, either. The sample was intended to represent typical girls in our metropolitan area (just east of San Francisco, California) with and without ADHD. Thus, girls with ADHD were recruited from local schools, mental health centers, pediatric practices, general medical settings, talks at self-help groups, and through direct advertisements. Girls without ADHD were recruited in a similar manner and were age- and ethnicity-matched to the group with ADHD.

A multi-gated screening and assessment process was used to identify, from among the approximately 1,200 initial callers, children who were eligible to participate. Program descriptions were mailed to those callers who met our age and gender criteria. Still-interested families (n = 709) participated in a phone screen, and then parents and teachers of still-eligible children completed ADHD (Swanson, Nolan, and Pelham Rating Scale, SNAP-IV; Swanson, 1992) and problem behavior (Child Behavior Checklist, CBCL, and Teacher Report Form, TRF, Achenbach 1991a and 1991b) rating scales, reflecting the girl's behavior off medication. We intentionally set criteria for ADHD symptomatology low at this stage, requiring only five (rather than six) relevant symptoms of either inattention or hyperactivity–impulsivity, in order not to rule out prematurely any potentially eligible participants. For comparison girls, scores had to be below these cutoffs. Rating scales were returned by 450 families, and 62% (278) met initial criteria for participation. Thus, our multi-gated system guarded against false-positive inclusions.

Next, these families were invited for a diagnostic evaluation during which parents were administered the Diagnostic Interview Schedule for Children, 4th edition, or DISC-IV (Shaffer, Fisher, Lucas, Dulcan, & Schwab-Stone, 2000), and girls were administered, off medication, the Wechsler Intelligence Scale for Children (3rd ed., WISC-III; Wechsler, 1991). Here, regarding the DISC, we required that full diagnostic criteria for ADHD must be met for inclusion in the ADHD group. At this point, 33 were screened out, and 17 of those who met criteria for study inclusion declined to participate. Ultimately, 140 girls met diagnostic criteria for ADHD on the DISC-IV (supplemented with up to two symptoms from the teacher SNAP-IV). Our comparison group comprised 88 girls who did not meet either parent- or teacher-based criteria for ADHD. The sample was ethnically diverse (53% White, 27% African American, 11% Latina, 9% Asian American) and reflected the population of the San Francisco East Bay Area. By design, the ADHD and comparison groups did not differ on age or ethnic status. They also did not differ with respect to maternal income, family education, percentage receiving public assistance, or percentage living in a single-parent household (Hinshaw, 2002).

Ninety-three of the 140 girls with ADHD met criteria for ADHD-C and 47 met criteria for ADHD-I. In order to have maximum power for ADHD-C versus ADHD-I contrasts, the few girls with ADHD-predominantly hyperactive/impulsive type were excluded. Girls also were excluded if they had a full-scale IQ below 70, psychosis or overt neurological disorder, evidence of a pervasive developmental disorder, lack of English spoken in the home, and/or medical problems precluding summer camp participation. Common comorbidities were allowed, in order to ensure a sample representing girls with ADHD in the community, where comorbid conditions are plentiful (e.g., Angold, Costello, & Erkanli, 1999).

Regarding medication status, at W1, 71 of the 140 girls with ADHD had taken stimulant medication at some point prior to the summer program. At W2, 46 girls (all with a childhood ADHD diagnosis) were taking a stimulant medication and 67 were taking a psychotropic medication of some kind, including stimulants (65 of these had a childhood diagnosis of ADHD and two were from our comparison group). At W3, 49 young women were taking a stimulant medication (47 with a childhood diagnosis of ADHD and one without); 32 were taking a nonstimulant psychotropic medication (22 with childhood ADHD and seven without). Of these, 15 women were taking both a stimulant and a nonstimulant psychotropic medication. As would be expected in a naturalistic investigation in which selection factors obscure medication effects, continued medication use was not significantly associated with either better or worse outcome.

MEASURES

At each of the three assessment points, data were collected in 11 primary domains (see Table 7.1, in which domains are listed in roughly chronological order, according to when they were included as part of our assessment battery): demographic, ADHD diagnosis and symptoms, externalizing problems, internalizing problems, global impairment, neuropsychological performance, school achievement, well-being, peer relations, service utilization, and parenting (i.e., parenting behaviors and styles as well as parenting stress). Height and weight also were measured. In addition, at W1, we assessed perinatal problems and child prosocial behavior, as well as parental drinking history, symptoms of ADHD and depression, and social support. At W2, but not W3, we continued to assess prosocial behavior,

TABLE 7.1

ALL CONSTRUCT DOMAINS ASSESSED AT ANY TIME POINT

Domain	W1	W2	W3
Demographics	X	X	X
ADHD symptoms and diagnoses	X	X	X
Externalizing and internalizing symptoms and diagnoses	X	X	X
Global impairment	X	X	X
Neuropsychological performance	X	X	X
School achievement	X	X	X
Well-being	X	X	X
Peer relations	X	X	X
Service utilization	X	X	X
Parenting behavior/style/and perceived stress	X	X	X
Perinatal problems	X		
Prosocial behavior	X	X	
Parental drinking history	X		
Parental ADHD and depressive symptoms	X		X
Social support	X		X
Coping		X	
Pubertal timing		X	
Substance use and disorders		X	X
Self-harm		X	X
Eating pathology		X	X
Medication history		X	X
Personality		X	X
Life events		X	X
Parental marital conflict		X	X
Driving behavior			X
Emotion regulation			X
Online communications			X
Sexual behavior			X
Attitudes regarding mental health stigma			X
Attachment to parents			X

and added measures of personal coping and pubertal timing. At W2 and W3, our battery expanded to tap a variety of developmentally relevant constructs and outcomes, including substance use, eating pathology, medication history, personality, life events, and parental marital conflict. At W3, but not before, we also measured driving behavior, self-harm, emotion regulation, online communication, sexual behavior, attitudes regarding mental health stigma, and attachment to parents. At W3, as at W1, we also assessed parental symptoms of ADHD and depression, as well as social support.

As shown in Table 7.2, emphasis was placed on obtaining data from multiple informants (e.g., parent, teacher, self, peers, observers). At W1 and W2, parent measures were given to primary caregivers (usually mothers), as well as secondary caregivers (usually fathers), with 71% of secondary caregivers providing data at W1 and 54% providing data at W2.

Table 7.3 lists the key measures used in each of the 10 primary psychosocial domains investigated at all three assessment points. Demographic and service-use information was collected using extensive project-derived questionnaires. ADHD symptoms and diagnoses were assessed using the DISC-IV (Shaffer et al., 2000) and the SNAP-IV (Swanson, 1992); the DISC-IV also was used to assess co-occurring psychiatric problems (note that the extension of this measure, the DISC-Young Adult version, was used at W3). Additional measures of co-occurring pathology included the Achenbach scales (CBCL and TRF, Achenbach, 1991a and 1991b; Adult Behavior Checklist and Adult Self Report, Achenbach & Rescorla, 2003), either the Child Depression Inventory (Kovacs, 1992) or the Beck Depression Inventory-II (Beck, Steer, Ball, & Ranieri, 1996), and behavior observations during the summer camps and video-recorded parent–child interactions. Global impairment was assessed with the Columbia Impairment Scale (Bird, 1999). School achievement was assessed using the Wechsler Individual Achievement Test (WIAT; Wechsler, 1992). Well-being was assessed with the Harter scales (at W1, the Perceived Competence Scale for Children, Harter, 1982; at W2 and W3, the Self-Perception Profile, Harter, 1988). Peer relations were assessed (a) at W1 with sociometric nominations, as well as with observer report, (b) at W2 via

TABLE 7.2

INFORMANTS IN 10 PRIMARY PSYCHOSOCIAL DOMAINS ASSESSED AT ALL TIME POINTS

	Informant	W1	W2	W3
Demographics	Parent	X	X	X
	Participant			X
ADHD symptoms and diagnoses	Parent	X	X	X
	Teacher	X	X	
	Participant		X	X
Externalizing symptoms and diagnoses	Parent	X	X	X
	Teacher	X	X	
	Participant		X	X
	Observer	X	X	
	Peers	X		
Internalizing symptoms and diagnoses	Parent	X	X	X
	Teacher	X	X	
	Participant	X	X	X
	Observer	X		
Global impairment	Parent	X	X	X
	Participant			X
	Observer			X
School achievement	Teacher	X	X	
	Objective testing	X	X	X
Well-being	Participant	X	X	X
Peer relations	Parent	X	X	
	Teacher	X	X	
	Participant			X
	Observer and Peers	X		
Service use	Parent	X	X	X
	Participant			X
Parenting behavior/style/perceived stress	Parent	X	X	X
	Participant	X	X	
	Observer	X	X	

TABLE 7.3

KEY INSTRUMENTS USED IN THE 10 PRIMARY PSYCHOSOCIAL DOMAINS

Domains	Measure	W1	W2	W3
Demographics, Service use	Background Information Questionnaire (W1), Family Information Profile (W2/W3)	X	X	X
ADHD	Diagnostic Interview Scale for Children—IV	X	X	X
	Swanson, Nolan, and Pelham Rating Scale—IV	X	X	X
Externalizing	Diagnostic Interview Scale for Children—IV	X	X	X
	Swanson, Nolan, and Pelham Rating Scale—IV	X	X	
	Child/Adult Behavior Checklist	X	X	X
	Teacher Report Form	X	X	
	Adult Self Report			X
	Self-reported Delinquency		X	X
	Observations	X		
Internalizing	Diagnostic Interview Scale for Children–IV	X	X	X
	Child/Adult Behavior Checklist	X	X	X
	Teacher Report Form	X	X	
	Adult Self Report			X
	Child/Beck Depression Inventory—II	X	X	X
	Observations	X		
Global impairment	Columbia Impairment Scale	X	X	X
School achievement	Wechsler Individual Achievement Test	X	X	X
Well-being	Harter scales	X	X	X
Peers	Sociometrics	X		
	Dishion Social Preference Scale	X	X	
	Social Relationship Questionnaire	X	X	
	Inventory of Peer Attachment			X
Parental behavior and adjustment	Alabama Parenting Questionnaire	X	X	
	Ideas About Parenting	X	X	X
	Parental Stress Index	X	X	X
	Beck Depression Inventory	X		X
	Conners' Adult ADHD Rating Scale	X		X

parent and teacher report on the project-developed Social Relationships Questionnaire, as well as teacher report on the Dishion Social Preference Scale (Dishion, 1990), and (c) at W3 via self-report on the Inventory of Peer Attachment (Armsden & Greenberg, 1987). Key parenting measures included the Alabama Parenting Questionnaire (Shelton, Frick, & Wootton, 1996), the Ideas About Parenting scale (Heming, Cowan, & Cowan, 1990), and the Parental Stress Index (Abidin, 1997). At W1 and W2, parent–child interactions in semistructured situations were video recorded and coded.

Other selected psychosocial measures included the Social Skills Rating System (Gresham & Elliot, 1990) at W2; the Substance Use Questionnaire (Molina & Pelham, 2003), Eating Attitudes Test (Garner, Olmstead, Bohr, & Garfinkel, 1982), Eating Disorder Inventory (Garner, 1991), and Self-Injury Questionnaire (Claes, Vandereycken, & Vertommen, 2001) at W2 and W3; and the Driving Behavior Questionnaire at W3 (Barkley, Murphy, & Kwasnik, 1996). Finally, the Conners' Adult ADHD Rating Scale (CAARS, Conners, Erhardt, & Sparrow, 2004) was administered at W1 and W3 to parents about their own behavior, at W3 to parents about their daughters, and at W3 to participants about themselves.

Neuropsychological functioning at each wave was assessed via objective testing. The battery of neuropsychological tests was designed to tap a variety of executive functioning (EF) and intellectual difficulties and deficits commonly exhibited by boys with ADHD. These tests were administered while participants were off any stimulant medications. At W1 the neuropsychological battery included the following tests: the WISC-III (Wechsler, 1991), the WIAT (Wechsler, 1992), the Rey-Osterrieth Complex Figure Design (ROCF; Osterrieth, 1944), the Continuous Performance Test (CPT; Conners, 1995), the Porteus Maze Test (PM; Porteus, 1973), the Time-to-Do 20 Motor Battery (TTD-20; Denckla, 1974), the Grooved Pegboard (GPB; Knights & Norwood, 1979), the Rapid Automatized Naming test (RAN; Denckla & Rudel, 1974), and the Cancel Underlining test (CUL; Rourke & Orr, 1977). At W2, the neuropsychological battery was similar to, but shorter than that administered at W1. At W2 the CPT, RAN, and CUL were administered as they were at W1. Only the Digit

Span subtest of the WISC-III was administered and the Taylor Complex Figure Test (Taylor, 1969) was added instead of the ROCF. At W3, the neuropsychological battery included the CUL, CPT, and ROCF, as well as the Digit Span and Letter-Number Sequencing subtests of the Wechsler Adult Intelligence Scale-III (WAIS-III; Wechsler, 1997), and Conditions 2 and 4 of the Trail Making Test (Delis, Kaplan, & Kramer, 2001). Details about the particular scores obtained and analyzed from these neuropsychological tests are beyond the scope of this chapter; interested readers should consult the original publications (e.g., Hinshaw, Carte, Fan, Jassy, & Owens, 2007; Hinshaw, Carte, Sami, Treuting, & Zupan, 2002; Miller, Ho, & Hinshaw, 2012; Miller, Montenegro-Nevado, & Hinshaw, 2012; Miller, Loya, & Hinshaw, 2013).

Currently, a fourth wave of data collection (W4) is occurring with a battery very much like the W3 battery, notwithstanding the following notable differences: (1) W4 involves one half-day assessment for the young adult participant, supplemented by at-home questionnaires; (2) a parent is mailed questionnaires; (3) when possible, a romantic partner or a peer, along with a work supervisor are asked to complete questionnaires by mail; (4) we no longer administer a structured diagnostic interview intended to assess ADHD; and (5) there is expanded measurement of self-injury, borderline personality disorder, and depressive disorders.

RESULTS: INITIAL STATUS AND DEVELOPMENTAL OUTCOMES

Our key initial aim was to describe baseline characteristics and developmental outcomes among girls diagnosed with ADHD as children (6 to 12 years old), compared to similar girls without ADHD. Six published articles ("core papers") have addressed this primary objective. Three core papers have concerned psychosocial functioning (Hinshaw, 2002; Hinshaw, Owens, Sami, & Fargeon, 2006; Hinshaw, Owens, Zalecki, Huggins, Montenegro-Nevado, Schrodek, & Swanson, 2012), and three have focused on neuropsychological performance (Hinshaw et al., 2007;

Hinshaw et al., 2002; Miller, Ho et al., 2012). As described subsequently, a number of additional papers have focused on more specific domains of functioning and/or on mediator pathways that attempt to explain core developmental outcomes.

Childhood Functioning: Wave 1

The W1 psychosocial findings, in domains that also were examined during adolescence and young adulthood, are presented in Table 7.4 (compiled from tables originally published in Hinshaw, 2002) and generated using a series of ANOVAs for continuous dependent variables and X^2 tests for dichotomous dependent variables. (Note that in this and the papers described below, we paid close attention to issues of familywise alpha protection—for example, with initial multivariate analyses, given the many dependent measures included in the analyses.) Briefly, girls with ADHD demonstrated substantial psychiatric comorbidities; they showed cognitive performance that, although in the average range, was lower than that of comparison girls; and they demonstrated noteworthy peer rejection. Additionally, findings not displayed showed that the girls with ADHD displayed higher rates of maltreatment (abuse and neglect), adoption, speech/language problems, and use of educational services than the girls without ADHD, and their parents showed a small but significant tendency to employ authoritarian discipline styles. There were no demographic differences, however, between the groups (see Hinshaw, 2002 for these specific findings regarding demographic, background, and parenting variables). Effect sizes associated with significant contrasts were of medium-to-very-large size.

Inattentive versus comparison subtype contrasts were not commonly significant. Subtypes were equivalent on most background characteristics and rates of previous treatment, levels of inattention, IQ and academic achievement, positive peer nominations, and parenting practices. Exceptions included higher rates of previous maltreatment, summer-program peer rejection, and rates and levels of comorbid externalizing problems among

TABLE 7.4

FUNCTIONING AT WAVE 1 ACROSS DOMAINS

	Comparison (0)	Inattentive (1)	Combined (2)		Effect Sizes[b]		
	M (SD)	*M (SD)*	*M (SD)*	*p*[a]	*0–1*	*0–2*	*1–2*
ADHD SXS ($F_{86,448}$ = 121.54**)							
P CBCL Attention	52.2 (4.6)	74.0 (9.1)	74.8 (8.7)	< .01	1.65*	1.71*	0.06
P SNAP Inattention	0.4 (0.9)	7.7 (1.5)	7.5 (2.1)	< .01	1.90*	1.85*	0.05
P SNAP HI	0.2 (0.6)	3.0 (2.2)	6.7 (2.3)	< .01	0.82*	1.90*	1.08*
T SNAP Inattention	0.3 (1.0)	6.3 (2.4)	6.8 (2.0)	<.01	1.67*	1.81*	0.14
T SNAP HI	0.1 (0.5)	2.0 (2.2)	5.1 (2.5)	< .01	0.64*	1.73*	1.09*
COMORBIDITIES ($F_{10,424}$ = 10.15**)							
P DISC ODD (%)	6.8	46.8	71.0	< .01	12.0*	32.9*	2.7*
P DISC CD (%)	0.0	10.6	26.9	< .01		3.0*	
P DISC Anx (%)	3.4	19.1	31.1	< .01	6.7*	12.8*	1.9
P DISC Dep (%)	0.0	4.3	10.3	< .01	2.3		
Reading disorder	4.5	14.9	11.1	ns	3.7	2.6	0.7
EXTERNALIZING BEHAVIORS ($F_{14,438}$ = 16.46**)							
P CBCL Externalizing	45.9 (8.2)	58.6 (11.0)	68.7 (8.2)	< .01	0.94*	1.69*	0.75*
P SNAP ODD	0.3 (1.0)	2.3 (2.6)	4.6 (2.5)	< .01	0.72*	1.52*	0.80*
T SNAP ODD	0.0 (0.2)	1.6 (2.3)	3.9 (2.9)	< .01	0.61	1.51	0.90
S DBR Overt Agg	0.05 (0.07)	0.18 (0.38)	0.71 (0.94)	< .01	0.19	0.96*	0.77*
S DBR Covert antisocial behavior	0.04 (0.06)	0.09 (0.16)	0.34 (0.38)	< .01	0.17	1.03*	0.86*

(continued)

TABLE 7.4

CONTINUED

	Comparison (0)	Inattentive (1)	Combined (2)		Effect Sizes[b]		
	M (SD)	*M (SD)*	*M (SD)*	*p*[a]	*0–1*	*0–2*	*1–2*
S DBR Relational agg	0.22 (0.26)	0.45 (0.44)	1.14 (0.77)	< .01	0.33	1.31*	0.99*
S Observed noncompliance	0.042 (.038)	0.072 (.056)	0.145 (.095)	< .01	0.36*	1.23*	0.87*
S Observed agg	0.002 (.005)	0.005 (.012)	0.013 (.017)	< .01	0.23	0.85*	0.62*
INTERNALIZING BEHAVIORS ($F_{12,434} = 13.52^{**}$)							
P CBCL Internalizing	47.4 (11.2)	60.2 (10.2)	60.8 (10.3)	< .01	1.03*	1.08*	0.05
Y CDI Total	4.6 (4.8)	8.9 (5.9)	8.9 (6.7)	< .01	0.69*	0.70*	0.01
Y MASC T score	51.0 (15.7)	52.6 (16.4)	54.5 (18.6)	ns	0.09	0.21	0.11
S DBR withdrawn	1.50 (1.22)	2.06 (1.31)	1.52 (1.11)	ns	0.46	0.02	0.45
S DBR anx/dep	1.36 (1.03)	2.76 (1.58)	3.85 (2.78)	< .01	0.61*	1.08*	0.47
S Observed isolation	0.023 (.027)	0.038 (.036)	0.024 (.020)	< .01	0.56*	0.04	0.52*
PEER RELATIONSHIPS ($F_{4,450} = 17.28^{**}$)							
Sociometric positive nominations	0.161 (.098)	0.104 (.083)	0.100 (.096)	< .01	0.58*	0.61*	0.03
Sociometric negative nominations	0.028 (.047)	0.103 (.108)	0.220 (.223)	< .01	0.67*	1.10*	0.43*
IQ/ACHIEVEMENT ($F_{12,424} = 4.99^{**}$)							
WISC-III Verbal Comprehension	113.7 (13.3)	102.8 (16.5)	100.6 (13.3)	< .01	0.72*	0.86*	0.14
WISC-III Perceptual Organization	108.9 (14.3)	10[illegible].1 (13.9)	100.7 (14.8)	< .01	0.69*	0.55*	0.04
WISC-III Freedom from Distractibility	109.6 (10.9)	9[illegible].3 (11.9)	98.0 (13.5)	< .01	0.97*	0.86*	0.11

WISC-III Processing Speed	108.1 (14.3)	99.4 (15.3)	100.2 (16.1)	.01	0.55*	0.50*	0.05
WIAT Basic Reading	112.0 (12.6)	101.1 (14.2)	102.1 (14.6)	< .01	0.75*	0.68*	0.07
WIAT Math Reasoning	109.1 (13.8)	97.9 (14.6)	97.3 (14.2)	< .01	0.74*	0.78*	0.04

NOTE: * $p < .05$, ** $p < .01$, *** $p < .001$; P = Parent, T = Teacher, Y = Youth, S = Staff; SNAP = Swanson, Nolan, & Pelham rating scale; HI = hyperactivity/impulsivity; DISC-IV = Diagnostic Interview Schedule for Children 4.0; CBCL = Child Behavior Checklist; TRF = Teacher Report Form; ODD = Oppositional Defiant Disorder; CD = Conduct Disorder; DBR = daily behavior ratings; CDI = Child Depression Inventory; MASC = Multidimensional Anxiety Scale for Children; WISC = Weschsler Intelligence Scale for Children; WIAT = Wechsler Individual Achievement Test; agg = aggression; anx = anxiety; dep = depression; sxs = symptoms.

[a] Significance: One-way ANOVA for continuous variables; Pearson chi-square statistic for categorical variables.

[b] Cohen's *d* for continuous variables; odds ratios for categorical variables; Tukey's test for each pairwise comparison.

girls with ADHD-C versus girls with ADHD-I. Additionally, although teacher-, parent-, and self-rated internalizing problems did not differ significantly between the subtypes, observer-reported internalizing differences did: (a) girls with ADHD-I experienced more social isolation, and (b) girls with ADHD-C had higher levels of anxiety/depression. Except in the parenting domain, every difference between (i) girls with ADHD and comparison girls and (ii) girls with ADHD-C and ADHD-I, even including dimensional measures of disruptive behavior, survived covariation of comorbid ODD/CD and age. In the parenting domain, however, group differences on most variables were partially explained by ODD/CD comorbidity.

At W1, neuropsychological tests were chosen to assess EF, motor speed, and language processing. All 10 neuropsychological variables analyzed showed significant differences across groups, with 8 of 10 ADHD-C versus comparison contrasts significant (average effect size medium) and 6 of 10 ADHD-I versus comparison contrasts significant (average effect size small to medium), but only 2 of 10 ADHD-C versus ADHD-I contrasts significant (effect sizes small). Thus, there were performance deficits for girls with ADHD relative to comparisons, whereas girls with the various subtypes of ADHD showed mostly equivalent performance. The subtype exceptions were for the ROCF error proportion score, a measure of planning (a key executive function), and for the CPT commissions score, a measure of response inhibition. In both cases the girls with ADHD-I demonstrated somewhat better neuropsychological functioning than those with ADHD-C. All results were robust to statistical control of demographic variables and comorbidities; most results continued to hold when child IQ also was included as a covariate.

Adolescent Outcomes: Wave 2

Between W1 and W2, ADHD diagnoses based on DSM-IV diagnostic criteria were moderately stable for the girls originally diagnosed with ADHD-I (63% maintained this classification at W2), and less stable for the girls with ADHD-C (39% maintained this classification at W2), typically because of abatement of hyperactivity/impulsivity (HI) symptoms, common in ADHD samples (e.g., Barkley, Murphy, & Fischer, 2008; Hart, Lahey, Loeber, Applegate, & Frick, 1995). The difference in diagnostic persistence between the subtypes was statistically significant. Overall, of those with childhood ADHD who were followed up during adolescence, 69% continued to meet DSM-IV diagnostic criteria for some form of ADHD.

The W2 findings regarding psychosocial symptoms and impairments are presented in Table 7.5 (a different version of which was originally published in Hinshaw et al., 2006). As at W1, the analysis strategy involved ANOVAs (and ANCOVAs) for continuous dependent variables and X^2 tests (with follow-up logistic regressions including covariates) for dichotomous dependent variables. According to both parent and teacher report, girls with childhood-diagnosed ADHD continued to show greater psychiatric symptomatology across multiple domains (ADHD, externalizing, internalizing, substance abuse and dependence) and larger functional impairments (global, social skills, peer relations, academic performance, and service utilization rates) than did comparison girls, but not for every single parent- or teacher-reported outcome measure. Girls with childhood ADHD self-reported lower academic and social competence and higher levels of eating disorder and depressive symptoms at W2, but their self-reported substance use, delinquent behavior, and number of delinquent peers were equivalent to reports from the comparison girls. Effect sizes associated with significant contrasts were medium to large. As expected, given that functioning was measured five years later, these effect sizes were slightly smaller, overall, than those at W1, when ADHD status and functioning were examined concurrently. The functional deficits and problematic symptom profiles were apparent at W2 among the girls with ADHD even though on most measures they showed improvement across time relative to the comparison girls. On the other hand, the age-standardized WIAT Math scores of girls with childhood ADHD-C declined from W1 to W2, whereas comparison scores improved; math scores for girls with childhood ADHD-I were stable.

TABLE 7.5

FUNCTIONING AT WAVE 2 ACROSS DOMAINS BY WAVE 1 DIAGNOSTIC STATUS

	No Covariates							*Covariates*
	Comp (0)	**Inattentive (1)**	**Combined (2)**		**Effect Sizes[b]**			
	M (SD)	***M (SD)***	***M (SD)***	***p*[a]**	***0–1***	***0–2***	***1–2***	***p*[c]**
ADHD SXS ($F_{8, 278}$ = 19.49***)								
P SNAP Inattention	0.5 (0.5)	2.1 (0.7)	1.9 (0.8)	.000	1.62*	1.46*	0.15	.000
P SNAP HI	0.1 (0.2)	0.8 (0.5)	1.2 (0.8)	.000	0.83*	1.41*	0.58*	.000
T SNAP Inattention	0.4 (0.5)	1.2 (0.8)	1.2 (0.8)	.000	1.01*	0.95*	0.06	.004
T SNAP HI	0.1 (0.2)	0.4 (0.4)	0.7 (0.8)	.000	0.41	0.91*	0.51*	.055
EXTERNALIZING SXS ($F_{10,280}$ = 8.23***)								
P DISC ODD (%)	7.4	51.2	50.6	.000	13.1*	12.8*	1.0	.010
P DISC CD (%)	1.2	4.9	17.6	.001	4.1	17.2*	4.2*	.008
P CBCL Externalizing	45.8 (9.9)	58.8 (8.4)	63.0 (12.4)	.000	0.98*	1.29*	0.32	.000
T TRF Externalizing	49.0 (8.3)	55.3 (9.0)	58.3 (11.1)	.000	0.60*	0.89*	0.29	.033
Y SRD Total	0.8 (1.3)	1.1 (1.8)	0.9 (1.9)	.712	0.16	0.07	0.09	—
INTERNALIZING SXS ($F_{10,282}$ = 4.02***)								
P DISC Anx (%)	2.5	9.8	10.6	.103	4.3	4.7	1.1	—
P DISC Dep (%)	3.7	9.8	11.8	.154	14.9	3.4	1.3	—
P CBCL Internalizing	45.7 (10.9)	56.7 (9.8)	56.6(12.0)	.000	0.89*	0.87*	0.02	.005

T TRF Internalizing	49.8 (8.7)	54.5 (10.4)	54.8 (8.3)	.006	0.51*	0.54*	0.03	.519
Y CDI Total	5.3 (5.7)	6.5 (4.0)	7.8 (6.5)	.016	0.21	0.43*	0.22	.412
SUBSTANCE USE ($F_{4,400}$ = 2.62*)								
P DISC Sub. A/D (%)	1.2	0.0	7.1	.047	—	6.1	—	.266
Y SUQ Severity	-0.1 (0.6)	0.2 (1.1)	0.0 (1.0)	.160	0.33	0.11	0.22	—
EATING DISORDER SXS ($F_{8,398}$ = 2.31*)								
Y EAT Total	45.5 (11.2)	45.3 (11.2)	53.1(24.6)	.012	0.01	0.42*	0.43	.005
Y EDI Bulimia	9.8 (2.9)	10.2 (3.3)	11.7 (5.0)	.005	0.10	0.47*	0.37	.081
Y EDI Drive for thinness	12.6 (5.6)	13.4 (4.8)	15.8 (8.0)	.007	0.12	0.48*	0.36	.060
Y EDI Body dissatisfaction	21.1 (8.9)	24.4 (8.7)	24 .7(11.2)	.046	0.33	0.36	0.03	.370
GENERAL IMPAIRMENT ($F_{2,208}$ = 42.11***)								
P CIS	0.6 (0.5)	1.4 (0.5)	1.5 (0.8)	.000	1.07*	1.20*	0.13	.020
SOCIAL SKILLS ($F_{4,294}$ = 12.93***)								
P SSRS Total	1.5 (0.2)	1.2 (0.3)	1.1 (0.3)	.000	0.88*	1.18*	0.29	.014
T SSRS Total	1.6 (0.3)	1.3 (0.3)	1.3 (0.4)	.000	0.73*	0.73*	0.00	.002
PEER RELATIONSHIPS ($F_{8,268}$ = 7.70***)								
T Dishion Social preference	3.1 (1.3)	2.3 (1.6)	1.3 (2.6)	.000	0.37	0.83*	0.46*	.041
Y SRI Delinquent peers	3.2 (5.5)	4.6 (7.7)	3.1 (4.1)	.329	0.25	0.02	0.27	—
P SRQ “Friendship”	1.0 (0.4)	0.5 (0.6)	0.3 (0.7)	.000	0.76*	1.08*	0.32	.169
P SRQ “Peer conflict”	0.1 (0.2)	0.4 (0.4)	0.7 (0.7)	.000	0.44*	1.07*	0.6*2	.002

(*continued*)

TABLE 7.5

CONTINUED

	No Covariates							*Covariates*
	Comp (0)	**Inattentive (1)**	**Combined (2)**		**Effect Sizes**[b]			
	M (SD)	*M (SD)*	*M (SD)*	*p*[a]	*0–1*	*0–2*	*1–2*	*p*[c]
ACHIEVEMENT ($F_{6,294} = 11.34^{***}$)								
WIAT Math	112.9(14.2)	95.6 (15.5)	93.5 (16.8)	.000	0.96*	1.08*	0.12	.001
WIAT Reading	107.7 (8.2)	97.8 (13.1)	98.1 (11.5)	.000	0.85*	0.82*	0.03	.073
T TRF Academic	54.0 (9.5)	44.1 (8.4)	43.8 (8.2)	.000	0.99*	1.02*	0.03	.070
SELF-PERCEPTIONS ($F_{6,402} = 4.92^{***}$)								
Y Harter Self-worth	3.4 (0.5)	3.3 (0.6)	3.2 (0.7)	.054	0.16	0.32	0.16	—
Y Harter Social	3.4 (0.5)	3.2 (0.5)	3.1 (0.7)	.011	0.33	0.50*	0.17	.299
Y Harter Scholastic	3.2 (0.6)	2.8 (0.5)	2.8 (0.6)	.000	0.62*	0.62*	0.00	.107
SERVICE UTILIZATION ($F_{4,404} = 28.25^{***}$)								
P School services (%)	13.4	82.1	78.6	.000	29.5*	23.7*	0.8	.000
P Nonschool services (%)	31.7	71.8	70.2	.000	5.5*	5.1*	0.9	.703

NOTE: * $p < .05$, *** $p < .001$; P = Parent, T = Teacher, Y = Youth. ADHD = attention-deficit/hyperactivity disorder; SNAP = Swanson, Nolan, & Pelham rating scale; Comp = Comparison; HI = hyperactivity/impulsivity; sxs = symptoms; anx = anxiety; dep = depression; DISC = Diagnostic Interview Schedule for Children-IV; CBCL = Child Behavior Checklist; TRF = Teacher Report Form; ODD = Oppositional Defiant Disorder; CD = Conduct Disorder; SRD = Self-Reported Delinquency; CDI = Child Depression Inventory; Sub. A/D = Substance Abuse/Dependence; SUQ = Substance Use Questionnaire; EAT = Eating Attitudes Test; EDI = Eating Disorders Inventory; CIS = Columbia Impairment Scale; SSRS = Social Skills Rating System; SRI = Social Relationships Interview; SRQ = Social Relationships Questionnaire; WIAT = Wechsler Individual Achievement Test.

[a] Significance: One-way ANOVA for continuous variables; Pearson chi-square statistic for categorical variables.

[b] Cohen's *d* for continuous variables; odds ratios for categorical variables; Tukey's test for each pairwise comparison.

[c] Significance: One-way ANCOVA for continuous variables; Wald statistic from logistic regression for categorical variables. Baseline covariates included age, family income, maternal education, child IQ, ODD or CD diagnosis (except for externalizing problems) any anxiety or depressive diagnosis (except for internalizing problems), reading disorder (except for reading achievement), and medication status.

During adolescence, ADHD-C versus ADHD-I differences were rarely significant and almost always small. Overall, there were even fewer ADHD-C versus ADHD-I differences at W2 than there were at W1. Across 35 measures, only five showed significant differences, with medium effects: girls with childhood ADHD-C showed higher rates of comorbid CD, lower levels of peer social preference, and higher mother-reported conflict with peers (as well, of course, as higher levels of parent- and teacher-rated hyperactivity/impulsivity) than girls with childhood ADHD-I. These few differences are consistent with relevant literature and with BGALS findings from childhood. Our interpretation is that there are real, albeit rare, differences in functioning across girls with the various subtypes of ADHD.

Finally, in order to ascertain whether group differences at W2 were related to W1 ADHD status or associated conditions, we repeated our group contrasts covarying a comprehensive set of W1 variables: age, family income, maternal education, child IQ, ODD/CD diagnosis (except when predicting externalizing problems), any anxiety or depressive diagnosis (except when predicting internalizing problems), reading disorder (except when predicting reading achievement), and medication status. Most W2 group differences survived control for this stringent set of covariates and, therefore, could be reasonably attributed to childhood ADHD status. ADHD-comparison group differences, however, were reduced to marginal or non-significance for three of four eating pathology variables, reading achievement, teacher report of academic performance, substance use/abuse disorders, self-perceptions of competence, non-school services, and some measures of internalizing problems. Additional analyses suggested that Wave 1 ODD/CD was likely to be responsible for such attenuation of group differences.

The W2 neuropsychological battery was more circumscribed than that at W1 and focused primarily on aspects of EF. Findings were highly similar to those obtained during childhood. During adolescence, the girls with childhood ADHD displayed significant deficits on most measures. Comparison girls showed better performance than girls with ADHD-I on six of eight measures (effect sizes small-to-medium) and better performance than girls with ADHD-C on seven of eight measures (effect sizes small-to-medium). All ADHD-I versus ADHD-C contrasts were negligible or small and statistically nonsignificant. Most differences withstood statistical control of W1 age, demographic variables, and comorbidities. Additional control of child IQ eliminated the significant association between childhood ADHD and adolescent performance (which may be an instance of "overcontrol"). Secondary analyses using W2 (rather than W1) ADHD status, however, revealed strong concurrent neuropsychological differences between those with and without adolescent ADHD, even covarying IQ.

Young-Adult Outcomes: Wave 3

Our published findings regarding diagnostic stability were calculated using DSM-IV criteria, because that was the manual in use both at the time of the baseline assessments and when the follow-up papers were published. According to DSM-IV criteria, over half (58%) of the girls with childhood diagnoses of ADHD retained a diagnosis, of either subtype, at W3. A minority (39%) of girls with childhood ADHD-I retained this classification at W3. Twenty-two percent met criteria for ADHD-C, and 39% no longer met criteria for ADHD. Of the girls with initial diagnoses of ADHD-C, 39% retained this classification at W3, 17% met criteria for ADHD-I, and 44% no longer met criteria for ADHD. Using DSM-V (American Psychiatric Association, 2013) criteria specifying that five symptoms (as opposed to the six required by DSM-IV) are required for the diagnosis in individuals 17 years and older, 76.6% of those in the BGALS with a childhood diagnosis of ADHD retained the diagnosis during young adulthood. Thus, by either criterion set, the majority of girls met full DSM criteria for ADHD during young adulthood. Expectedly, diagnostic stability between W2 and W3 was somewhat higher: approximately two thirds of those diagnosed with ADHD at W2 (65% of those with ADHD-I and 74% of those with ADHD-C) retained an ADHD diagnosis at W3, using DSM-IV criteria at both time points.

The findings regarding symptomatology and impairment at W3 are presented in Table 7.6, a version of which was originally published in Hinshaw et al. (2012). The analytic strategy employed was parallel to those used at W1 and W2. Across most domains during young adulthood, girls with Wave 1 ADHD diagnoses were significantly more symptomatic and impaired than the comparison group, with effect sizes ranging from medium to very large. As was true at W2, parent- or objective-report of outcome yielded significant group differences more often than did self-report. According to parent report, young adult women with childhood diagnoses of ADHD had higher levels of ADHD and externalizing symptoms, higher rates of ODD/CD comorbidity, higher levels of internalizing problems, greater global impairment and service utilization, and fewer years of education than girls without childhood diagnoses of ADHD. According to objective testing, girls with childhood ADHD had lower academic achievement in math and reading in young adulthood than girls without childhood diagnoses of ADHD. In addition, girls with ADHD self-reported lower levels of academic competence and greater rates of suicide attempts and self-injury. There were, however, no significant group differences, according to self-report, with respect to social competence, internalizing symptoms, substance use severity, eating pathology, delinquent behavior, or problematic driving.

Significant ADHD-C versus ADHD-I differences at W3 were rarely found, with the important exception of self-injury and suicide attempts, which predominated in the childhood-diagnosed combined type. Specifically, 22% of girls with childhood ADHD-C reported a previous suicide attempt, versus 8% of girls with childhood ADHD-I and 6% of comparison girls. Rates of nonsuicidal self-injurious behavior (NSSI) were parallel: over half of the originally diagnosed girls with ADHD-C had engaged in moderate to severe levels by W3, significantly higher than the rates for the subgroup with ADHD-I (29%) or the comparison girls (19%). The only other dependent variables evidencing a significant difference between girls with ADHD-C and ADHD-I were parent report of externalizing problems, comorbid conduct disorder, and hyperactivity/impulsivity, each of which demonstrated an effect of moderate size (with ADHD-C participants scoring higher, as expected).

TABLE 7.6

FUNCTIONING AT WAVE 3 ACROSS DOMAINS BY WAVE 1 DIAGNOSTIC STATUS

	No Covariates							*Covariates*
	Comp (0)	**Inattentive (1)**	**Combined (2)**		**Effect Sizes[b]**			
	M (SD)	***M (SD)***	***M (SD)***	p^a	***0-1***	***0-2***	***1-2***	p^c
ADHD SXS ($F_{8,310}$ = **15.89**, P = **.000**)								
P SNAP Inattention	0.4 (0.5)	1.6 (0.9)	1.8 (0.8)	.000	1.27*	1.46*	0.19	.000
P SNAP HI	0.1 (0.2)	0.6 (0.6)	1.0 (0.8)	.000	0.69*	1.33*	0.64*	.000
Y SNAP Inattention	0.6 (0.5)	1.0 (0.7)	1.1 (0.7)	.000	0.60*	0.73*	0.14	.029
Y SNAP HI	0.4 (0.4)	0.7 (0.5)	0.9 (0.6)	.000	0.47*	0.89*	0.43	.014
EXTERNALIZING SXS ($F_{8,324}$ = 10.25, P = .000)								
P DISC ODD/CD (%)	4.7	48.8	40.7	.000	19.5*	14.1*	0.7	.009
P ACBL Externalizing	46.7 (9.0)	56.8 (9.0)	62.3 (10.9)	.000	0.84*	1.30*	0.46*	.000
Y ASR Externalizing	50.2 (10.2)	56.8 (12.6)	57.6 (12.5)	.000	0.54*	0.61*	0.07	.042
Y SRD Total	1.8 (2.1)	1.7 (1.8)	1.8 (2.1)	.980	0.03	0.00	0.04	N/A
INTERNALIZING SXS ($F_{10,322}$ = 4.85, P = .000)								
P DISC Dep (%)	7.0	19.5	21.2	.024	3.2*	3.6*	1.1	.858
P DISC Anx (%)	10.5	34.1	32.2	.001	4.4*	4.1*	0.9	.066
P ACBL Internalizing	44.9 (10.8)	55.2 (10.1)	59.3 (13.1)	.000	0.77*	1.08*	0.31	.113
Y ASR Internalizing	51.8 (11.7)	54.7 (13.2)	55.2 (13.0)	.189	0.23	0.27	0.04	N/A
Y BDI Total	8.2 (10.5)	10.1 (10.6)	11.6 (10.1)	.094	0.19	0.33	0.15	N/A

(*continued*)

TABLE 7.6

CONTINUED

	No Covariates							*Covariates*
	Comp (0)	**Inattentive (1)**	**Combined (2)**		**Effect Sizes**[b]			
	M (SD)	***M (SD)***	***M (SD)***	p^a	***0-1***	***0-2***	***1-2***	p^c
SUBSTANCE USE								
Y SUQ Severity	-0.05 (0.8)	0.09 (1.0)	0.01 (0.9)	.703	0.16	0.06	0.10	N/A
EATING DISORDER SXS ($F_{8,384}$ = 0.90, P = .519)								
Y EAT Total	50.8 (17.4)	49.8 (14.0)	54.9 (18.4)	.199	0.06	0.23	0.30	N/A
Y EDI Bulimia	12.8 (5.4)	12.7 (6.0)	13.3 (5.4)	.828	0.02	0.08	0.10	N/A
Y EDI Drive for thinness	17.3 (8.1)	15.7 (7.4)	18.5 (8.3)	.195	0.19	0.16	0.35	N/A
Y EDI Body dissatisfaction	26.6 (9.9)	26.5 (12.0)	29.2 (10.3)	.223	0.01	0.25	0.26	N/A
Global Impairment								

P CIS	0.5 (0.5)	1.3 (0.7)	1.5 (0.9)	.000	0.98*	1.14*	0.16	.033
ACADEMIC ACHIEVEMENT ($F_{6.404}$ = 9.38, P = .000)								
WIAT Math	105.9(12.5)	91.0 (15.8)	91.3 (16.3)	.000	0.91*	0.89*	0.02	.193
WIAT Reading	108.8 (8.5)	97.2 (15.9)	97.3 (14.7)	.000	0.83*	0.83*	0.00	.012
Years of education	13.1 (1.6)	12.7 (1.0)	12.4 (1.5)	.004	0.30	0.53*	0.23	.135
SELF-PERCEPTIONS ($F_{6,390}$ = 3.01, P = .007)								
Y Harter Self-worth	3.2 (0.7)	3.0 (0.7)	3.0 (0.7)	.076	0.27	0.35	0.07	N/A
Y Harter Social	3.3 (0.7)	3.1 (0.6)	3.1 (0.7)	.085	0.34	0.30	0.04	N/A
Y Harter Scholastic	3.1 (0.7)	2.7 (0.7)	2.7 (0.7)	.000	0.59*	0.58*	0.01	.581
SERVICE UTILIZATION ($F_{8,398}$ = 12.65, P = .000)								
Any school services(%)	21.3	61.9	66.7	.000	6.0*	7.4*	1.2	.000
Any mental health tx(%)	51.3	71.4	73.6	.006	2.4*	2.6*	1.1	.072
Any stimulant (%)	1.2	43.9	58.1	.000	62.6*	111.1*	1.8	.000

(continued)

TABLE 7.6

CONTINUED

	No Covariates							Covariates
	Comp (0)	Inattentive (1)	Combined (2)		Effect Sizes[b]			
	M (SD)	*M (SD)*	*M (SD)*	p^a	*0-1*	*0-2*	*1-2*	p^c
Any other med (%)	18.5	17.1	32.6	.053	0.9	2.1*	2.3	.168
SELF-HARM ($F_{4,384}$ = 5.51, P = .000)								
Y Suicide attempts (%)	6.0	7.7	22.4	.004	1.3	4.5*	3.5*	.020
Y Self-injury (%)	19.0	28.9	50.6	.000	1.7	4.4*	2.5*	.028
DRIVING								
Y DBQ	1.4 (1.1)	1.6 (1.1)	1.3 (1.0)	.593	0.12	0.10	0.22	N/A

NOTE: Y = young adult self-report; P = parent's report on young adult. SNAP = Swanson, Nolan, & Pelham; Comp = Comparison; HI = hyperactivity/impulsivity; sxs = symptoms; anx = anxiety; dep = depression; DISC = Diagnostic Interview Schedule for Children-IV; ACBL = Adult Behavior Checklist; ASR = Adult Self-Report; SRD = Self-Report of Delinquency; BDI = Beck Depression Inventory-II; SUQ = Substance Use Questionnaire; EAT = Eating Attitudes Test; EDI = Eating Disorder Inventory-2; CIS = Columbia Impairment Scale; WIAT = Wechsler Individual Achievement Test-II; SIQ = Self-Injury Questionnaire; Med hx = medication history; Other = nonstimulant psychotropic medication; DBQ = Driving Behavior Questionnaire; N/A = not applicable (i.e., no ANCOVA because of lack of significance of ANOVA).

[a] Significance: One-way ANOVA for continuous variables; Pearson chi-square statistic for categorical variables.

[b] Cohen's *d* for continuous variables; odds ratios for categorical variables; Tukey's test for each pairwise comparison; * $p < .05$.

[c] Covariates: W1 age, W1 maternal education, W1 family income, W1 child FSIQ, W1 comorbid ODD/CD (from P DISC),W1 comorbid anxiety or depression (from P DISC),W1 reading disorder, medication status (any stimulants or other psychotropic medication taken between W2 and W3). With medication status and nonschool treatments as outcomes, we did not covary medication status. With W3 externalizing variables as outcomes, we did not covary comorbid ODD/CD. With W3 internalizing variables as outcomes, we did not covary comorbid depression/dysthymia or anxiety. With W3 achievement variables as outcomes, we did not covary W1 reading disorder.

For most domains, ADHD-related deficits survived stringent statistical control of W1 age, family income, maternal education, child IQ, comorbid diagnoses, and medication status (i.e., whether or not any psychotropic medication had been taken between W2 and W3). Therefore, it is reasonable to assume significant group differences can be attributed specifically to childhood ADHD status. However, differences at W3 in rates of mental health treatment (but not school services), self-reported well-being, internalizing symptoms, years of education, and math achievement were no longer significant once the potential confounds were considered.

The W3 neuropsychological battery was quite comparable to that used at W2, measuring various components of EF. Overall, girls with childhood-diagnosed ADHD, relative to comparisons, displayed significant neuropsychological deficits during young adulthood. Results were highly similar to those reported at W1 and W2. At W3, girls with ADHD-I and ADHD-C performed less well than comparisons on six of eight measures. Effect sizes for ADHD-I contrasts were small-to-large and for ADHD-I contrasts were small-to-medium. All ADHD-I versus ADHD-C contrasts were small and nonsignificant. Significant group differences held with covariation of W1 age, demographic variables, and comorbidities. Additional control of childhood IQ eliminated some associations. However, group differences for CPT commissions, CUL, and Letter-Number Sequencing were still significant, suggesting that differences in response inhibition and working memory were independent of IQ.

Secondary analyses using ADHD diagnostic persistence (rather than Wave 1 ADHD status) as the predictor also were conducted. In these analyses, neuropsychological performance during young adulthood was determined across three groups of girls: those without an ADHD diagnosis at either W1 or W3, those with ADHD at W1 but not W3 (remitted ADHD), and those with ADHD at both W1 and W3 (persistent ADHD). According to these analyses, similar neuropsychological deficits were evident among all girls with childhood ADHD, whether or not their ADHD had remitted by young adulthood.

RESULTS: PREDICTORS OF OUTCOME

Findings from our prospective investigation and from other large, longitudinal studies of children with ADHD are converging on an increasingly consistent narrative of substantial psychiatric problems and functional impairments among both boys and girls with ADHD as they mature into adolescence and adulthood (e.g., Barkley et al., 2008; Biederman et al., 2010; Klein et al., 2012; Weiss & Hechtman, 1993). However, the typical or average outcome is, of course, not experienced by each child with ADHD. Wide interindividual variability exists with respect to later symptomatology and impairment. Understanding this variability is imperative, because it informs both developmental theory and treatment efforts intended to target those most at risk.

Ongoing work in our lab is intended to elucidate predictors or moderators of developmental outcomes, as well as mediators that help to explain the relation between ADHD status or severity and outcomes. Predictors are baseline characteristics that show associations with outcome, regardless of initial ADHD status. Moderators are baseline characteristics on which the association between initial ADHD and outcome depends. Mediators are temporally intervening, explanatory variables that might account for different developmental outcomes. Thus far, our BGALS findings, summarized below, have primarily concerned whether outcome is predicted, moderated, or mediated by aspects of ADHD (e.g., subtype, persistence, severity), psychiatric comorbidity, EF, and/or peer relationships.

Of note, the majority of our longitudinal analyses have employed data from the entire sample, which includes girls with and without ADHD. Although we typically have not tested the predictive utility of variables specifically among the subgroup of girls with ADHD, the findings nevertheless apply to both girls with ADHD and to girls without ADHD. Exceptions to this interpretation involve instances in which we have found evidence of moderation by diagnostic status, that is, when association between a predictor and an outcome differs among girls with and without ADHD. We note these instances below.

Attention Deficit Hyperactivity Disorder Subtype, Persistence, and Severity

Subtype differences in outcome were investigated in depth in the primary adolescent (W2; Hinshaw et al., 2006) and young-adult (W3; Hinshaw et al., 2012) outcome papers, with findings described above. To review, besides expectable differences in levels of hyperactivity/impulsivity, very few childhood ADHD-C/ADHD-I differences were found at W2 or W3. Only comorbid externalizing problems, peer problems during adolescence, and the presence of self-injury and suicide attempts during young adulthood differed by subtype. Subsequently, Swanson et al. (2014) extended these analyses and also documented ADHD-C versus ADHD-I differences in both the variety and severity of self-injurious acts by young adulthood. Mikami et al. (2008) also demonstrated ADHD-C versus ADHD-I differences in pathological eating during adolescence, using a different measure than used in Hinshaw et al. (2006). In each of these specific instances, girls with the initial ADHD-C diagnoses fared somewhat more poorly (effect sizes were medium) during adolescence and young adulthood than did the girls with initial ADHD-I diagnoses. Overall, however, subtype was not a particularly salient predictor of most developmental outcomes, except in the key domain of self-injury and in the domains of externalizing and peer problems.

The persistence of ADHD is another aspect of the disorder that may predict outcome. Three BGALS investigations considered whether transient (diagnosed during childhood but then remitted) versus persistent (diagnosed at W1 and W3) ADHD is related to outcome. As noted above, Miller, Ho et al. (2012) found girls with transient and persistent ADHD to show equivalent neuropsychological performance during young adulthood. In contrast, Swanson et al. (2014) found that three measures of nonsuicidal self-injury indicated greater impairment among those with persistent versus transient ADHD (effect sizes were medium). Similarly, in Guendelman, Ahmad et al. (2016), those with persistent ADHD experienced more intimate partner violence by young adulthood than those whose ADHD was transient. Additional work will be done with the

BGALS dataset to answer questions about the relation between ADHD persistence and adult outcome, particularly when W4 data become available.

Domain-specific (hyperactive/impulsive, or HI, versus inattentive, or IA) symptom severity is another aspect of ADHD that may be related to later outcome. BGALS analyses have addressed this issue, although thus far they have employed only a circumscribed set of outcomes. Regarding adolescent outcome, HI and IA symptoms seem equally but differentially predictive. Specifically, childhood impulsivity, but not inattention, significantly predicted adolescent eating pathology (Mikami et al., 2008), but the effect size was quite small. In Lee and Hinshaw (2006), childhood HI symptoms predicted adolescent conduct problems, substance use, and internalizing problems, whereas IA symptoms predicted school suspensions and expulsions as well as low academic achievement, covarying many potential confounds. Effect sizes for HI and IA symptoms were equivalent. These predictions from HI symptoms *may* reflect heterotypic continuity of impulsivity across childhood and adolescence, but this explanation does not readily account for the relation between IA symptoms and school disciplinary actions.

Concerning young-adult outcome, BGALS findings again show different associations for childhood HI versus IA symptoms that probably depend on the outcome in question and the analytic method used. Thus far, and somewhat counterintuitively, IA symptoms appear to outperform HI symptoms in the prediction of certain risky behaviors. In particular, IA (but not HI) symptoms directly (and indirectly) predicted young adult driving outcomes, although HI symptoms did predict accidents only for those with low deviant peer affiliation (Cardoos, Loya, & Hinshaw, 2013). Regarding nicotine use, although childhood HI symptoms predicted daily smoking during young adulthood, IA symptoms predicted daily smoking, smoking severity, having ever tried a cigarette, and age of first cigarette. When tested along with HI symptoms and early conduct problems, only IA symptoms uniquely predicted nicotine use (Cardoos & Hinshaw, 2013). One tentative explanation, consistent with other literature (Burke, Loeber, & Lahey, 2001), is that rather than behavioral disinhibition prompting cigarette use, children with inattention might be self-medicating with a widely accessible stimulant.

On the other hand, in Miller, Loya, and Hinshaw (2015), HI symptoms predicted three young adult outcomes (internalizing problems, academic achievement, and global functioning), whereas IA symptoms predicted only global functioning. Of note, however, is the fact that these direct associations were tested by their inclusion in structural equation models in which adolescent EF was modeled as a mediator. This data analytic method was different from that used in Cardoos and Hinshaw (2013), which may partially account for the discrepant findings. Overall, HI and IA symptoms seem differently associated with various adolescent and young adult outcomes, but overall their predictive power may be essentially equivalent.

Comorbidity and Co-occurring Emotional and Behavioral Problems

In the BGALS, behavioral and emotional problems co-occurring with ADHD predicted outcome during both adolescence and young adulthood. As shown in Lee and Hinshaw (2006), noncompliance observed during the summer camp predicted school suspensions and expulsions, internalizing and conduct problems, and substance use during adolescence, covarying for family income and child age, ADHD symptoms, negative peer status, and antisocial behavior. Covert antisocial behavior, measured with a laboratory task, predicted adolescent internalizing problems, also with covariation of an extensive list of possible confounds. Somewhat surprisingly, overt, observed aggression was not a predictor of adolescent outcomes, but this finding may relate to the low base rate of overt aggression among girls, especially in comparison with their rates of noncompliance. Like noncompliance and covert antisocial behavior, childhood irritability also predicted adolescent externalizing and internalizing problems among girls with and without ADHD (Mullin & Hinshaw, 2007), but only the association with externalizing problems withstood control of ADHD status, peer rejection, and overt aggression.

Co-occurring externalizing and internalizing problems also are associated with young adult outcomes in BGALS. In Owens and Hinshaw (2015), childhood and adolescent symptoms of ODD/CD both predicted overall functioning during young adulthood, specifically among girls with childhood ADHD, with the association between childhood ODD/CD and later functioning mediated by adolescent internalizing problems. Relatedly, Swanson et al. (2014) showed (a) adolescent internalizing problems to mediate the relation between childhood ADHD and suicide attempts made by young adulthood, and (b) adolescent externalizing problems (along with a neuropsychological measure of response inhibition) to mediate the relation between childhood ADHD and severity of nonsuicidal self-injury by young adulthood.

Executive Functioning

Executive functions comprise a set of cognitive processes, including aspects of attention, planning, and inhibition, involved in organizing and modifying behavior. EF problems commonly co-occur with ADHD; they are thought of by some as a central feature of the disorder (Barkley, 2015; Brown, 2013). In BGALS, certain childhood measures of EF have been associated with adolescent outcome. In Miller and Hinshaw (2010), performance on two out of four neuropsychological tests of EF (the CPT and ROCF) predicted adolescent academic achievement and/or peer acceptance in the entire sample, covarying diagnostic status or IQ. Effect sizes were small. ROCF scores also predicted global functioning during adolescence specifically and only among girls with ADHD. Similarly, in Rinsky and Hinshaw (2011), both childhood response inhibition (measured by the CPT) and planning (measured by the ROCF) negatively predicted social functioning during adolescence, covarying childhood diagnostic status. Again, effect sizes were small. Poor planning positively predicted internalizing/externalizing comorbidity, especially among girls diagnosed with ADHD-C; it also predicted internalizing problems only and specifically among girls with ADHD-C.

Regarding outcomes assessed during young adulthood, Miller et al. (2013) showed that changes in global EF predicted changes in HI and IA symptoms. Specifically, greater reduction in global executive dysfunction was associated with greater reduction of HI and IA symptoms between childhood and young adulthood. Furthermore, specifically among girls with ADHD, working memory deficits were associated with lower levels of later reading achievement and impaired global EF was related to later school suspensions/expulsions (Miller, Nevado-Montenegro et al., 2012). Across the entire sample, working memory and global EF were related to later occupational functioning. In Meza, Owens, and Hinshaw (2015) childhood response inhibition predicted suicidal ideation, suicide attempts, and nonsuicidal self-injury measured during young adulthood. Finally, in Miller et al. (2015), a latent measure of global adolescent EF mediated longitudinal associations between childhood ADHD symptoms (both HI and IA) and young adult academic achievement (both reading and math) and overall functioning.

Peer Relationships and Other Risk Factors

Peer relationships also may be associated with certain outcomes among girls with and without ADHD. Both Lee and Hinshaw (2006) and Mikami and Hinshaw (2006) showed that childhood peer rejection or negative peer status predicted academic problems (low achievement; school suspensions/expulsions) during adolescence, over and above variance accounted for by potential confounds. Meza, Owens, and Hinshaw (2015) and Cardoos et al. (2013) each showed adolescent peer relationships to mediate associations between childhood risk factors and young adult outcomes. Specifically, in Meza et al. (2015) the associations between childhood response inhibition and both suicidal ideation and attempts were partially mediated by teacher-rated social preference during adolescence; the link between response inhibition and later NSSI was partially mediated by self-report of peer victimization during adolescence. Similarly, self-report of deviant peer affiliation mediated the relation between adolescent IA symptoms and young adult driving outcomes (accidents and citations) in Cardoos et al. (2013).

Finally, two other BGALS reports have identified predictors of outcome among girls with ADHD. In Guendelman, Owens et al. (2016), girls with childhood ADHD who also were maltreated (neglected or abused) were significantly more impaired as young adults than non-maltreated girls with ADHD. Specifically, they reported greater rates of suicide attempts, higher levels of internalizing and eating-disorder symptomatology, and lower self-worth, all with medium effect sizes. Gard, Owens, and Hinshaw (2015) showed prenatal tobacco smoke exposure to positively predict HI symptom levels, but not IA symptom levels, during both adolescence and adulthood.

DISCUSSION

The primary take-home message from these BGALS findings is that during childhood, adolescence, and young adulthood, in almost every psychosocial and neuropsychological domain we investigated, females with ADHD show sizable disadvantages and deficits relative to females without ADHD. The sheer range of negative outcomes is noteworthy. Our findings affirm the public health significance of ADHD in girls, given the likelihood of persisting symptoms and (especially) impairment in crucial domains. Overall, our core conclusion is that childhood ADHD in girls portends noteworthy problems during both adolescence and young adulthood.

In particular, compared with girls without ADHD, girls with childhood ADHD in the BGALS had, on average, a greater range and higher levels of later psychiatric symptoms, greater overall impairment, more peer rejection, increased service utilization, lower educational achievement, and poorer performance on neuropsychological tests. Furthermore, even with covariation of key potential confounds, most diagnostic group differences remained significant during childhood and adolescence (except for internalizing problems during adolescence), suggesting their specific association with early ADHD and not with common co-occurring features. During young adulthood, inclusion of potential confounds reduced some additional findings to nonsignificance. However, even if variation in certain adult outcomes might have been attributed to common co-occurring features like psychiatric comorbidities, ADHD status is nevertheless indirectly implicated in the prediction of these detrimental outcomes precisely because it is counterfactual to separate common co-occurring features from ADHD itself.

Gender and Long-term Outcomes

BGALS findings regarding increased risk for later psychiatric comorbidities are quite consistent with findings from the other major longitudinal study of girls (Biederman, Monuteaux, Mick, Spencer, Wilens, Klein et al., 2006; Biederman et al., 2010) and boys with ADHD (e.g., Barkley Fischer, Edelbrock, & Smallish, 1990; Biederman, Faraone, Milberger, & Guite, 1996; Biederman, Monuteaux, Mick, Spencer, Wilens, Silva et al., 2006; Bussing, Mason, Bell, Porter, & Garvan, 2010; Fischer, Barkley, Smallish, & Fletcher, 2002; Klein et al., 2012; Lee, Lahey, Owens, & Hinshaw, 2008; Mannuzza, Klein, Abikoff, & Moulton, 2004; Weiss & Hechtman, 1985), although increased risk for later internalizing problems among boys is not uniformly found (e.g., Klein et al., 2012; Mannuzza, Klein, Bessler, Malloy, & LaPadula, 1998). Among samples either exclusively or predominantly male in nature, longitudinal findings of greater overall impairment (Barkley & Fischer, 2011; Klein et al., 2012), lower academic and educational attainment (Barkley, Fischer, Smallish, & Fletcher, 2006; Klein et al., 2012; Lee et al., 2008; Mannuzza, Klein, Bessler, Malloy, & Hynes, 1997), and poorer neuropsychological functioning (Barkley & Fischer, 2011; Halperin, Trampush, Carlin, Marks, & Newcorn, 2008; Seidman, 2006) are also quite similar to BGALS findings. Furthermore, comorbid ODD/CD during childhood seems to be a potent predictor of later functioning in boys (e.g., Barkley et al., 1990, 2006; Chilcoat & Breslau, 1999;

Mannuzza & Klein, 2000; Molina & Pelham, 2003; Realmuto et al., 2009), just as it is in the BGALS (Owens & Hinshaw, 2015).

The dissimilarities between the BGALS findings and those from studies of boys appear to lie in the substance use and delinquency domains, as well as self-harm. Most studies of boys show that childhood ADHD increases risk for later delinquency (Bussing et al., 2010; Klein et al., 2012; Satterfield & Schell, 1997; Sibley et al., 2011), even though it may well be the case that associated externalizing problems are the more specific predictors. Some research (e.g., Biederman, Monuteax, Mick, Spencer, Wilens, Silva et al., 2006; Molina et al., 2013), but not all (e.g., Biederman et al., 1996), demonstrates increased risk for substance use. It may be that risk is increased for only certain substances or substance use patterns (Barkley et al., 1990; Klein et al., 2012; Molina & Pelham, 2003). In contrast, we have not found later delinquency and substance use severity differences across girls with and without childhood ADHD. As noted below, however, this "negative" finding may be due to our reliance on self-report of these constructs. In addition, we have thus far focused our efforts on global measures. Certain findings (Cardoos & Hinshaw, 2013) do show that childhood ADHD is a risk factor for more specific substance use outcomes, such as nicotine use. In the substance use and delinquency domains, outcome differentiated by childhood diagnostic status may be revealed as we look more closely at specific, as opposed to global, measures of these constructs. We also are investigating whether developmental aspects of substance use (i.e., timing and acceleration) vary for girls with and without ADHD. Finally, the extraordinarily high rates of self-harm (suicide attempts and nonsuicidal self-injurious behavior) among the BGALS participants, particularly those with initial ADHD-C, have not been found among males with ADHD in prior research.

Persistence of Attention Deficit Hyperactivity Disorder

BGALS findings also have important implications for what is known about the stability versus discontinuity of ADHD. Perennial questions are: "Do children with ADHD grow out of it?" and "How do ADHD symptoms change over time?" Clearly, and in parallel with similar findings from samples of boys (e.g., Barkley, Fischer, Smallish, & Fletcher, 2002; Biederman, Mick, & Faraone, 2000), BGALS participants did not typically grow out of their ADHD. As noted above, 69% of those with childhood ADHD diagnoses retained a diagnosis during adolescence, and 58% retained a diagnosis during young adulthood. Biederman and colleagues used a slightly less conservative estimate of diagnostic persistence in their longitudinal female sample and found ADHD retention rates of 82% in adolescence (Biederman, Monuteaux, Mick, Spencer, Wilens, Klein et al., 2006) and 62% during young adulthood (Biederman et al., 2010). Furthermore, when we operationalized persistence using DSM-V criteria, which require only five symptoms for the diagnosis in adults, 76.6% of the girls with a childhood diagnosis of ADHD retained the diagnosis during young adulthood. In addition to the lower symptom threshold, this high rate of diagnostic persistence also reflected our primary reliance on parent-report of continuing symptoms (Barkley et al., 2002; Sibley et al., 2015). In addition, we utilized a sample rigorously diagnosed with ADHD as children, rather than sampling participants who simply surpassed rating scale cut-offs for ADHD symptoms.

In the BGALS, parent- and teacher-reported inattention and hyperactivity/impulsivity symptoms during adolescence and young adulthood were also significantly higher, with large or very large effects, among those with childhood ADHD versus those without. Even with the tendency for girls with ADHD to under-report symptoms and impairment, they self-reported significantly higher levels of symptoms during adolescence and young adulthood than did girls without ADHD, and the differences were of at least moderate size. These findings suggest that many girls with a childhood diagnosis, even if they no longer meet strict diagnostic criteria for ADHD, still exhibit problematic ADHD symptoms as they mature into adulthood.

Informant and Long-term Outcome

As just noted, impairments among girls and women with ADHD were particularly salient in the BGALS when outcomes were reported by parents or teachers and were less likely when self-reported. Some of the surprising null findings in the substance use, delinquency, and driving domains may be due to such reliance on self-report. Relatedly, if we had used youth-report on the DISC-IV to diagnose ADHD during young adulthood, only about one fifth of the girls originally diagnosed with ADHD would have retained that diagnosis, in comparison with the well over half who did when based primarily on parent-report on the DISC-IV. These results cohere with Barkley et al. (2002) and Sibley et al. (2015) who each reported that rates of adult ADHD diagnoses among probands who were followed longitudinally vary dramatically as a function of informant.

Predictors and Long-term Outcome

ADHD subtype is the only predictor about which we have enough information to reach any kind of conclusion. During each developmental period, girls with childhood-diagnosed ADHD-C and ADHD-I appeared quite similar in terms of psychiatric symptoms (except, of course, for symptoms of hyperactivity/impulsivity) and impairment. There were no significant subtype differences with respect to internalizing symptoms or disorders, eating disorder symptoms, substance use, perceptions of self-competence, general impairment, academic achievement, service use, or driving behavior. The key subtype distinctions were higher rates of externalizing and peer problems during childhood and adolescence, and higher rates of self-harm during young adulthood, among those with ADHD-C compared with those with ADHD-I. Of note, to our knowledge, ours is the only long-term study in which developmental outcomes have been compared for children with different subtypes of ADHD. Even though a discernible pattern is apparent in our data, these findings await replication before definitive statements can be made.

In most cases, group and subtype differences survived control of a stringent set of covariates, suggesting that differences were due to ADHD status per se and not to associated conditions or potential confounds.

Thus, socioeconomic status (SES) and race were unrelated to outcome, as was child IQ (except for academic achievement and neuropsychological outcomes). In no case did inclusion of these demographic and cognitive covariates impact relations between predictors and outcome. Of course, the BGALS sample is sufficiently small that demographic or SES effects—apparent in the general population—may not be visible.

Regarding the identification of other predictors of long-term outcomes, the primary message from the BGALS is essentially that we have a lot more to learn. Mixed findings from BGALS indicate that the jury is still out regarding the predictive significance of HI versus IA symptoms. We have tested the importance of transient versus persistent ADHD for only a few outcomes, and results have not been uniform. We know that comorbid disruptive disorders portend poor outcome overall, but we do not know which specific outcomes are more or less related to disruptive comorbidity. Indeed, we have just begun to investigate relations among many possible predictors of many adolescent and adult outcomes.

Limitations and Future Directions

The population to which our findings can be generalized is an important consideration. We did not recruit a truly representative sample; our participants do not fully represent girls with ADHD in the United States, or even in our region. Our goal was to intensively study psychiatric symptoms, a wide variety of associated impairments, social relationships, cognitive functioning, and family interactions in a large, diverse, and well-characterized sample of girls with ADHD, which precluded recruitment of the large number of participants needed to represent adequately the complete population of girls with ADHD. The population to which our findings can be generalized is one composed of ethnically and socioeconomically diverse girls who have either been suspected of having ADHD or who have been previously diagnosed, and whose families are seeking and willing to participate in a no-cost summer program.

Another limitation was our suboptimal understanding of girls' peer relationships during adolescence. We had to rely on parent and teacher report during this developmental period because it was difficult to conceive of a means of privately obtaining valid and reliable measures of peer acceptance and friendships in the middle school or high school context. Also, because we chose to assess thoroughly a wide variety of domains from multiple perspectives during various developmental periods, we were not able to obtain many measures repeatedly over shorter intervals, which may have facilitated more sensitive measurement of change.

In the future, in addition to better delineating which particular predictors are associated with which particular developmental outcomes among children with ADHD, a few key questions deserve consideration. First, to what extent are identified predictors equifinal or multifinal (Cicchetti & Rogosch, 1996)? In other words, do certain predictors portend a variety of outcomes, and/or is a particular outcome associated with a variety of predictors? Second, are certain predictors especially hazardous, or is there a nonspecific, cumulative effect of multiple predictors associated with detrimental outcomes (e.g., Shaw, Vondra, Hommerding, Keenan, & Dunn, 1994)? Third, do particular variables actually moderate outcome, that is, are they associated with outcome among children with ADHD but not (or significantly less so) among children without ADHD? Finally, after we achieve a better understanding of which predictors (or moderators) are associated with different outcomes among children with ADHD, we will need to understand the reasons for the associations. We must understand mediators, causal processes, and true mechanisms, rather than simply accumulating data that support or disconfirm predictive models. Given the range and impact of the many long-lasting, negative outcomes for girls with childhood diagnoses of ADHD, this search for explanation is a clinical and scientific priority.

REFERENCES

Abidin, R. (1997). Parenting Stress Index: A measure of the parent-child system. In C. P. Zalaquett & R. J. Wood (Eds.), *Evaluating Stress: A Book of Resources* (pp. 277–291). Lanham, MD: Scarecrow Education.

Achenbach, T. M. (1991a). *Manual for the Child Behavior Checklist for ages 4–18 and 1991 Profile*. Burlington, VT: University Associates in Psychiatry.

Achenbach, T. M. (1991b). *Manual for the Teacher's Report Form and 1991 Profile*. Burlington, VT: University Associates in Psychiatry.

Achenbach T. M., & Rescorla, L. A. (2003). *Manual for the ASEBA Adult Forms & Profiles*. Burlington, VT: University of Vermont, Research Center for Children, Youth, & Families.

American Psychiatric Association. (1994). *Diagnostic and Statistical Manual of Mental Disorders* (4th ed.). Washington, DC: Author.

American Psychiatric Association. (2013). *Diagnostic and Statistical Manual of Mental Disorders* (5th ed.). Washington, DC: Author.

Angold, A., Costello, E. J., & Erkanli, A. (1999). Comorbidity. *Journal of Child Psychology and Psychiatry*, *40*, 57–87.

Armsden, G. C., & Greenberg, M. T. (1987). The Inventory of Parent and Peer Attachment: Individual difference and their relationship to psychological well-being in adolescence. *Journal of Youth and Adolescence*, *16*, 427–454.

Arnold, L. G. (1996). Sex differences in ADHD: Conference summary. *Journal of Abnormal Child Psychology*, *24*, 555–569.

Barkley, R. A. (2015). Executive functioning and self-regulation viewed as an extended phenotype: Implications of the theory for ADHD and its treatment. In R. A. Barkley (Ed.), *Attention-Deficit Hyperactivity Disorder: A Handbook for Diagnosis and Treatment* (4th ed.) (pp 405–434). New York: Guilford.

Barkley, R. A., & Fischer, M. (2011). Predicting impairment in major life activities and occupational functioning in hyperactive children as adults: Self-reported executive function (EF) deficits versus EF tests. *Developmental Neuropsychology*, *36*, 137–161.

Barkley, R. A., Fischer, M., Edelbrock. C. S., & Smallish, L. (1990). The adolescent outcome of hyperactive children diagnosed by research criteria: I. An 8-year prospective follow-up study. *Journal of the American Academy of Child and Adolescent Psychiatry*, *29*, 546–557.

Barkley, R. A., Fischer, M., Smallish, L., & Fletcher, K. E. (2002). The persistence of attention-deficit/hyperactivity disorder into young adulthood as a function of reporting source and definition of disorder. *Journal of Abnormal Psychology*, *111*, 279–289.

Barkley, R. A., Fischer, M., Smallish, L., & Fletcher, K. E. (2006). Young adult outcome of hyperactive children: Adaptive functioning in major life activities, *Journal of the American Academy of Child and Adolescent Psychiatry*, *45*, 192–202.

Barkley, R. A. Murphy, K. R., & Fischer, M. (2008). *ADHD in Adults: What the Science Says*. New York: Guilford Press.

Barkley, R. A. Murphy, K. R., & Kwasnik, D. (1996). Motor vehicle driving competencies and risks in teens and young adults with attention deficit hyperactivity disorder. *Pediatrics*, *98*, 1089–1095.

Beck, A. T., Steer, R. A., Ball, R., & Ranieri, W. F. (1996). Comparison of Beck Depression Inventories-IA and II in psychiatric outpatients. *Journal of Personality Assessment*, *67*, 588–597.

Biederman, J., Faraone, S., Milberger, S., & Guite, J. (1996). A prospective 4-year follow-up study of attention-deficit hyperactivity disorder. *Archives of General Psychiatry*, *53*, 437–446.

Biederman, J., Mick, E., & Faraone, S. V. (2000). Age-dependent decline of symptoms of attention deficit hyperactivity disorder: Impact of remission definition and symptom type. *American Journal of Psychiatry, 157*, 816–818.

Biederman, J., Monuteaux, M. C., Mick, E., Spencer, T., Wilens, T. E., Klein, K. L., . . . Faraone, S.V. (2006). Psychopathology in females with attention-deficit/hyperactivity disorder: A controlled, five-year prospective study. *Biological Psychiatry, 60*, 1098–1105.

Biederman, J., Petty, C. R., Monuteaux, M. C., Fried, R., Byrne, D., Mirto, T., . . . Faraone, S. V. (2010). Adult psychiatric outcomes of girls with attention deficit hyperactivity disorder: 11-year follow-up in a longitudinal case-control study. *American Journal of Psychiatry, 167*, 409–417.

Biederman, J., Monuteaux, M. C., Mick, E., Spencer, T., Wilens, T. E., Silva, J. M., . . . Faraone, S. V. (2006). Young adult outcome of attention deficit hyperactivity disorder: A controlled 10-year follow-up study. *Psychological Medicine, 36*, 167–179.

Bird, H. R. (1999). The assessment of functional impairment. In D. Shaffer, C. P. Lucas, & J. E. Richters (Eds.), *Diagnostic Assessment in Child and Adolescent Psychopathology* (pp. 209–229). New York: Guilford.

Brown, T. E. (2013). *A New Understanding of ADHD in Children and Adults: Executive Function Impairments.* New York: Routledge.

Burke, J. D., Loeber, R., & Lahey, B. B. (2001). Which aspects of ADHD are associated with tobacco use in early adolescence? *Journal of Child Psychology and Psychiatry, 42*, 493–502.

Bussing, R., Mason, D. M., Bell, L., Porter, P. & Carvan, C. (2010). Adolescent outcomes of childhood attention-deficit/hyperactivity disorder in a diverse community sample. *Journal of the American Academy of Child and Adolescent Psychiatry, 49*(6), 595-605.

Cardoos, S., & Hinshaw, S. (2013, October). *Childhood predictors of cigarette smoking in young adult women with and without ADHD.* Paper presented at the meeting of the American Academy of Child and Adolescent Psychiatry, Orlando, FL.

Cardoos, S., Loya, F., & Hinshaw, S. P. (2013). Adolescent girls' ADHD symptoms and young adult driving: The role of perceived deviant peer affiliation. *Journal of Clinical Child and Adolescent Psychology, 42*, 232–242.

Chilcoat, H. D., & Breslau, N. (1999). Pathways from ADHD to early drug use. *Journal of the American Academy of Child and Adolescent Psychiatry, 38*, 1347–1354.

Cicchetti, D., & Rogosch, F. A. (1996). Equifinality and multifinality in developmental psychopathology. *Development and Psychopathology, 8*, 597–600.

Claes, L., Vandereycken, W., & Vertommen, H. (2001). Self-injurious behavior in eating-disordered patients. *Eating Behaviors, 2*, 263–272.

Conners, C. K. (1995). *Conners' Continuous Performance Test and Computer Program User's Manual.* Toronto, Canada: Multi-Health Systems, Inc.

Conners, C. K., Erhardt, D., & Sparrow, E. (2004). Conners' Adult ADHD Rating Scale. North Tonawanda, NY: Multi-Health Systems, Inc.

Denckla, M. B. (1974). Development of motor co-ordination in normal children. *Developmental Medicine and Child Neurology, 16*, 729–741.

Denckla, M. B., & Rudel, R. (1974). Rapid "automatized" naming of pictured objects, colors, letters, and numbers by normal children. *Cortex, 10*, 186–202.

Delis, D. C., Kaplan, E., & Kramer, J. (2001). *Delis-Kaplan Executive Function System*. San Antonio, TX: The Psychological Corporation.

Dishion, T. (1990). The peer context of troublesome child and adolescent behavior. In P. E. Leone (Ed.), *Understanding Troubled and Troubling Youth* (pp. 128–153). Thousand Oaks, CA: Sage.

Fischer, M., Barkley, R. A., Smallish, L., & Fletcher, K. E. (2002). Young adult follow-up of hyperactive children: Self-reported psychiatric disorders, comorbidity, and the role of childhood conduct problems and teen CD. *Journal of Abnormal Child Psychology*, *30*, 463–475.

Gard, A. M., Owens, E. B., & Hinshaw, S. P. (2015). Prenatal smoke exposure differentially predicts ADHD symptom domains in adolescence and young adulthood. Manuscript submitted for publication.

Gaub, M., & Carlson, C. L. (1997). Gender differences in ADHD: A meta-analysis and critical review. *Journal of the American Academy of Child and Adolescent Psychiatry*, *36*, 1036–1046.

Garner, D. M. (1991). *Eating Disorder Inventory* (2nd ed.). Odessa, FL: Psychological Assessment Resources.

Garner, D. M., Olmstead, M. P., Bohr, Y., & Garfinkel, P. E. (1982). The Eating Attitudes Test: Psychometric features and clinical correlates. *Psychological Medicine*, *12*, 871–878.

Gershon, J. (2002). A meta-analytic review of gender differences in ADHD. *Journal of Attention Disorders*, *5*, 143–154.

Gresham, F. M., & Elliott, S. N. (1990). *Social Skills Rating System—Parent, Teacher, and Child Forms*. Circle Pines, MN: American Guidance Systems.

Guendelman, M., Owens, E. B., Galan, C., Gard, A., & Hinshaw, S. P. (2016). Early-adult correlates of maltreatment in girls with attention-deficit/hyperactivity disorder: Increased risk for internalizing symptoms and suicidality. *Development and Psychopathology*, *28*, 1–14.

Guendelman, M., Ahmad, S., Meza, J. I., Owens, E. B., & Hinshaw, S. P. (2016). Childhood attention- deficit/hyperactivity disorder predicts intimate partner victimization in young women. *Journal of Abnormal Child Psychology*, *44*, 155–166.

Halperin, J. M., Trampush, J. W., Carlin, J., Marks, D. J., Newcorn, J. H. (2008). Neuropsychological outcome in adolescents/young adults with childhood ADHD: Profiles of persisters, remitters, and controls. *Journal of Child Psychology and Psychiatry*, *49*(9), 958–966.

Hart, E. L., Lahey, B. B., Loeber, R., Applegate, B., & Frick, P. J. (1995). Developmental change in attention-deficit hyperactivity disorder in boys: A four-year longitudinal study. *Journal of Abnormal Child Psychology*, *23*, 729–749.

Harter, S. (1982). The Perceived Competence Scale for Children. *Child Development*, *53*, 87–97.

Harter, S. (1988). *Manual for the Self-Perception Profile for Adolescents*. Unpublished manuscript, University of Denver.

Heming, G., Cowan, P., & Cowan, C. P. (1990). Ideas about parenting. In J. Touliatos, B. F. Perlmutter, & M. A. Straus (Eds.), *Handbook of Family Measurement Techniques* (pp. 382–383). Thousand Oaks, CA: Sage Publications.

Hinshaw, S. P. (2002). Preadolescent girls with attention-deficit/hyperactivity disorder: I. Background characteristics, comorbidity, cognitive and social functioning, and parenting practices. *Journal of Consulting and Clinical Psychology, 70*, 1086–1098.

Hinshaw, S. P., Carte, E. T., Fan, C., Jassy, J. S., & Owens, E. B. (2007). Neuropsychological functioning of girls with attention-deficit/hyperactivity disorder followed prospectively into adolescence: Evidence for continuing deficits? *Neuropsychology, 21*, 263–273.

Hinshaw, S. P., Carte, E. T., Sami, N., Treuting, J. J., & Zupan, B. A. (2002). Preadolescent girls with attention-deficit/hyperactivity disorder: II. Neuropsychological performance in relation to subtypes and individual classification. *Journal of Consulting and Clinical Psychology, 70*, 1099–1111.

Hinshaw, S. P., Owens, E. B., Sami, N., & Fargeon, S. (2006). Prospective follow-up of girls with attention-deficit/hyperactivity disorder into adolescence: Evidence for continuing cross-domain impairment. *Journal of Consulting and Clinical Psychology, 74*, 489–499.

Hinshaw, S. P., Owens, E. B., Zalecki, C., Huggins, S. P., Montenegro-Nevado, A., Schrodek, E., & Swanson, E. N. (2012). Prospective follow-up of girls with attention-deficit hyperactivity disorder into young adulthood: Continuing impairment includes elevated risk for suicide attempts and self-injury. *Journal of Consulting and Clinical Psychology, 80*, 1041–1051.

Horn, W., Wagner, A., & Ialongo, N. (1989). Sex differences in school-age children with pervasive attention deficit hyperactivity disorder. *Journal of Abnormal Child Psychology, 17*, 109–125.

Klein, R. G., Mannuzza, S., Olazagasti, M. A. R., Roizen, E., Hutchinson, J. A., Lashua, E. C., & Castellanos, F. X. (2012). Clinical and functional outcome of childhood attention-deficit/hyperactivity disorder 33 years later. *Archives of General Psychiatry, 69*, 1295–1303.

Knights, R. M., & Norwood, J. A. (1979). *A Neuropsychological Test Battery for Children: Examiner's Manual*. Ottawa, Canada: Knights Psychological Consultants.

Kovacs, M. (1992). *Manual: Children's Depression Inventory*. Toronto, Canada: Multi-Health Systems Inc.

Lahey, B. B., Applegate, B., McBurnett, K., Biederman, J., Greenhill, L., Hynd, G. W., . . . Shaffer, D. (1994). DSM–IV field trials for attention deficit hyperactivity disorder in children and adolescents. *American Journal of Psychiatry, 151*, 1673–1685.

Lee, S. S., & Hinshaw, S. P. (2006). Predictors of adolescent functioning in girls with attention-deficit/hyperactivity disorder: The role of childhood ADHD, conduct problems, and peer status. *Journal of Clinical Child and Adolescent Psychology, 35*, 356–368.

Lee, S. S., Lahey, B. B., Owens, E. B., & Hinshaw, S. P. (2008). Few preschool boys and girls with ADHD are well-adjusted during adolescence. *Journal of Abnormal Child Psychology, 38*, 132–143.

Mannuzza, S., & Klein, R. G. (2000). Long-term prognosis in attention-deficit/hyperactivity disorder. *Child and Adolescent Psychiatric Clinics of North American, 9*, 711–726.

Mannuzza, S., Klein, R. G., Abikoff, J., & Moulton, J. L. (2004). Significance of childhood conduct problems to later development of conduct disorder among children with ADHD: A prospective follow-up study. *Journal of Abnormal Child Psychology, 32*, 565–573.

Mannuzza, S., Klein, R. G., Bessler, A., Malloy, P., & Hynes, M. E. (1997). Educational and occupational outcome of hyperactive boys grown up. *Journal of the American Academy of Child and Adolescent Psychiatry, 36*, 1222–1227.

Mannuzza, S., Klein, R. G., Bessler, A., Malloy, P., & LaPadula, M. (1998). Adult psychiatric status of hyperactive boys grown up. *American Journal of Psychiatry, 155*, 493–498.

Meza, J., Owens, E. B., & Hinshaw, S. P. (2015). *Response inhibition, peer preference and victimization, and self-harm: Longitudinal associations in young adult women with and without ADHD.* Manuscript submitted for publication.

Mikami, A. Y., & Hinshaw, S. P. (2006). Resilient adolescent adjustment among girls: Buffers of childhood peer rejection and attention-deficit/hyperactivity disorder. *Journal of Abnormal Child Psychology, 34*, 825–839.

Mikami, A. Y., Hinshaw, S. P., Patterson, K. A., & Lee, J. C. (2008). Eating pathology among adolescent girls with attention-deficit/hyperactivity disorder. *Journal of Abnormal Psychology, 117*, 225–235.

Miller, M., Ho, J., & Hinshaw, S. P. (2012). Executive functions in girls with ADHD followed prospectively into young adulthood. *Neuropsychology, 26*, 278–287.

Miller, M., Montenegro-Nevado, A. J., & Hinshaw, S. P. (2012). Childhood executive function continues to predict outcomes in young adult females with and without childhood diagnosed ADHD. *Journal of Abnormal Child Psychology, 40*, 657–668.

Miller, M., Loya, F., & Hinshaw, S. P. (2013). Executive functions in girls with and without childhood ADHD: Developmental trajectories and associations with symptom change. *Journal of Child Psychology and Psychiatry, 54*, 1005–1015.

Miller, M., Loya, F., & Hinshaw, S. P. (2015). *Adolescent executive function mediates longitudinal associations between childhood ADHD symptoms and young-adult outcomes.* Manuscript submitted for publication.

Miller, M., & Hinshaw, S. P. (2010). Does childhood executive function predict adolescent functional outcomes in girls with ADHD? *Journal of Abnormal Child Psychology, 38*, 315–326.

Molina, B. S. G., Hinshaw, S. P., Arnold, L. E., Swanson, J. M., Pelham. W. E., Hechtman, L.,. . .Marcus, S. (2013). Adolescent substance us in the Multimodal Treatment Study of Attention-Deficit/Hyperactivity Disorder (ADHD) (MTA) as a function of childhood ADHD, random assignment to childhood treatments, and subsequent medication. *Journal of the American Academy of Child and Adolescent Psychiatry, 52*, 250–263.

Molina, B. S. G., & Pelham, W. E. (2003). Childhood predictors of adolescent substance use in a longitudinal study of children with ADHD. *Journal of Abnormal Psychology, 112*, 497–507.

Mullin, B., & Hinshaw, S. P. (2007, March). *Is Irritability a Unique Predictor of Multifinality in ADHD and Healthy Adolescent Girls?* Poster presented at the biennial meeting of the Society for Research in Child Development, Boston.

Nadeau, K. G., Littman, E. B, & Quinn, P. O. (1999). *Understanding Girls with AD/HD.* Silver Spring, MD: Advantage Books.

Osterrieth, P.A. (1944). Le test de copie d'une figure complex [A test of copying a complex figure]. *Achives de Psychologie*, 30, 206–256.

Owens, E. B., & Hinshaw, S. P. (2015). *Childhood conduct problems, adolescent internalizing problems and adult functioning among women with childhood ADHD.* Manuscript submitted for publication.

Pelham, W. E., Walker, J. L., Sturgis, B. S., & Hoza, B. (1989). Comparative effects of methylphenidate on ADD girls and ADD boys. *Journal of the American Academy of Child and Adolescent Psychiatry, 28*, 882–887.

Porteus, S. D. (1973). *Porteus Maze Test: Fifty Years' Application.* Palo Alto, CA: Pacific Books.

Realmuto, G. M., Winters, K. C., August, G. J., Lee, S., Fahnhorst, T., & Botzet, A. (2009). Drug use and psychosocial functioning of a community-derived sample of adolescent with childhood ADHD. *Journal of Child and Adolescent Substance Abuse, 18*, 172–192.

Rinsky, J., & Hinshaw, S. P. (2011). Linkages between childhood executive functioning and adolescent social functioning and psychopathology in girls with ADHD. *Child Neuropsychology, 17*, 368–390.

Rourke, B. P., & Orr, R. R. (1977). Prediction of reading and spelling performance of normal and retarded readers: A four-year follow-up. *Journal of Abnormal Child Psychology, 5*, 9–20.

Satterfield, J. H., & Schell, A. (1997). A prospective study of hyperactive boys with conduct problems and normal boys: Adolescent and adult criminality. *Journal of the American Academy of Child and Adolescent Psychiatry, 36*, 1726–1735.

Seidman, L. (2006). Neuropsychological functioning in people with ADHD across the lifespan. *Clinical Psychology Review, 26*, 466–485.

Shaffer, D., Fisher, P., Lucas, C. P., Dulcan, M. K., & Schwab-Stone, M. E. (2000). NIMH Diagnostic Interview Schedule for Children, Version IV (NIMH DISC-IV): Description, differences from previous versions, and reliability of some common diagnoses. *Journal of the American Academy of Child and Adolescent Psychiatry, 39*, 28–38.

Shaw, D. S., & Vondra, J. I., Hommerding, K. D., Keenan, K., & Dunn, M. (1994). Chronic family adversity and early child behavior problems: A longitudinal study of low income families. *Journal of Child Psychology and Psychiatry, 35*, 1109–1122.

Shelton, K. K., Frick, P. J., & Wootton, J. (1996). Assessment of parenting practices in families of elementary school-age children. *Journal of Clinical Child Psychology, 25*, 317–329.

Sibley, M. H., Pelham, W. E., Molina, B. S. G., Gnagy, E. M., Waschbusch, D. A., Biswas, A., . . . Karch, K. M. (2011). The delinquency outcomes of boys with ADHD with and without comorbidity. *Journal of Abnormal Child Psychology, 39*, 21–32.

Sibley, M. H., Swanson, J., Arnold, L. E., Hechtman, L., Owens, E. B., Mitchell, J. . . . and the MTA Group. (2015). Defining symptomatic ADHD persistence into adulthood: Source, method, and symptom threshold effects. Manuscript submitted for publication.

Swanson, J. M. (1992). *School-based Assessments and Interventions for ADD students.* Irvine, CA: K. C. Press.

Swanson, E. N., Owens, E. B., & Hinshaw, S. P. (2014). Pathways to self-harmful behaviors in young women with and without ADHD: A longitudinal investigation of mediating factors. *Journal of Child Psychology and Psychiatry, 44,* 505–515.

Taylor, L. B. (1969). Localization of cerebral lesions by psychological testing. *Clinical Neurosurgery, 16,* 269–287.

Wechsler, D. (1991). *Wechsler Intelligence Scales for Children* (3rd ed.). San Antonio, TX: Psychological Corporation.

Wechsler, D. (1992). *Wechsler Individual Achievement Test.* San Antonio, TX: Psychological Corporation.

Wechsler, D. (1997).*Wechsler Adult Intelligence Scale* (3rd ed.). San Antonio, TX: Psychological Corporation.

Weiss, G., & Hechtman, L. (1985). Psychiatric status of hyperactives as adults: A controlled prospective 15-year follow-up of 63 hyperactive children. *Journal of the American Academy of Child Psychiatry, 24,* 211–220.

Weiss, G., & Hechtman, L. (1993). *Hyperactive Children Grown Up: ADHD in Children, Adolescents, and Adults* (2nd ed.). New York: Guildford Press.

8

The Multimodal Treatment of Children with ADHD (MTA) Follow-up Study

Outcomes and Their Predictors

ARUNIMA ROY AND LILY HECHTMAN

The Multimodal Treatment of Children with ADHD (MTA) study, at the time of its inception, was the first of its kind for assessing and comparing psychiatric treatment modalities. To date, the MTA remains one of the largest ever clinical trials conducted for ADHD. The study began in 1994 with the primary goal of delineating the best possible treatment for ADHD, a disorder that was then, among all mental health problems, considered the most amenable to treatment (Richters et al., 1995). Over the course of the next 19 years that this study continued it produced some important results that not only improved therapeutic strategies for the management of ADHD, but also challenged the prevailing notions of the time. This chapter focuses on the results gathered from this immense, ground-breaking study, and discusses the findings from the follow-ups at childhood, adolescence, and adulthood.

OBJECTIVES

The initial idea for a randomized clinical trial to assess treatments for ADHD originated in the 1990s (Richters et al., 1995). At this time, the definitiveness of ADHD as a separate diagnostic entity already had been firmly established and the *Diagnostic and Statistical Manual of Mental Disorders-III* (DSM-III) had been in existence for three years, categorizing ADHD as a disorder in its own right. Although the confusion around changing ADHD criteria and the disorder's status as a separate entity had been resolved, other questions were yet unanswered. Foremost was the wide discrepancy in the literature regarding the treatment of ADHD, which translated to difficulty in treatment guidelines for clinical practice. It was unknown how many children received medications for ADHD. The differences in efficacy among the commonly used medications, namely, dextroamphetamine, methylphenidate, and pemoline were not well established, and it was difficult to decide on appropriate dosage standards. Apart from stimulants, studies at that time also had shown the utility of a variety of other medications such as antidepressants, clonidine, and neuroleptics. To what extent these medications were effective over and above stimulants was not known. Most importantly, the long-term efficacy of stimulants and other treatment modalities was yet to be established (Greenhill et al., 1996; Richters et al., 1995).

A major objective of the MTA trial was to establish specific treatment strategies and assess the relative effectiveness of such strategies (Arnold et al., 1997; Greenhill et al., 1996; Richters et al., 1995). At the time, several questions remained unanswered regarding response to ADHD treatments. First, it was not known to what extent age, sex, or preexisting comorbidities affected treatment response. Second, studies previously had established that therapeutic strategies produced domain specific improvements such that either symptomatology or functioning problems (academic, social, emotional, behavioral) improved. The reasons for such differential improvement with different therapeutic strategies were not known. Thus, one of the goals was to determine the best treatment combination that could improve both symptomatology and functioning in multiple domains. Third, response to existing treatments was erratic, and reasons for such were unknown. For example, aggressive behaviors could be reasonably managed by treatments. However, peer status—determined to a large extent by presence or absence of aggressive behaviors—did not improve in concert with a reduction in aggression. Fourth, it was unknown whether, and to what extent, behavior improvement in one sphere of life (classroom, playground, or family) was transferred to improvements in other spheres.

The core objectives of the MTA were thus: to determine the best possible treatment/combination of treatments that was effective in reducing ADHD symptoms as well as academic, social, and emotional problems; and, to determine whether treatment strategies should be tailored on a case-by-case basis, depending on patient characteristics such as age, gender, and preexisting comorbidities. To answer these questions, the National Institute of Mental Health funded a two-year study into assessing and comparing various treatment modalities for ADHD. After a long competitive process, six proposals were selected, based on the best, most innovative research ideas. Leading researchers from six sites across the United States and Canada set out to design this large-scale study, which began after a few months of planning, deliberating, and designing.

DESIGN

The study was designed for a two-year period during which the first 14 months were to focus on treatment regimens (telephone interviews were conducted at three and nine months into treatment), with an end-of-treatment assessment at 14 months and a follow-up 10 months after the end-of-treatment assessment (or 24 months from baseline). A total of 579 children (20% girls) with ADHD were included, aged seven to nine years, and residing with the same primary caretaker for a minimum of six preceding months. Participants were recruited from a variety of sources including mental health settings, pediatric referrals, advertisements, and school notices. All children were assessed for ADHD combined type (DSM-IV) at study entry using the parent-reported Diagnostic Interview Schedule (DISC 3.0). For cases falling below the diagnostic threshold, an additional assessment was made using teacher-reported symptomatology. Because one important aim of the study included understanding the effects of treatments on comorbidities, no attempts were made to exclude participants with comorbid oppositional defiant (ODD), conduct (CD), or anxiety disorders (Arnold et al., 1997; Hinshaw et al., 1997). Please see Figure 8.1 for further details on sample sizes at each assessment wave.

Participants were randomly assigned to one of the following treatment conditions: (1) medication management; (2) behavior therapy (This included parent training, child-focused treatment in a summer treatment program, and school-based interventions. Further details are included in the following section.); (3) Combination of medication and behavioral therapy; and (4) community care. Treatments continued for a total of 14 months. Assessments of ADHD symptomatology as well as functioning were made using self-, teacher- and parent-reports at baseline, at three months (during treatment phase), at nine months (during treatment phase), at 14 months (end of treatment), and at 24 months (10 months after treatment completion). At the end of two years, additional funding became available, allowing a naturalistic follow-up of all participants on a longer term. It was decided that continuation of the follow-ups could provide important knowledge and several benefits. As all participants were entering early adolescence—a period marked by increasing complexity of social functioning, higher risks for mental health problems and substance abuse—follow-ups could provide additional knowledge on coping during this period and also inform about the long-term effects of medications. These follow-up assessments were carried out periodically

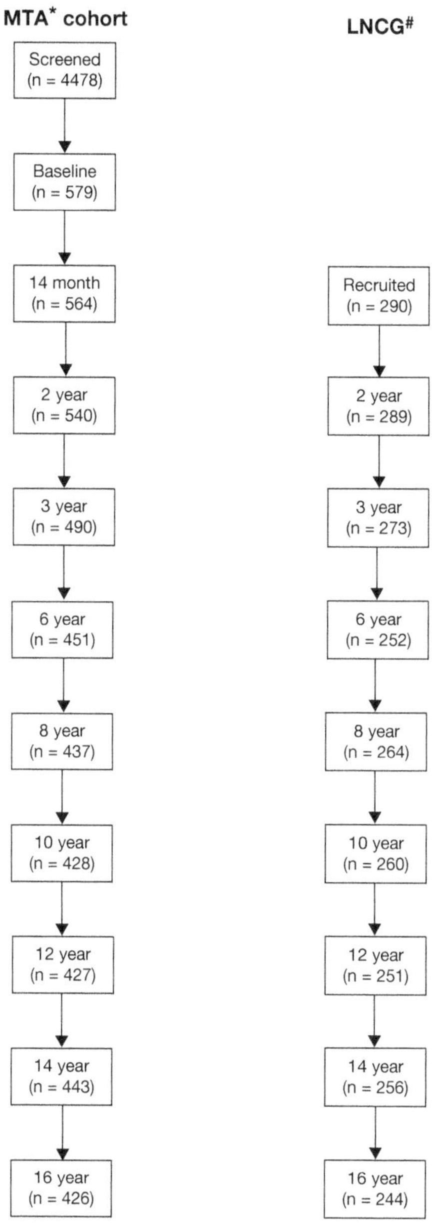

Figure 8.1 Overview of sample sizes across all assessment waves in the MTA study.
* Multimodal Treatment of ADHD.
# Local Normative Comparative Group.

during childhood at 3 years after baseline, during adolescence at 6, 8, and 10 years after baseline, and during adulthood at 12, 14, and 16 years after baseline (Arnold et al., 1997; Greenhill et al., 1996; Hinshaw et al., 1997; Jensen, 1999; MTA Cooperative Group, 1999a; MTA Cooperative Group, 1999b).

At the end of the 14-month treatment it also was decided to include an age- and sex-matched control sample: children from the same classrooms as the ADHD group but without ADHD to compare with the treatment groups. Thus, at the 24-month assessment, the Local Normative Comparative Group (LNCG) including 290 subjects was recruited. These subjects were often classmates of the participants with ADHD and were matched for age and gender. About 31 children in this group were diagnosed with ADHD and were consequently excluded. The LNCG (N = 259) group also was followed-up at similar intervals as the original MTA group.

In addition to the measures described, two additional assessments were made at a few selected sites. First, peer-nominated data on social functioning was collected from three sites at baseline and from all sites at 14 months and 24 months. The peer-nominated assessments were made on 165 children with ADHD and the same-sex classmates of each participant (n = 1,298, 21% girls) at baseline. At the 14-month and two-year assessments, sociometric measures were collected from 285 children with ADHD and the same-sex classmates of each participant with ADHD (n = 2232, 21% girls). All children were asked to name three same-sex classmates they liked most (positive nominations) and disliked most (negative nominations). In addition, children were asked to rate every peer on a 5-point scale rating from 1 = "really like" to 5 = "really dislike." Second, structural and functional brain scans were acquired from 129 participants at four sites at the 14- and 16-year follow-ups. After observing a 24-hour washout period for medications, participants underwent detailed cognitive assessments and a T1/T2-weighted Magnetic Resonance Imaging (MRI) scan. Qualitative interviews also were conducted with 125 MTA participants and 58 LNCG (n = 183) participants from four sites at the 14- and 16-year follow-ups.

TREATMENT PROTOCOL

The treatment protocol employed by the MTA was unique and based decisions on information from previous studies. Each treatment arm was designed as a management strategy (Arnold et al., 1997; Greenhill et al., 1996; Hinshaw et al., 1997; MTA Cooperative Group, 1999b; Murray et al., 2008; Vitiello et al., 2001; Wells et al., 2000; Wells, 2001). Provisions also were made to address clinical emergencies/nonattendance with a reserve capacity of eight treatment sessions per participant. Further, efforts were made to enhance compliance by providing encouragement to families and by monitoring adherence (through attendance records, salivary measurements of methylphenidate and monthly pill counts).

The medication management arm (for both medication only and combined treatment groups) required thrice daily dosing (as long-acting medications were not available at the time) and monthly monitoring through half-hour medication visits. Initially, a 28-day, double-blind titration regimen was established. Post-titration, parent- and teacher-rated ADHD symptoms were reviewed by clinicians to establish dosage requirements on a per participant basis. Methylphenidate was the drug of choice and only with nonresponse were participants titrated to other drugs (in the following order—dextroamphetamine, pemoline, imipramine). However, only methylphenidate and dextroamphetamine needed to be used.

The behavioral management arm (for both behavioral therapy only and combined groups) consisted of three distinct components: parent training, child-focused treatment, and school-based intervention. The parent-training component included 27 group sessions plus eight individual sessions with a therapist–consultant, initially on a weekly basis. The child-focused component comprised an eight-week summer treatment program that included interventions for eight hours per day, five days per week. In the summer treatment program, the first half of each day was spent in a classroom setting where academic and organizational skills were taught. The second half of the day was spent in sport with an emphasis on social skills. The school-based intervention component comprised a daily report card, which was completed by the teacher as well as assessed and re-evaluated by the parents at home. Additionally, paraprofessional aid (usually by counsellors from the summer treatment program) was provided in the classroom for half a day, five days per week. The trained paraprofessional aides assisted children in implementing the social and organizational skills learned during the summer treatment program in their actual school settings.

The combined management arm required additional considerations to make the therapies comparable to the medication only and behavioral only treatments. This involved integrating the medication and behavioral therapies with adjustment of dosage levels, and regular communication among the various treatment providers (teachers, consultants, and pharmacotherapists).

Participants randomized to the community care group received whichever treatment parents preferred or arranged for their children in the community. All participants in this arm received a list of community mental health resources and reports on their initial study assessments. About 67% of participants in this group received some form of ADHD medication from their community health provider during the MTA treatment phase.

RESULTS

Childhood Outcomes

Results from the childhood assessments showed that up to a third of the MTA sample already had received psychoactive medication prior to being randomized. Comorbidity was also high at the time of entry among participants; using the Diagnostic Interview Schedule for Children (DISC), it was revealed that 40% suffered from additional Oppositional Defiant Disorder (DSM-IV), 14% from Conduct Disorder (DSM-IV), and 34% from anxiety disorders (DSM-III-R) (Table 8.1) (Jensen et al., 2001; C. G. MTA., 1999; Swanson, Arnold, Kraemer, Hechtman, Molina, Hinshaw, Vitiello, Jensen, Steinhoff, Lerner, and Greenhill, MTA Cooperative Group, 2008a; Swanson, Arnold, Kraemer, Hechtman, Molina, Hinshaw,

TABLE 8.1

BASELINE CHARACTERISTICS OF PARTICIPANTS IN THE FOUR RANDOMIZED GROUPS

	Randomly Assigned Treatment Groups			
Variables	Medication Management n = 144	Behavioral Management n = 144	Combined Therapy n = 145	Community Care n = 146
Age (in years), Mean ± SD	8.6 ± 0.8	8.3 ± 0.8	8.4 ± 0.8	8.5 ± 0.5
Girls, N (%)	26 (18)	30 (21)	31 (21)	27 (19)
INATTENTION[1], MEAN ± SD				
Parent-reported	2.03 ± 0.64	1.99 ± 0.63	2.07 ± 0.61	2.05 ± 0.65
Teacher-reported	2.27 ± 0.61	2.28 ± 0.64	2.16 ± 0.67	2.19 ± 0.69
HYPERACTIVITY/IMPULSIVITY[1], MEAN ± SD				
Parent-reported	1.89 ± 0.62	1.89 ± 0.64	1.91 ± 0.69	1.95 ± 0.67
Teacher-reported	2.08 ± 0.71	2.05 ± 0.75	1.89 ± 0.77	1.93 ± 0.81
COMORBIDITY[2], N (%)				
Anxiety Disorders	52 (36)	50 (35)	50 (35)	42 (29)
Conduct Disorder	23 (16)	18 (13)	20 (14)	22 (15)
Oppositional Defiant Disorder	55 (38)	60 (42)	53 (37)	63 (43)
Affective problems	5 (3)	5 (4)	5 (4)	7 (5)
Tics	11 (8)	14 (10)	19 (13)	19 (13)
Mania/hypomania	2 (1)	6 (4)	5 (4)	0 (0)

[1] Assessed with the Swanson, Nolan, & Pelham scale (SNAP).

[2] Assessed with the Diagnostic Interview Schedule for Children (DISC 3.0).

Vitiello, Jensen, Steinhoff, Lerner, and Greenhill, MTA Cooperative Group, 2008b).

Initial analyses included assessments of outcomes through four time-points: baseline, three months into treatment, nine months into treatment, and at the end of treatment (14 months after baseline). The effects of treatment were assessed on outcomes of ADHD symptoms (Swanson,

Nolan, & Pelham scale or SNAP), behaviors (Classroom Observation Code or COC), oppositional/aggressive symptoms (SNAP), internalizing problems (Social Skills Rating System or SSRS/Multidimensional anxiety scale or MASC), parent–child relationships (Parent–Child Relationship Questionnaire or PCRQ), social skills (SSRS), and academic achievement (Wechsler Individual Achievement Test or WIAT).

Early results (between baseline and 14-month follow-up) showed that all participants improved in ADHD symptomatology and functioning over time. Participants differed, however, in the extent to which they improved and this was determined by their treatment groups. Children in the medication management and combined therapy groups showed the largest improvement in symptoms of hyperactivity and inattention. A closer examination revealed that combination therapy was slightly superior to medication management alone; combined treatments provided greater improvements in oppositional/aggressive symptoms, internalizing symptoms, reading achievement, and parent child relations. Importantly, combined therapy achieved similar ADHD symptom improvement as medication management at lower stimulant dosages. Results further showed that behavioral therapy alone did not provide substantial symptom improvement, but was superior to community care in improving parent–child relations.

Up to two thirds of participants in the community care group received medication. Nevertheless, the community care group showed less improvement in ADHD symptoms and functioning outcomes than the combined care and medication management groups. Additional analyses were carried out to understand how the combined and medication therapy arms proved superior to community care despite participants in community care receiving medications for ADHD. These analyses showed that children receiving medications in the community care group showed greater symptom improvement than children not receiving medications in community care. Further, the medicated community care subgroup showed similar improvements as the behavior management only group, but yet was inferior to the medication management group. It was speculated that the superiority of the MTA management over usual community care may have been contributed by the following: medication was often not well titrated in the community with usually no input from the school, and little to no monitoring after initial prescription to adjust dosages and deal with side effects. Furthermore, the tailored dosage regimens and intense thrice per day dosing in the combined and medicated groups also may have contributed to the differences noted (Jensen, 1999; MTA Cooperative Group, 1999a; Pelham, 1999).

Analyses were carried out to assess the influence of medication adherence and several other baseline variables on treatment effects. First, medication adherence was defined for two groups: those receiving treatment at "as-intended" or "below-intended" levels. Cut-offs for as-intended treatment in the medicated group were established with a minimum of 80% family attendance for the monthly medication visits, and with prescriptions written and delivered to families during these visits. For the behavioral treatment, "as-intended" cut-offs were established for a minimum of 75% attendance. Results revealed that as-intended treatments were superior to below-intended treatments (in both combined and medication management groups) in improving ADHD symptoms. Second, influences of gender, prior medication status, comorbidities, and use of public assistance on treatment effects were determined. Participants' gender, use of medications prior to randomization, and presence of comorbid ODD/CD did not influence effects of treatments. Presence of comorbid anxiety, however, moderated the effects of treatment such that ADHD and internalizing symptom improvement produced by medication only and combined management groups was comparable to that of behavioral therapy (in comorbid anxious subgroups). A comparison of participants with comorbid ODD and comorbid ODD plus anxiety showed differential response to treatments—while children with comorbid ODD responded best to medication management, those with comorbid anxiety plus ODD responded best to combined therapy. Finally, use of public assistance also influenced the effects of treatment groups. Participants in the combined therapy group who received public assistance showed an improvement in their social skills (MTA Cooperative Group, 1999; Owens et al., 2003).

At 24 months (ten months after end of treatment), 93% of the original sample was reassessed for effects of treatments on ADHD symptomatology and functioning outcomes (MTA Cooperative Group, 2004a; Murray et al., 2008). None of the treatments had an effect on academic achievement or social skills. ADHD and ODD symptom scores, however, differed among the four groups. The initial symptom improvements noticed in all four groups had diminished in intensity by this time point. Instead, only children in the combined and medication management arms continued to show significant ADHD symptom improvements, albeit with reduced effects: differences in effect sizes between the medicated and nonmedicated groups were halved as compared to effects at the 14-month assessments. The marginal superiority of the combined therapy over medication management, seen at 14 months, disappeared by this time. Furthermore, the superiority of behavioral therapy over community care also had disappeared by 24 months (MTA Cooperative Group, 2004b).

Assessments at 24 months also showed a pattern of increasing medication use in groups not previously medicated, namely, community care and behavioral therapy arms. On the other hand, participants randomized to receive medications (combined and medication management groups) reduced medication consumption. Despite a reduction, rate of medication use by participants and dosages prescribed were higher in the combined and medication management groups than in the community care and behavior therapy groups. This partly contributed to the enduring superiority of combined care and medication management groups in reducing ADHD and ODD symptoms. Additional analyses showed that previously unmedicated children, upon beginning medication, improved significantly in their symptoms. Conversely, previously medicated children either continuing or stopping medications showed a moderate-to-severe deterioration in their symptoms. Analyses of medication use in this manner also revealed a serious side effect—consistently medicated children showed growth suppression, while children with ADHD who never received medications had normal growth levels (MTA Cooperative Group, 2004b).

At 36 months after baseline, 83.8% of the original MTA sample was reassessed for ADHD symptoms, ODD symptoms, reading ability, social skills, and a measure of overall functional impairment (Jensen et al., 2007). The effects of combined, medication, and psychosocial therapy disappeared completely and none of the treatment arms showed any differences in ADHD symptomatology. Instead all four treatment groups showed similar improvements between baseline and the 36-month follow-up in domains of ADHD symptoms, ODD symptoms, reading ability, and social skills. Additionally, all treatment groups showed a reduction in comorbidity rates between baseline and three years. To further understand these effects, the use of medications after the MTA treatment was ascertained, and the effects of such medication use were assessed. It was found that taking medications continuously, as opposed to not taking any medications, was likely to reduce ADHD symptoms. The effects of continuous medication on symptoms occurred irrespective of initial randomization and across all groups. Additional findings at the 36-month follow-up related to the effects of sex, public assistance use, and parental inattention on outcomes. Across all treatment groups, boys and participants on public assistance were less likely to improve in their ADHD/ODD symptoms and social skills than girls and children not on assistance. Similarly, children of parents with inattention problems did not improve in their ADHD symptoms and reading abilities, irrespective of initial treatment group assignment.

Apart from effects of medications on ADHD symptomatology, assessments also focused on substance use patterns, aggressive–delinquent behaviors, and social functioning among children with ADHD. Also between the 14- and 36-month outcomes, details of the LNCG group became available, allowing direct comparisons of the MTA group with children without ADHD. It was found that approximately a fifth of children with ADHD reported illicit substance use as opposed to less than a tenth of children from the LNCG. Between a quarter to a third of children from the MTA group had engaged in delinquent behavior, while less than a tenth of children from the LNCG reported delinquency (Molina et al., 2007). Sociometric data revealed that children with ADHD were more likely to be perceived negatively by peers, to have a lower peer status, and to have fewer friends than same-sex classmates (Hoza et al., 2005; Hoza et al., 2005). Further, rejection and negative peer imbalance (difference between peer scores given to others as opposed to scores received) distinguished between children with and without ADHD (Mrug et al., 2009). Randomized treatments were found to have no effect on substance use, delinquency, or peer-nominated social functioning measures at 36 months post baseline (Hoza et al., 2005; Hoza et al., 2005; Jensen et al., 2001; Molina et al., 2007).

Medications did not seem to affect function and symptom severity beyond 24 months (Arnold et al., 2004; Jensen et al., 2007), but did have more persistent effects on children's growth (Swanson et al., 2007). Height and weight of children receiving medications was lower than those not receiving any medications, and did not catch up to normal levels after treatments were completed. The largest growth suppression was present in children who were consistently medicated starting before randomization. Growth of children newly started on medications lagged by approximately 2 cm fewer and 2.7 kg less than unmedicated children.

Adolescent Outcomes

Assessments between six and ten years after baseline included 80% participants from the original MTA cohort and 90% from the LNCG (mean age 13–18 years). Initially assigned groups did not differ in medication use by six to eight years and about a third of all participants were receiving stimulants for at least 50% of the days in a year. No effects of initial MTA treatments on ADHD symptomatology were found at these follow-ups. Assessments of comorbidity, reading achievement, and social skills also did not differ among the four assigned treatment groups. Adolescents from the MTA groups continued to show significant impairment in several functioning domains as compared with adolescents from the LNCG group, suggesting that normalization of symptoms did not occur by this age (Molina et al., 2009). Further, participants who had consistently taken medications for their symptoms were shorter in stature than unmedicated participants with a childhood history of ADHD.

Changes in adolescents' self-perceived symptomatology and functioning were assessed and these showed significantly positive and biased estimations. Participants from the MTA had a high self-perceived social functioning that did not change much between childhood and adolescence. Participants from the LNCG, on the other hand, accurately estimated their social standing with only slightly biased assessments at early adolescence. It was suggested that the positively biased opinions were self-protective. Further, for children with ADHD, biased self-estimations of social standing was related to aggressive behaviors. It was speculated that behavioral problems, such as aggression, may lead to self-protective biases about social functioning. Contrary to the social domain, however, positively biased estimations of behavior competence in childhood had normalized by adolescence in the MTA sample. It was suggested, in line with the self-protection theory, that only developmentally important domains (social and not behavioral functioning in adolescence) show biased estimations. Positively biased self-estimations also proved to increase the risk for aggressive behaviors and did not protect against depression at adolescence (Hoza et al., 2010).

By early adolescence, participants with ADHD were approximately twice as likely to consume substances (alcohol, tobacco, marijuana and to a lesser extent opioids, narcotics, hallucinogens, etc.) than participants in the LNCG group. The risk for substance use was high for both boys and girls with ADHD. Among the participants in the MTA group, none of the four original treatment subgroups differed in substance use patterns at adolescence. Initial treatments did not affect substance use between six and ten years at follow-up. Substance use patterns were reanalyzed after regrouping adolescents based on medication use since baseline. Medication use (including prior to and after randomization) did not influence substance use patterns at adolescence (Molina et al., 2013).

Adulthood Outcomes

At 12, 14, and 16 years after baseline, 82% participants from the MTA group and 93% participants from the LNCG group were reassessed for ADHD symptomatology and a variety of other functioning outcomes. Because all participants were more than 18 years (mean age 27.4 years) of age, questionnaires were modified for adult assessments. An observer (parent) as well as self-rated Conner's Adult ADHD Rating Scale (CAARS) showed continuing ADHD symptoms in participants from the MTA group (Sibley et al., submitted; Swanson et al., submitted). Importantly, using DSM-5 criteria, only half of all individuals in the original MTA treatment groups remitted while the other half presented with symptomatic ADHD. Groups were defined as persistent or remitted via either self- or observer- (usually parent) reported CAARS scores, only when information from both sources was present. As found in the childhood and adolescent follow-ups, severity of ADHD symptoms assessed with self- and parent- (or observer-) reports showed a wide divergence (Swanson et al., submitted). The discrepancy between self- and observer-rated ADHD symptoms has been well established for children and adolescents. It was speculated, however, that these differences would diminish by adulthood. Contrary to these expectations, adults with ADHD continued to under-report their symptoms. Parent-reported symptomatology, on the other hand, remained higher than self-reports and correlated well with functional impairments. Further, initial treatment group randomization did not seem to influence symptoms in adulthood. More interestingly, the age-related improvement in ADHD symptoms, seen in childhood, also was not sustained. Thus, adults (at least half of the sample) continued to be symptomatic.

As in the childhood and adolescent follow-ups, no effects of initial randomized treatments were found on symptomatology or functioning. In adulthood, differences between the MTA and the LNCG groups were found consistently. LNCG adults achieved higher educational attainments, had higher incomes, were less often without employment, were less likely to have substance use problems (substance use disorders from the Diagnostic Interview Schedule for Children–Youth Assessment), had fewer run-ins with law enforcement, and showed less emotional lability (Conners' Adult ADHD Rating Scale—emotional/lability subscale and Neo-Five Factor Inventory—Neuroticism subscale) than the MTA participants (Hechtman et al., submitted). Further, a childhood diagnosis of ADHD was associated with poor cognitive functioning at adulthood, especially in domains of working memory, verbal memory, decision-making, and response inhibition (Tamm et al., 2013). In terms of mood and anxiety problems, however, both LNCG and MTA adults fared equally well (Hechtman et al., submitted). Further, differences in adulthood functioning were present between those with and without concurrent ADHD symptoms, and three consistent patterns of adulthood functioning were found upon comparing symptom persistent, remittent, and LNCG participants (Hechtman et al., submitted).

The first, most common pattern was one in which the LNCG group fared the best, the symptom persistent ADHD subgroup the worst, and the symptom remittent ADHD subgroup performed in-between the LNCG and the persisters. (Please see Figure 8.2, Figure 8.3, and Figure 8.4 for examples of the three functioning patterns.) Thus, the largest effect sizes (of differences) were found between the LNCG and the symptom persistent ADHD subgroup. This pattern was found for outcomes of educational,

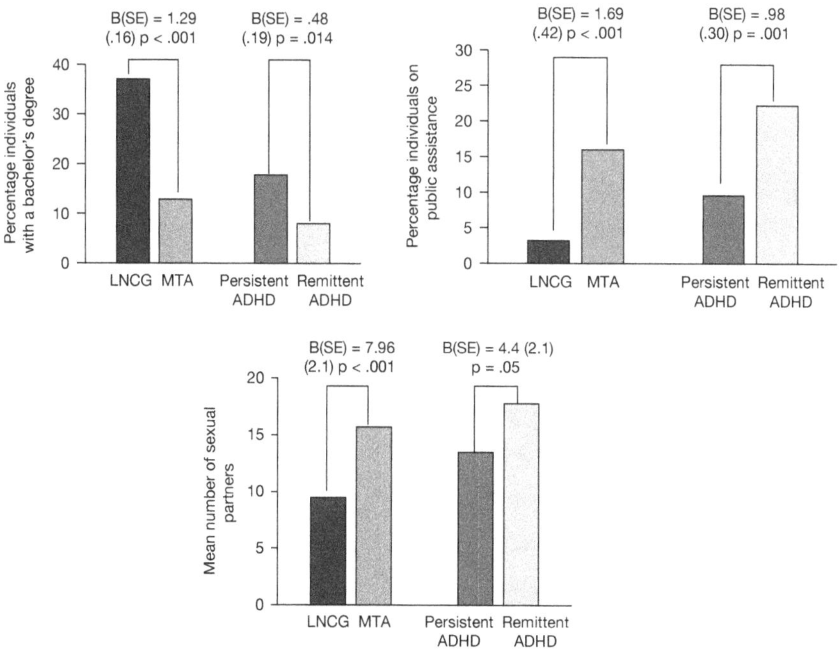

Figure 8.2 Patterns of adult outcomes—type 1: comparison of adult outcomes in MTA versus LNCG groups and in persistent versus remitted participants with childhood ADHD. See also color plate section.

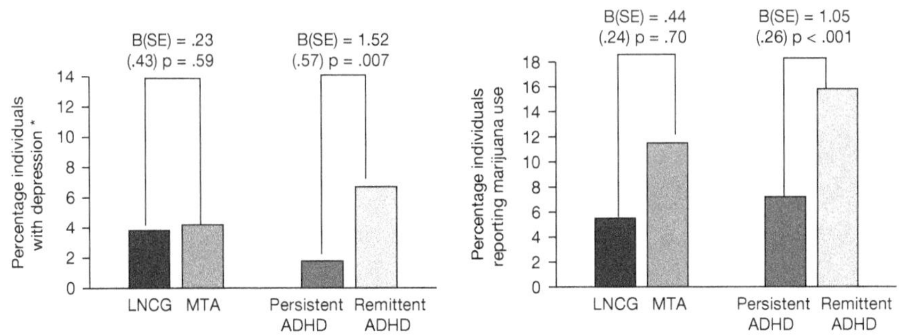

Figure 8.3 Patterns of adult outcomes—type 2: comparison of adult outcomes in MTA versus LNCG groups and in persistent versus remitted participants with childhood ADHD. See also color plate section.

occupational, and sexual functioning. In the educational domain, 37.1% of the participants from the LNCG group obtained a bachelor's degree compared with 17.8% from the symptom remittent subgroup and only 8% from the symptom persistent subgroup. For the occupational domain, participants from the symptom persistent subgroup had the highest rates of quitting their jobs/being fired, the lowest income levels, and were most likely to be on public assistance, as opposed to participants from the symptom remittent and LNCG subgroups. For example, 22.6% of the symptom persistent ADHD subgroup was on public assistance as compared with 9.6% of the symptom remittent subgroup and 3.2% of the LNCG group. In the sexual functioning domains, ADHD was associated with younger age at first intercourse, a higher number of sexual partners, increased risk

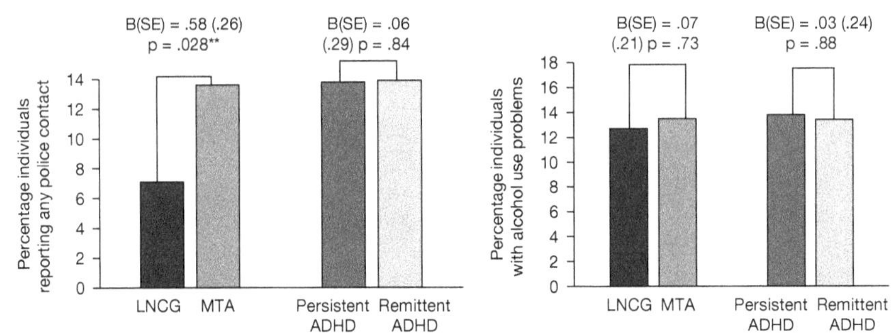

Figure 8.4 Patterns of adult outcomes—type 3: comparison of adult outcomes in MTA versus LNCG groups and in persistent versus remitted participants with childhood ADHD. See also color plate section.

of pregnancy, and greater numbers of offspring by age 18 than the LNCG group. The symptom persistent and remittent subgroups differed significantly in age at first sexual intercourse and differed marginally in number of partners. Effect sizes were small to medium. This pattern illustrates that even if symptoms remit, the negative impact of early ADHD symptoms is still seen even though the functional effects are much less marked than with symptom persistence.

The second pattern was one in which the LNCG and symptom-desistent groups showed comparable outcomes and both differed from the symptom persistent group. This pattern was seen for outcomes of emotional lability, neuroticism, and anxiety, mood, and substance-use disorders. For example, the ADHD group as a whole (including persisters and remitters) performed worse than the LNCG group in impulsivity/emotional lability and neuroticism, but not in mood or anxiety problems. The symptom persistent ADHD subgroup, however, performed worse than the symptom desistant group on assessments of impulsivity/emotional lability and neuroticism and also endorsed higher rates of mood (7.8% vs. 1.8%) and anxiety problems (14.2% vs. 5%). Participants from the symptom desistant group, in turn, performed comparable to the LNCG participants in the same outcome domains. For substance use, however, the LNCG and ADHD groups (including persisters and remitters) did not differ significantly. Nevertheless, the symptom persistent subgroup differed significantly from the remittent and LNCG subgroups; persisters as compared to remitters showed higher rates of marijuana use problems (26.7% vs. 14%), other substance use problems (8.3% vs. 1.9%), and any substance use problem (38.5% vs. 28.7%). The symptom remittent subgroup, in turn, was comparable to the LNCG subgroup. The second pattern suggests that persistent ADHD symptoms continue to have an impact on emotional and substance use, but past ADHD symptoms may not have any residual effects on functioning in these domains. This illustrates the value of differentiating between persisters and remitters in examining functional outcomes.

The third pattern was characterized by a lack of any significant differences among the three subgroups. This pattern was seen for outcomes of police contact, jail time, and alcohol use disorder. The total number of police contacts as well as time spent in jail was comparable between the ADHD and LNCG groups. Alcohol use, common at this age (young adulthood), also did not differ among participants.

Lastly and though not statistically significant, the ADHD group faced a higher number of deaths (three suicides, four homicides, two deaths due to driving under influence, one hit and run; total ten deaths) than the LNCG group (one suicide). This higher death rate in the ADHD group is a serious concern, which needs further research and must be clinically addressed.

Predictors of Attention Deficit Hyperactivity Disorder Symptom Severity and Persistence

Symptoms of ADHD showed different patterns with time among subgroups of the MTA sample. Three classes of children could be defined based on symptom changes between baseline, through the treatment phase, and up to the 36-month follow-up. The first class of children constituted a third of the total sample and were characterized by a gradual and linearly improving symptom profile over time. The second class, the largest and representing half of the sample, showed a dramatic symptom improvement by end of treatment followed by maintenance of symptoms at the same level till 36 months. The third and smallest class, constituting about a seventh of the entire sample, showed an initial symptom improvement followed by deterioration and return to pretreatment ADHD symptom levels. Each of these three classes differed in a number of baseline characteristics. The largest proportion of the sample with dramatic and significant symptom improvement (and which was maintained over time) was characterized by low ADHD symptomatology and psychopathology and fewer problem behaviors at baseline. Further, children in this class had higher birth weights, IQ, and social skills than children from the other groups. This class also had a preponderance of participants on combined and medication therapies as opposed to behavioral and community care therapies. Thus, assignment to combined management or medication management groups increased chances of having significant and sustained symptom improvement. The smallest class, with post-treatment symptom worsening, was associated with higher baseline ADHD symptoms, lower IQ, and poorer social skills than the other two groups (Jensen et al., 2007; Swanson, Hinshaw et al., 2007).

Despite initial improvements across all three classes, ADHD symptom levels in these children were higher than those seen in the LNCG group. Similar to the previous analysis, randomized treatments were associated with symptom improvement in all three classes at 14 months. Further, and again similar to previous results, symptom improvements with randomly assigned treatments were halved in all three classes at the 24-month time-point. At 36 months though, the effects of treatments on ADHD symptoms differed among the three latent classes. About a third of the children from class one (gradual and linearly improving profile) continued to benefit from the MTA treatments at the 36-month follow-up. For the other two classes though, and as seen before, no effects of treatments remained at the 36-month assessment. A closer examination of these differences revealed that actual medication use* also continued to benefit children from class 1 but not children from class 2 or class 3 at the 36-month assessment (Swanson, Hinshaw et al., 2007).

These three childhood-symptom based classes were more accurate at predicting adolescent ADHD severity than the other randomized treatment variables. Children from the second class with the largest childhood improvement continued having lower symptom scores than the other two classes. Children in the smallest class, with a rebound in their symptoms, performed worst in terms of symptom severity at adolescence (Molina et al., 2009).

Predictors of Functioning Difficulties

Symptom Severity

ADHD symptom severity in childhood showed three distinct patterns or classes (Swanson, Hinshaw et al., 2007), which were further associated with

* Use of medication, or lack thereof, was not strictly adhered to according to the random group assignment during 14 months of treatment. The actual use of medication between baseline and the 36-month assessments was determined using the Services for Children and Adolescents Parent Interview or SCAPI.

functioning in adolescence. Children with dramatic symptom improvement in childhood showed low ODD scores, aggression problems, police contact, use of school service, or grade retention. Children with the least improvement in ADHD symptoms showed the worst functioning in the above mentioned domains at adolescence, while those with a linearly improving ADHD profile had functioning scores intermediate to those of the other two classes (Molina et al., 2009).

Social Functioning

Social functioning of children with ADHD during childhood was found to be an important indicator of functioning in later life. Children with ADHD who were peer rejected were likely to suffer from delinquency, substance abuse, and anxiety problems at mid adolescence, and had poorer ratings on global functioning measures than children with (near) normal social standing. Friendships did not seem to protect from the detrimental effects of childhood peer rejection (Mrug et al., 2012).

Positive Illusory Bias

A positive self-illusory bias was another indicator of poor adjustment among MTA participants. Positively biased estimations of behavior (in childhood) was associated with driving problems such as driving infraction, receiving tickets, or having one's license revoked. Further, positively biased estimations of behavioral and academic competence partly mediated the relationship between childhood ADHD and risky sexual behaviors at adolescence (Hoza et al., 2013).

Effects of positive social biases on childhood functioning were examined, keeping in consideration actual competence levels (McQuade et al., 2014). As none of the four treatment arms had an effect on children's positive biases, participants from all treatment groups were assessed as a group and compared with the LNCG (Hoza et al., 2004). A high perception of social competence was associated with aggression among children with ADHD, especially for those who had a high peer standing. However, high social success combined with moderate self-perceptions protected against aggressive behaviors in childhood. The association of positive bias with depressive outcomes also was moderated by levels of actual competence. Positive social biases protected against childhood depression only among children with ADHD whose actual social competence was low. Conversely, children without a positive bias and with low social competence showed high levels of depression. For children in the LNCG group, however, self-perceptions of social competence did not seem to affect depressive scores (McQuade et al., 2014).

Other Predictors

Apart from social functioning and ADHD severity, other baseline factors influenced outcomes and are worthy of mention. First, perinatal problems, such as infant breathing difficulties and early labor, increased risk for childhood comorbid depression (Owens & Hinshaw, 2013). Next, baseline factors such as a higher parental education level, good homework management, and higher teacher-rated classroom performance was associated with higher school grades. Academic functioning, however, as measured by the Wechsler Individual Achievement Test (WIAT) was unrelated to most factors that predicted good school grades. Apart from classroom performance, a low family income, low IQ, requirement for special education services, and inattention symptoms were associated with low scores on the WIAT. It was suggested that skill sets required to attain school grades differed widely from those that contributed to good achievement test scores. School performance also was found to be moderated by sex, such that girls with ADHD performed somewhat worse than boys with ADHD (Langberg et al., 2011).

CONCLUSIONS

The most important conclusions to be drawn from the MTA study relate to the use of medications in the management of ADHD. Medications alone or a combination of medication and behavioral therapy produced dramatic improvements in symptoms while functioning in academic, social, and emotional domains was influenced most by combined therapy (MTA Cooperative Group, 1999a; MTA Cooperative Group, 1999b). The effects of these treatments wore off after cessation of therapy (Jensen et al., 2007), most likely due to discontinuation of long-term treatment adherence. The treatment strategy used in the MTA was an improvement over interventions commonly available at the time. Further, suspicions of stimulant medications influencing substance use/abuse were put to rest (Molina et al., 2013). Previous to the MTA, it was well established that ADHD symptoms increased risk of substance abuse. It was hypothesized at the time that treatment with stimulants, which reduced ADHD symptoms, should reduce the risk of substance use, too. A second line of hypothesis suggested that stimulant medication actually may increase risk for substance abuse. Both were shown to be incorrect because medications neither contributed to nor attenuated the risk for substance abuse at adolescence (Molina et al., 2013).

Effectiveness of medications, at least in the short-term, was dependent on the intensity and duration of such therapy (MTA Cooperative Group, 1999a; MTA Cooperative Group, 1999b). As results showed, the higher and repeated dosing schedule used in the MTA was superior to the medication management used in community care. Further, regular monitoring of medication adherence, with assessments of effectiveness and side effects produced greater benefits. Importantly, effectiveness of treatment depended on existing comorbidity (MTA Cooperative Group, 1999a). Children with ODD responded best to medication management. Among children with comorbid anxiety, however, behavior therapy alone was beneficial. Children with comorbid ODD plus anxiety responded best to interventions that combined medication and behavior therapy.

Although medications produced the best outcomes among all other forms of therapy, a few disadvantages were evident. First, long-term and persistent improvements in symptoms did not occur (Jensen et al., 2007; Swanson, Hinshaw et al., 2007; Swanson et al., submitted). This may have ensued due to a lack of effective medication treatment; after 14 months, that is, at the end of treatment, all participants in the medication group were treated in the community where optimal titration and monitoring for adherence and side effects did not occur. Further, the use of medications decreased over time to 8% by adulthood. Second, significant growth suppression occurred with use of medications (Greenhill et al., submitted;

Swanson et al., 2007). Growth suppression was exacerbated when medication was started early and was consistently adhered to without interruptions (Greenhill et al., submitted). Conversely, intermittent medication resulted in fewer growth suppression problems. Third, it was found difficult to maintain adherence to medications in the long-term (Molina et al., 2009; Pappadopulos et al., 2009).

The MTA study with its multiple, longitudinal follow-ups over 16 years produced some important insights into time-dependent changes in ADHD symptomatology and long-term functioning. An age-dependent reduction in ADHD symptomatology was present in all affected individuals (Swanson et al., submitted). There was, however, a divergence in individual profiles of improvement between adolescence and adulthood. Only half of all individuals with childhood ADHD improved sufficiently and normalized. For the other half, symptoms persisted into adulthood (Sibley et al., submitted; Swanson et al., submitted). The results from this study pertain to early adulthood, and it is possible that a longer follow-up will show further changes in these profiles. Future studies may assess the normalization of ADHD symptoms into mid- and late-adulthood to determine whether symptom changes occur throughout life and are not resistant to change later in adulthood.

The longitudinal follow-ups were also informative regarding age-dependent changes in positive illusory biases, which differed according to the affected functioning domain. Although behavioral biases declined between childhood and adolescence, social biases continued into adolescence and were self-protective in nature (Hoza et al., 2013). Biases regarding ADHD symptomatology, too, continued long-term into adulthood, and a high discrepancy was found between self- and observer-rated ADHD symptom score in the adulthood follow-ups (Swanson et al., submitted). Further, observer ratings of symptomatology correlated well with functioning problems. This has important implications for clinical decisions such that the under-reporting of symptoms by adults with ADHD must be considered while making diagnostic and treatment decisions. Moreover, there may be a need for additional observer evidence to determine true functioning levels. The implications of persistent biases in social functioning and symptoms are yet to be understood in detail and the effects of such biases on long-term mental health and functioning should be explored in future studies.

In sum, our current understanding of the long-term outcomes of ADHD leaves much to be desired: in terms of interindividual variability as well as time-dependent changes seen in various functioning domains. Improved insights into the natural course of this disorder are necessary for development of efficient therapies that can provide enduring benefits. ADHD is a chronic condition that requires regular, consistent, and ongoing treatment that is titrated and monitored for side effects. Furthermore, an effective treatment regimen requires inclusion of psychosocial therapy such as training for time management, organizational skills, social skills, and emotional regulation, in order to improve long-term outcomes. An early cessation of treatment (as with the 14-month treatment regimen in the MTA) may result in relapse of symptoms and impairment. The MTA study clearly showed that medication treatment in the community was not as effective as the multimodal treatment provided in the study, because the former lacked careful titration, monitoring, and dose adjustments for efficacy and side effects. Thus, after 14 months, when participants were no longer provided treatments in the MTA study, all children received treatment in the community. Consequently, differences in the initially randomized treatment groups (or improvement in ADHD symptoms) disappeared. In future, more studies are required to substantiate the benefits of long-term, well-monitored treatments for individuals with ADHD. Simultaneously, efforts must be made to develop newer treatment modalities that aim to reduce not only symptoms of ADHD but also the accompanying functioning difficulties that are all too common. Thus, treatments must be effective, multimodal, and ongoing in order to bring about more positive long-term outcomes.

REFERENCES

Arnold, L. E., Abikoff, H. B., Cantwell, D. P., Conners, C. K., Elliott, G., Greenhill, L. L., . . . Wells, K. C. (1997). National Institute of Mental Health collaborative Multimodal Treatment Study of Children with ADHD (the MTA). Design challenges and choices. *Archives of General Psychiatry*, *54*(9), 865–870.

Arnold, L. E., Chuang, S., Davies, M., Abikoff, H. B., Conners, C. K., Elliott, G. R., . . . Wigal, T. (2004). Nine months of multicomponent behavioral treatment for ADHD and effectiveness of MTA fading procedures. *Journal of Abnormal Child Psychology, 32*(1), 39–51.

Greenhill, L. L., Abikoff, H. B., Arnold, L. E., Cantwell, D. P., Conners, C. K., Elliott, G., . . . Wells, K. (1996). Medication treatment strategies in the MTA study: Relevance to clinicians and researchers. *Journal of the American Academy of Child and Adolescent Psychiatry, 35*(10), 1304–1313. doi:S0890-8567(09)63633-9 [pii]

Greenhill, L. L., Swanson, J. M., Waxmonsky, J., Hechtman, L., Arnold, L. E., Wigal, T., . . . Hinshaw, S. P. (2016). Long-term effects of stimulant medication treatment in the MTA: Longitudinal analyses of height velocity changes through the 10-year follow-up. Manuscript submitted for publication.

Hechtman, L., Swanson, J., Sibley, M. H., Stehli, A., Arnold, L. E., Owens, E. B., . . . Lakes, K. D. Functional adult outcomes 16 years after childhood diagnosis of attention-deficit/hyperactivity disorder: MTA results. (2016). Manuscript submitted for publication.

Hinshaw, S., March, J. S., Abikoff, H., Arnold, L., Cantwell, D., Conners, C., . . . Hechtman, L. (1997). Comprehensive assessment of childhood attention-deficit hyperactivity disorder in the context of a multisite, multimodal clinical trial. *Journal of Attention Disorders, 1*(4), 217–234.

Hoza, B., Gerdes, A. C., Hinshaw, S. P., Arnold, L. E., Pelham, W. E., Jr., Molina, B. S., . . . Wigal, T. (2004). Self-perceptions of competence in children with ADHD and comparison children. *Journal of Consulting and Clinical Psychology, 72*(3), 382–391. doi:10.1037/0022-006X.72.3.382 [doi]

Hoza, B., Gerdes, A. C., Mrug, S., Hinshaw, S. P., Bukowski, W. M., Gold, J. A., . . . Wigal, T. (2005). Peer-assessed outcomes in the Multimodal Treatment Study of Children with Attention Deficit Hyperactivity Disorder. *Journal of Clinical Child and Adolescent Psychology, 34*(1), 74–86. doi:10.1207/s15374424jccp3401_7 [doi]

Hoza, B., McQuade, J. D., Murray-Close, D., Shoulberg, E., Molina, B. S., Arnold, L. E., . . . Hechtman, L. (2013). Does childhood positive self-perceptual bias mediate adolescent risky behavior in youth from the MTA study? *Journal of Consulting and Clinical Psychology, 81*(5), 846–858. doi:10.1037/a0033536 [doi]

Hoza, B., Mrug, S., Gerdes, A. C., Hinshaw, S. P., Bukowski, W. M., Gold, J. A., . . . Arnold, L. E. (2005). What aspects of peer relationships are impaired in children with attention-deficit/hyperactivity disorder? *Journal of Consulting and Clinical Psychology, 73*(3), 411–423. doi:2005-06517-004 [pii]

Hoza, B., Murray-Close, D., Arnold, L. E., Hinshaw, S. P., Hechtman, L., & MTA Cooperative Group. (2010). Time-dependent changes in positively biased self-perceptions of children with attention-deficit/hyperactivity disorder: A developmental psychopathology perspective. *Development and Psychopathology, 22*(2), 375–390. doi:10.1017/S095457941000012X [doi]

Jensen, P. S. (1999). Fact versus fancy concerning the multimodal treatment study for attention-deficit hyperactivity disorder. *Canadian Journal of Psychiatry. Revue Canadienne De Psychiatrie, 44*(10), 975–980.

Jensen, P. S., Arnold, L. E., Swanson, J. M., Vitiello, B., Abikoff, H. B., Greenhill, L. L., . . . Hur, K. (2007). 3-year follow-up of the NIMH MTA study. *Journal of the*

American Academy of Child and Adolescent Psychiatry, *46*(8), 989–1002. doi:10.1097/CHI.0b013e3180686d48 [doi]

Jensen, P. S., Hinshaw, S. P., Swanson, J. M., Greenhill, L. L., Conners, C. K., Arnold, L. E., . . . Wigal, T. (2001). Findings from the NIMH multimodal treatment study of ADHD (MTA): Implications and applications for primary care providers. *Journal of Developmental and Behavioral Pediatrics*, *22*(1), 60–73.

Langberg, J. M., Molina, B. S., Arnold, L. E., Epstein, J. N., Altaye, M., Hinshaw, S. P., . . . Hechtman, L. (2011). Patterns and predictors of adolescent academic achievement and performance in a sample of children with attention-deficit/hyperactivity disorder. *Journal of Clinical Child and Adolescent Psychology*, *40*(4), 519–531. doi:10.1080/15374416.2011.581620 [doi]

McQuade, J. D., Vaughn, A. J., Hoza, B., Murray-Close, D., Molina, B. S., Arnold, L. E., & Hechtman, L. (2014). Perceived social acceptance and peer status differentially predict adjustment in youth with and without ADHD. *Journal of Attention Disorders*, *18*(1), 31–43. doi:10.1177/1087054712437582 [doi]

Molina, B. S., Flory, K., Hinshaw, S. P., Greiner, A. R., Arnold, L. E., Swanson, J. M., . . . Wigal, T. (2007). Delinquent behavior and emerging substance use in the MTA at 36 months: Prevalence, course, and treatment effects. *Journal of the American Academy of Child and Adolescent Psychiatry*, *46*(8), 1028–1040. doi:10.1097/chi.0b013e3180686d96 [doi]

Molina, B. S., Hinshaw, S. P., Eugene Arnold, L., Swanson, J. M., Pelham, W. E., Hechtman, L., . . . MTA Cooperative Group. (2013). Adolescent substance use in the multimodal treatment study of attention-deficit/hyperactivity disorder (ADHD) (MTA) as a function of childhood ADHD, random assignment to childhood treatments, and subsequent medication. *Journal of the American Academy of Child and Adolescent Psychiatry*, *52*(3), 250–263. doi:10.1016/j.jaac.2012.12.014 [doi]

Molina, B. S., Hinshaw, S. P., Swanson, J. M., Arnold, L. E., Vitiello, B., Jensen, P. S., . . . MTA Cooperative Group. (2009). The MTA at 8 years: Prospective follow-up of children treated for combined-type ADHD in a multisite study. *Journal of the American Academy of Child and Adolescent Psychiatry*, *48*(5), 484–500. doi:10.1097/CHI.0b013e31819c23d0 [doi]

Mrug, S., Hoza, B., Gerdes, A. C., Hinshaw, S., Arnold, L. E., Hechtman, L., & Pelham, W. E. (2009). Discriminating between children with ADHD and classmates using peer variables. *Journal of Attention Disorders*, *12*(4), 372–380. doi:10.1177/1087054708314602 [doi]

Mrug, S., Molina, B. S., Hoza, B., Gerdes, A. C., Hinshaw, S. P., Hechtman, L., & Arnold, L. E. (2012). Peer rejection and friendships in children with attention-deficit/hyperactivity disorder: Contributions to long-term outcomes. *Journal of Abnormal Child Psychology*, *40*(6), 1013–1026. doi:10.1007/s10802-012-9610-2 [doi]

MTA Cooperative Group. (2004a). National Institute of Mental Health multimodal treatment study of ADHD follow-up: 24-month outcomes of treatment strategies for attention-deficit/hyperactivity disorder. *Pediatrics*, *113*(4), 754–761.

MTA Cooperative Group. (2004b). National Institute of Mental Health multimodal treatment study of ADHD follow-up: Changes in effectiveness and growth after the end of treatment. *Pediatrics*, *113*(4), 762–769.

MTA Cooperative Group. (1999a). Moderators and mediators of treatment response for children with attention-deficit/hyperactivity disorder: The Multimodal Treatment Study of Children with Attention-Deficit/Hyperactivity Disorder. *Archives of General Psychiatry*, *56*(12), 1088–1096.

MTA Cooperative Group. (1999b). A 14-month randomized clinical trial of treatment strategies for attention-deficit/hyperactivity disorder. *Archives of General Psychiatry*, *56*(12), 1073–1086.

Murray, D. W., Arnold, L. E., Swanson, J., Wells, K., Burns, K., Jensen, P., . . . Strauss, T. (2008). A clinical review of outcomes of the Multimodal Treatment Study of Children with Attention-Deficit/Hyperactivity Disorder (MTA). *Current Psychiatry Reports*, *10*(5), 424–431.

Owens, E. B., & Hinshaw, S. P. (2013). Perinatal problems and psychiatric comorbidity among children with ADHD. *Journal of Clinical Child and Adolescent Psychology*, *42*(6), 762–768. doi:10.1080/15374416.2013.785359 [doi]

Owens, E. B., Hinshaw, S. P., Kraemer, H. C., Arnold, L. E., Abikoff, H. B., Cantwell, D. P., . . . Wigal, T. (2003). Which treatment for whom for ADHD? Moderators of treatment response in the MTA. *Journal of Consulting and Clinical Psychology*, *71*(3), 540–552.

Pappadopulos, E., Jensen, P. S., Chait, A. R., Arnold, L. E., Swanson, J. M., Greenhill, L. L., . . . Newcorn, J. H. (2009). Medication adherence in the MTA: Saliva methylphenidate samples versus parent report and mediating effect of concomitant behavioral treatment. *Journal of the American Academy of Child and Adolescent Psychiatry*, *48*(5), 501–510. doi:10.1097/CHI.0b013e31819c23ed [doi]

Pelham, W. E., Jr. (1999). The NIMH Multimodal Treatment Study for Attention-Deficit Hyperactivity Disorder: Just say yes to drugs alone? *Canadian Journal of Psychiatry. Revue Canadienne De Psychiatrie*, *44*(10), 981–990.

Richters, J. E., Arnold, L. E., Jensen, P. S., Abikoff, H., Conners, C. K., Greenhill, L. L., . . . Swanson, J. M. (1995). NIMH collaborative multisite multimodal treatment study of children with ADHD: I. background and rationale. *Journal of the American Academy of Child and Adolescent Psychiatry*, *34*(8), 987–1000. doi:S0890-8567(09)63342-6 [pii]

Sibley, M. H., Swanson, J. M., Arnold, L. E., Hechtman, L., Owens, E. B., Stehli, A., . . . Pelham, W. E. Defining ADHD symptom persistence in adulthood: Optimizing sensitivity and specificity. (2016). Manuscript submitted for publication.

Swanson, J., Arnold, L. E., Kraemer, H., Hechtman, L., Molina, B., Hinshaw, S., . . . MTA Cooperative Group. (2008a). Evidence, interpretation, and qualification from multiple reports of long-term outcomes in the Multimodal Treatment Study of Children with ADHD (MTA): Part I: Executive summary. *Journal of Attention Disorders*, *12*(1), 4–14. doi:10.1177/1087054708319345 [doi]

Swanson, J., Arnold, L. E., Kraemer, H., Hechtman, L., Molina, B., Hinshaw, S., . . . MTA Cooperative Group. (2008b). Evidence, interpretation, and qualification from multiple reports of long-term outcomes in the multimodal treatment study of children with ADHD (MTA): Part II: Supporting details. *Journal of Attention Disorders*, *12*(1), 15–43. doi:10.1177/1087054708319525 [doi]

Swanson, J. M., Arnold, L. E., Molina, B. S., Sibley, M. H., Hechtman, L., Hinshaw, S. P., . . . Arcos-Burgos, M. Prospective 16-year follow-up of the multimodal treatment study of ADHD: Effects of medication, maturation, and source on symptom severity in adulthood. (2016). Manuscript submitted for publication.

Swanson, J. M., Elliott, G. R., Greenhill, L. L., Wigal, T., Arnold, L. E., Vitiello, B., . . . Volkow, N. D. (2007). Effects of stimulant medication on growth rates across 3 years in the MTA follow-up. *Journal of the American Academy of Child and Adolescent Psychiatry*, *46*(8), 1015–1027. doi:10.1097/chi.0b013e3180686d7e [doi]

Swanson, J. M., Hinshaw, S. P., Arnold, L. E., Gibbons, R. D., Marcus, S., Hur, K., . . . Wigal, T. (2007). Secondary evaluations of MTA 36-month outcomes: Propensity score and growth mixture model analyses. *Journal of the American Academy of Child and Adolescent Psychiatry*, *46*(8), 1003–1014. doi:10.1097/CHI.0b013e3180686d63 [doi]

Tamm, L., Epstein, J. N., Lisdahl, K. M., Molina, B., Tapert, S., Hinshaw, S. P., . . . Swanson, J. M. (2013). Impact of ADHD and cannabis use on executive functioning in young adults. *Drug and Alcohol Dependence*, *133*(2), 607–614.

Vitiello, B., Severe, J. B., Greenhill, L. L., Arnold, L. E., Abikoff, H. B., Bukstein, O. G., . . . Cantwell, D. P. (2001). Methylphenidate dosage for children with ADHD over time under controlled conditions: Lessons from the MTA. *Journal of the American Academy of Child and Adolescent Psychiatry*, *40*(2), 188–196. doi:S0890-8567(09)60368-3 [pii]

Wells, K. C. (2001). Comprehensive versus matched psychosocial treatment in the MTA study: Conceptual and empirical issues. *Journal of Clinical Child Psychology*, *30*(1), 131–135. doi:10.1207/S15374424JCCP3001_16 [doi]

Wells, K. C., Pelham, W. E., Kotkin, R. A., Hoza, B., Abikoff, H. B., Abramowitz, A., . . . Schiller, E. (2000). Psychosocial treatment strategies in the MTA study: Rationale, methods, and critical issues in design and implementation. *Journal of Abnormal Child Psychology*, *28*(6), 483–505.

9

Influences of Treatment on Long-term Outcome

LILY HECHTMAN

It is difficult to evaluate the influence of treatment on long-term outcome in ADHD because such long-term controlled treatment studies do not exist. Such studies do not exist because they would not be feasible or ethical. One could not randomly assign participants to treatment (whether medication or psychosocial treatment) or no treatment for five to ten years. So we are left with uncontrolled naturalistic studies from which to draw conclusions.

Naturalistic follow-up studies are problematic, however, because the participants who continue to take medication are not randomly assigned but may be self-selected for a number of reasons, which can affect the interpretation of findings. These reasons can include greater severity of initial symptoms, greater and more serious comorbidities and adversities, lower IQ, and lower socioeconomic status (SES)—which may preclude other interventions and so only ongoing medication treatment is given. All these factors may, in fact, override any possible effects of medication treatment. Consequently, the effects of treatment will not be seen because they are overshadowed by all these other intervening factors, which are not controlled for, evaluated, or taken into account.

The first Montreal cohort of hyperactive children was recruited in the early 1960s, before stimulants were widely used in Canada, and so generally did not receive medication (stimulant) treatment. In the late 1960s and early 1970s, a second cohort was recruited (Hechtman, Weiss, & Perlman, 1984). This group of hyperactive children received three to five years of sustained stimulant treatment in childhood. Comparison of the two hyperactive cohorts in adulthood showed that the stimulant-treated group was slightly older (21.8 vs. 19.6 years). The two groups were similar, however, with respect to IQ and socioeconomic status. There were few differences between the stimulant-treated and untreated hyperactives. Out of over 40 variables analyzed, treated hyperactives fared better only in a few areas: fewer car accidents, seeing childhood more positively, stealing less in elementary school, and having better social skills and better self-esteem.

This suggests that stimulant treatment in childhood may result in a more positive childhood experience, which has an impact on social functioning and self-esteem, but because medication treatment was limited to three to five years during childhood, it failed to impact most areas of adolescent and adult functioning.

LIMITED DURATION OF TREATMENT

A second difficulty in evaluating the influence of treatment on long-term outcome relates to the fact that treatment duration is usually limited to interventions for varying periods of time; for example, from several weeks to three to five years during childhood. Generally, there is a quite significant decrease in treatment adherence or involvement with the advent of adolescence, with further decreases in adulthood.

Thus, the New York Study began as a short-term treatment study of hyperactive children, comparing the effects of methylphenidate and thioridazine (Gittelman-Klein, Klein, Katz, Saraf, & Pollack, 1976), and a controlled trial of behavior modification and methylphenidate (Gittelman et al., 1980). It then continued as a follow-up study without systematic treatment after childhood.

The Milwaukee Study also started as a study that explored the effect of stimulant treatment on mother–child interactions (Barkley, Karlsson, Pollard, & Murphy, 1985; Barkley, Karlsson, Strzelecki, & Murphy, 1984) in childhood, and then continued as a follow-up study into adolescence and adulthood. At the adult follow-up (mean age 27 years), only 7%–14% of adults with childhood ADHD were taking medication (Barkley, Murphy, & Fischer, 2008).

A similar picture is seen in both the Pittsburgh (Pelham & Hoza, 1996) and the Berkeley Girls Study (Hinshaw, 2002). Both recruited their study subjects from summer day-programs in childhood. At that time, 50% or more of the subjects were receiving stimulant medication. In the Pittsburgh study, this number decreased to only 23.9% at mean age 17 years (Kuriyan et al., 2014), decreased to 33% in the Berkeley Girls study in adolescence (Hinshaw, Owens, Sami, & Fargeon, 2006), and further decreased in adulthood.

In the Multisite Multimodal Treatment of Attention-Deficit/Hyperactivity Disorder Study (the MTA Study), medication treatment also decreased significantly in later childhood and adolescence and was slightly less than 10% in the ADHD group at the 10-year follow-up (Molina et al., 2013).

Thus, a very consistent picture emerges wherein treatment, usually stimulant medication treatment in childhood is of short duration, three to five years at most, and then decreases markedly in adolescence to about 10% of the ADHD group and continues to decline even further in adulthood.

Therefore, one cannot truly evaluate the impact of brief childhood medication treatment on long-term outcomes, given that it is unrealistic to expect treatment in childhood to have an effect on an ongoing chronic condition such as ADHD, which continues into adulthood.

Only one study, the Massachusetts study, reported that stimulant treatment in childhood affected young adult outcome at the 10-year follow-up. ADHD children treated with stimulants were significantly less likely to repeat a grade; to subsequently develop mood, anxiety, and disruptive disorders (Biederman, Monuteaux, Spencer, Wilens, & Faraone, 2009); and to develop substance abuse disorders (Biederman et al., 2008). It is unclear why the findings in the Massachusetts study differ from those of all the other prospective follow-up studies (e.g., New York, Milwaukee, Pittsburgh, the Berkeley Girls Study, and the Multisite Multimodal Treatment of ADHD study [MTA]).

DISCONTINUATION OF TREATMENT IN ADOLESCENCE

One might well ask why medication treatment is so often discontinued in adolescence. There are three possible major explanations for this discontinuation. The first pertains to the adolescent stage of development. During this stage, adolescents want to become autonomous and not be controlled by their parents; taking medication often becomes an issue on which they take a stance. Secondly, adolescents do not want to feel that they are different from their peers. Taking daily medication makes them feel different and so they resist it. Finally, adolescents want to feel free to experiment with drugs and alcohol and they have been warned against combining medication with these substances. All these reasons contribute to a precipitous drop in adolescents' adherence to medication treatment.

LIMITATIONS OF COMMUNITY MEDICATION TREATMENT

A second reason for a significant decline in medication adherence over time includes the many limitations of community medication treatment documented in the Multisite Multimodal Treatment of ADHD study (MTA) (MTA Cooperative Group, 1999). Participants in the MTA were randomly assigned to four different treatment strategies for a 14-month duration: medication, behavioral treatment, a combination of these, and community treatment. The community treatment group consistently performed worst on many outcomes despite the fact that 66% of this group received medication in the community. However, medication in the community was rarely titrated to optimal dose, school information was not obtained, there was no regular monitoring to adjust dose or deal with side effects, and follow-up occurred infrequently (e.g., once every six months or once per year). This inadequate medication treatment often resulted in medication being discontinued when the dose and/or side effects were problematic.

The positive effects of medication have been well documented in many short-term studies and were evident during the 14 months of intensive treatment in the MTA (MTA Cooperative Group, 1999). The impact of this treatment was still seen (though to a decreased degree) at 24-month follow-up (MTA Cooperative Group, 2004), though the effect was about half that documented at 14 months.

At three-year follow-up (Jensen et al., 2007), no effect of the initial 14 months of medication treatment could be found and all four initially randomized treatment groups had similar outcomes in many domains.

SUMMARY OF LONG-TERM IMPACT OF MEDICATION TREATMENT

It is difficult to evaluate the long-term impact of medication treatment on adult outcome given that randomized long-term medication studies do not exist because they are not feasible or ethical. Naturalistic nonrandomized studies may involve a self-selection bias that makes interpretation of results difficult.

There is a precipitous decline in medication adherence in adolescence, followed by further decreases in adulthood, with less than 10% continuing to take medication as adults. Generally, receiving medication in childhood does not seem to have an impact on adult outcomes.

ADHD is a chronic condition that continues into adulthood in about 50% of subjects and requires continued carefully titrated and monitored medication treatment for most of these individuals to affect adult functioning.

IMPACT OF PSYCHOSOCIAL TREATMENTS ON LONG-TERM ADULT OUTCOMES

It has long been recognized that medication alone cannot address all the difficulties experienced by patients with ADHD. Thus, other psychosocial interventions have been developed to address deficits in social skills (Pfiffner, Villodas, Kaiser, Rooney, & McBurnett, 2013; Pfiffner et al., 2007), anger management, and organizational, time management, and study skills (Gallagher, Abikoff, & Spira, 2014). Interventions are directed either directly to the child (individually or in a small group setting) or through the parents via parent-training programs. These interventions have shown short-term benefits suggested by improvements in these areas immediately following the intervention and in some cases even six months or one year later (Gallagher et al., 2014). However, long-term impact of these psychosocial interventions during childhood has not been documented. In fact, in the MTA (MTA Cooperative Group, 1999) the superiority of the combined (medication and behavioral) treatment group after 14 months of treatment was markedly reduced at 24 months (MTA Cooperative Group, 2004) and not at all present by the 3-year follow-up (Jensen et al., 2007). Thus, the impact of the psychosocial treatments does not endure, and does not seem to affect functioning in adolescence and adulthood. It may well be that the strategies taught are not continued to be implemented or do not generalize to new situations that arise. Here again ongoing, less intensive, booster sessions may be needed to foster the continued implementation of psychosocial treatments and their adaptation to new challenges with which the individual may need to cope.

The efficacy of cognitive behavioral therapy in adolescents (Antshel, Faraone, & Gordon, 2014) and adults (Safren et al., 2010; Solanto et al., 2010) clearly suggest the need and usefulness of the intervention in addition to medication. However, the long-term impact of these interventions has not been documented and ongoing booster sessions to ensure continued use and adoption of the intervention may be needed.

SUMMARY

Medication and/or psychosocial treatment in childhood do not appear to have an impact on adult outcomes of individuals with ADHD.

This lack of impact suggests that ADHD is a chronic condition that requires ongoing medication and psychosocial treatment.

There is a marked decline, however, in medication adherence in adolescence, which continues into adulthood, when less than 10% of adults with ADHD continue to use medication. Too often, psychosocial treatments do not continue to be used or adapted to new challenges. Thus, ongoing regular follow-up may be needed to offer patients interventions (medication and psychosocial treatment) that they require and can implement to ensure more positive long-term outcomes.

REFERENCES

Antshel, K. M., Faraone, S. V., & Gordon, M. (2014). Cognitive behavioral treatment outcomes in adolescent ADHD. *Journal of Attention Disorders, 18*(6), 483–495. doi:10.1177/1087054712443155

Barkley, R. A., Karlsson, J., Pollard, S., & Murphy, J. V. (1985). Developmental changes in the mother–child interactions of hyperactive boys: effects of two dose levels of Ritalin. *Journal of Child Psychology and Psychiatry, 26*(5), 705–715.

Barkley, R. A., Karlsson, J., Strzelecki, E., & Murphy, J. V. (1984). Effects of age and Ritalin dosage on the mother–child interactions of hyperactive children. *Journal of Consulting and Clinical Psychology, 52*(5), 750–758.

Barkley, R. A., Murphy, K. R., & Fischer, M. (2008). *ADHD in Adults: What the Science says.* New York: Guilford Press.

Biederman, J., Monuteaux, M. C., Spencer, T., Wilens, T. E., & Faraone, S. V. (2009). Do stimulants protect against psychiatric disorders in youth with ADHD? A 10-year follow-up study. *Pediatrics, 124*(1), 71–78. doi:10.1542/peds.2008-3347

Biederman, J., Monuteaux, M. C., Spencer, T., Wilens, T. E., Macpherson, H. A., & Faraone, S. V. (2008). Stimulant therapy and risk for subsequent substance use disorders in male adults with ADHD: a naturalistic controlled 10-year follow-up study. *American Journal of Psychiatry*, *165*(5), 597–603. doi:10.1176/appi.ajp.2007.07091486

Gallagher, R., Abikoff, H. B., & Spira, E. G. (2014). *Organizational Skills Training for Children with ADHD: An Empirically Supported Treatment*. New York: Guilford Press.

Gittelman-Klein, R., Klein, D. F., Katz, S., Saraf, K., & Pollack, E. (1976). Comparative effects of methylphenidate and thioridazine in hyperkinetic children. I. Clinical results. *Archives of General Psychiatry*, *33*(10), 1217–1231.

Gittelman, R., Abikoff, H., Pollack, E., Klein, D. F., Katz, S., & Mattes, J. A. (1980). A controlled trial of behavior modification and methylphenidate in hyperactive children. In *Hyperactive Children: The Social Ecology of Identification and Treatment* (pp. 221–243). Orlando, Florida: Academic Press, Inc.

Hechtman, L., Weiss, G., & Perlman, T. (1984). Young adult outcome of hyperactive children who received long-term stimulant treatment. *Journal of the American Academy of Child Psychiatry*, *23*(3), 261–269.

Hinshaw, S. P. (2002). Preadolescent girls with attention-deficit/hyperactivity disorder: I. Background characteristics, comorbidity, cognitive and social functioning, and parenting practices. *Journal of Consulting and Clinical Psychology*, *70*(5), 1086–1098.

Hinshaw, S. P., Owens, E. B., Sami, N., & Fargeon, S. (2006). Prospective follow-up of girls with attention-deficit/hyperactivity disorder into adolescence: Evidence for continuing cross-domain impairment. *Journal of Consulting and Clinical Psychology*, *74*(3), 489–499. doi:10.1037/0022-006X.74.3.489

Jensen, P. S., Arnold, L. E., Swanson, J. M., Vitiello, B., Abikoff, H. B., Greenhill, L. L., . . . Hur, K. (2007). 3-year follow-up of the NIMH MTA study. *Journal of the American Academy of Child and Adolescent Psychiatry*, *46*(8), 989–1002. doi:10.1097/CHI.0b013e3180686d48

Kuriyan, A. B., Pelham, W. E., Jr., Molina, B. S., Waschbusch, D. A., Sibley, M. H., & Gnagy, E. M. (2014). Concordance between parent and physician medication histories for children and adolescents with attention-deficit/hyperactivity disorder. *Journal of Child and Adolescent Psychopharmacology*, *24*(5), 269–274. doi:10.1089/cap.2013.0081

Molina, B. S., Hinshaw, S. P., Eugene Arnold, L., Swanson, J. M., Pelham, W. E., Hechtman, L., . . . MTA Collaborative Group. (2013). Adolescent substance use in the multimodal treatment study of attention-deficit/hyperactivity disorder (ADHD) (MTA) as a function of childhood ADHD, random assignment to childhood treatments, and subsequent medication. *Journal of the American Academy of Child and Adolescent Psychiatry*, *52*(3), 250–263. doi:10.1016/j.jaac.2012.12.014

MTA Cooperative Group. (1999). A 14-month randomized clinical trial of treatment strategies for attention-deficit/hyperactivity disorder. The MTA Cooperative Group. Multimodal Treatment Study of Children with ADHD. *Archives of General Psychiatry*, *56*(12), 1073–1086.

MTA Cooperative Group. (2004). National Institute of Mental Health Multimodal Treatment Study of ADHD follow-up: 24-month outcomes of treatment strategies for attention-deficit/hyperactivity disorder. *Pediatrics*, *113*(4), 754–761.

Pelham, W. E., & Hoza, B. (1996). Intensive treatment: A summer treatment program for children with ADHD. In E. D. Hibbs & P. S. Jensen (Eds.), *Psychosocial Treatments for Child and Adolescent Disorders: Empirically Based Strategies for Clinical Practice* (pp. 311–340). New York: American Psychological Association Press.

Pfiffner, L. J., Villodas, M., Kaiser, N., Rooney, M., & McBurnett, K. (2013). Educational outcomes of a collaborative school–home behavioral intervention for ADHD. *School Psychology Quarterly*, *28*(1), 25–36. doi:10.1037/spq0000016

Pfiffner, L. J., Yee Mikami, A., Huang-Pollock, C., Easterlin, B., Zalecki, C., & McBurnett, K. (2007). A randomized, controlled trial of integrated home–school behavioral treatment for ADHD, predominantly inattentive type. *Journal of the American Academy of Child and Adolescent Psychiatry*, *46*(8), 1041–1050. doi:10.1097/chi.0b013e318064675f

Safren, S. A., Sprich, S., Mimiaga, M. J., Surman, C., Knouse, L., Groves, M., & Otto, M. W. (2010). Cognitive behavioral therapy vs. relaxation with educational support for medication-treated adults with ADHD and persistent symptoms: a randomized controlled trial. *Journal of the American Medical Association: JAMA*, *304*(8), 875–880. doi:10.1001/jama.2010.1192

Solanto, M. V., Marks, D. J., Wasserstein, J., Mitchell, K., Abikoff, H., Alvir, J. M., & Kofman, M. D. (2010). Efficacy of meta-cognitive therapy for adult ADHD. *American Journal of Psychiatry*, *167*(8), 958–968. doi:10.1176/appi.ajp.2009.09081123

10

Summary

LILY HECHTMAN

This chapter will summarize the similarities and differences in key adult outcome areas of the various prospective follow-up studies of children with ADHD into adulthood. It also will attempt to identify important predictors of these adult outcomes, particularly where consensus among studies exists. Finally, areas of controversy, which remain unresolved, also will be highlighted.

SUMMARY OF ADULT OUTCOMES

Educational Domain

There is general agreement that as adults, participants with childhood ADHD have lower educational attainments (Weiss, Hechtman, Milroy, & Perlman, 1985) when compared with matched control subjects. They have more academic difficulties (Hinshaw, Owens, Sami, & Fargeon, 2006; Robb et al., 2011), need to repeat more grades, and drop out of school more often

(Barkley, Fischer, Smallish, & Fletcher, 2006). Thus, they have fewer years of education (Barkley, Murphy, & Fischer, 2008; Hinshaw et al., 2012) and are less likely to complete high school. For example, in the Milwaukee study (Barkley et al., 2008), at age 27 years, 62%–67% of the ADHD group had completed high school versus 99% of the control group. The ADHD group is thus also less likely to go on to university. In the Milwaukee study (Barkley et al., 2008), at age 27, 9%–20% had attended college compared with 68% of the control group. Numbers were slightly better for college attendance in the Pittsburgh study (Kuriyan et al., 2013) with 29.5% of the ADHD group pursuing a bachelor's degree compared with 76.8% in the control group.

However, many attending college do not actually receive a degree. So, in the Montreal study (Weiss & Hechtman, 1993) only 5% of the ADHD subjects earned a university degree compared with 41% of the control subjects. Figures were slightly better in the New York study, with 15.6% of ADHD subjects versus 34.6% of the controls obtaining a bachelor's degree and 3.7% of the ADHD group versus 29.4% of the controls attaining a master's degree (Klein et al., 2012).

The Multisite Multimodal Treatment of ADHD study showed that at mean age 25 years educational levels attained are affected by persistence of ADHD symptoms (Hechtman et al., submitted). Thus 8% of the ADHD symptom-persistent group obtained a bachelor's degree compared with 17.5% of the symptom-desistent group and 37.1% of the control group.

Thus, in the educational domain, subjects with ADHD are more likely to drop out of high school, not attain high school graduation, not enter university, and not complete a university degree than matched control subjects. Persistence of ADHD symptoms has an impact on this educational picture. These educational limitations affect future occupational and income opportunities.

Occupational and Income Domains

Given the lower educational attainment in the ADHD group, it is not surprising that as adults the ADHD subjects have lower occupational status as measured by the Hollingshead (1975) socioeconomic status scale (Barkley et al., 2008; Biederman et al., 2012; Klein et al., 2012; Weiss & Hechtman, 1993). As seen in the Pittsburgh study, 72.5% of the ADHD subjects have unskilled jobs compared with 36% of the control subjects (Kuriyan et al., 2013). The ADHD group, however, also is rated by employees as showing poorer workplace performance both in the tasks they are required to perform and in their relationships with coworkers and supervisors (Barkley et al., 2008; Klein et al., 2012; Weiss et al., 1985). The ADHD group is thus more likely to be fired, laid off, or quit their jobs compared with the control group (Barkley et al., 2008; Hechtman et al., submitted; Weiss & Hechtman, 1993). More time is spent by the ADHD group unemployed and not in school compared with the control group (Hechtman et al., submitted). In the Pittsburgh study (Kuriyan et al., 2013), 16.6% of the ADHD group compared with 2.4% of the control group were neither employed nor in school. Persistence of ADHD symptoms in adulthood is more likely to result in unemployment (Barkley et al., 2008; Hechtman et al., submitted). These employment problems result in lower incomes in the ADHD group compared with the control group (Klein et al., 2012) and in a greater likelihood to be on public assistance. In the MTA study, 22% of the ADHD symptom-persistent group, compared with 9.6% of the ADHD symptom-desistent group and 3.2% of the Local Normative Community Group were on public assistance (Hechtman et al., submitted).

Emotional Domain

There is general agreement that the ADHD group has more emotional problems in adulthood than the control group. Thus, the Montreal Study showed that 33% of the control subjects had no psychiatric symptoms and received no psychiatric diagnosis compared with 11% of the ADHD subjects (Weiss et al., 1985).

The exact nature of these emotional problems, however, differs in different studies. Thus, the Massachusetts study (Biederman, Faraone, Keenan, & Tsuang, 1991) always has reported high rates of anxiety and depression in their ADHD group compared with their control group. The

Montreal (Weiss & Hechtman, 1993), New York (Klein et al., 2012), and Milwaukee (Barkley et al., 2008) studies did not. The Pittsburgh study suggested increased depressive symptoms in adulthood, particularly if ADHD symptoms persisted (Bagwell, Molina, Kashdan, Pelham, & Hoza, 2006), and the MTA (Hechtman et al., submitted) also documented higher rates of mood (7.8% vs. 1.8%, *OR* = 4.5) and anxiety (14.2% vs. 5%, *OR* = 3.12) disorders in the ADHD symptom-persistent versus -desistent groups. The latter group was similar to the Local Normative Comparison Group.

The Berkeley Girls study (Hinshaw et al., 2006) also showed that different informants presented very different pictures of emotional functioning. Thus, via parent report, the ADHD group showed more externalizing, oppositional defiant, and conduct problems, as well as internalizing difficulties compared with the control group. By self-report, however, no differences in these areas were reported between the two groups.

The Berkeley Girls study (Hinshaw et al., 2012) highlighted the area of suicide attempts and nonsuicidal self-injury and distinguished between ADHD combined (ADHD-C) and inattentive (ADHD-I) subtypes. Suicide attempts occurred in 22% of the ADHD-C, 8% of the ADHD-I, and 6% of the control group, while nonsuicidal self-injury occurred in 50% of the ADHD-C, 29% of the ADHD-I, and 19% of the control group.

In the Montreal study (Weiss et al., 1985), there were six suicide attempts in the ADHD group versus zero in the control group.

Even though the numbers are relatively small, there is some concern about the higher rate of suicide in the ADHD group as compared with the control group. Specifically, there were three suicides in the New York study (Klein et al., 2012) in the ADHD group and none in the control group. Similarly in the MTA study (Hechtman et al., submitted), there were three suicides in the ADHD group and one in the control group. The combination of poor functioning, increased despondency, and greater substance abuse and impulsivity may all result in a lethal situation.

High rates of Bipolar I disorder are unique to the Massachusetts study (Biederman et al., 2006) and may reflect diagnostic criteria problems in the *Diagnostic and Statistical Manual of Mental Disorders–IV* (DSM-IV) for the Bipolar I diagnosis, which may have been addressed in DSM-5 with the introduction of the Severe Mood Dysregulation Disorder diagnosis.

In general, the ADHD group has more emotional problems than the control group, and this is particularly evident when the ADHD symptoms persist.

Antisocial Behavior

The rate of oppositional defiant and conduct disorder in children with ADHD is high. In some cases, but not all, this comorbidity contributes to antisocial personality disorder in adulthood. In the Montreal study (Weiss & Hechtman, 1993; Weiss et al., 1985), 23% of the ADHD group met criteria for the antisocial personality disorder diagnosis versus 2.4% of the control group. Similarly, in the New York study (Klein et al., 2012), 16% of the ADHD group met criteria for this diagnosis compared with 0% of the control group.

In the Milwaukee study (Barkley et al., 2008) most of the antisocial personality diagnosis occurred in the ADHD group with persistent symptoms (ADHD+H) at 38.9% versus the ADHD group without persistent symptoms (ADHD–H) at 16.5% versus the control group at 8%.

The delinquent acts documented in the Milwaukee study (Barkley et al., 2008) included breaking and entering, stealing, assault, carrying an illegal weapon, selling drugs, and disorderly conduct. An increased number of arrests, convictions, and incarcerations occurred in the ADHD group compared with the control group and this was particularly true for the ADHD+H where symptoms persisted, with 50% of that group experiencing arrests and incarcerations.

The New York study (Mannuzza, Klein, & Moulton, 2008) also documented more arrests, convictions, and incarcerations in the ADHD group versus the control group. Furthermore, the effects of antisocial personality disorder (ASP) and substance use disorder (SUD) were implicated in multiple arrests. The pattern of ASP disorder influenced substance abuse, which, in turn, resulted in arrests that were documented in 69% of the cases. Rates of multiple arrests in ADHD subjects were comparable to controls in the absence of ASP disorder or SUD.

In the Berkeley Girls study (Hinshaw et al., 2012), however, there were no differences in antisocial or delinquent behavior between the ADHD and control groups. However, the ADHD combined subgroup versus the inattentive subgroup had more externalizing disorders with conduct disorders.

Finally, in the MTA study (Hechtman et al., submitted), there were no differences in police involvement or jail time between the ADHD persistent, desistent, or non-ADHD control groups.

These differences in levels of antisocial behavior among the various studies may be a function of the particular location, subject composition (e.g., all girls), and time when the study was carried out, given that crime rates have declined significantly in recent years.

Substance Use

The picture regarding alcohol and other substance use disorders in adults with childhood ADHD versus controls differs among studies.

Alcohol Use

In the Montreal study (Hechtman & Weiss, 1986), the ADHD group reported more alcohol use compared with the control group. Similarly, increases in alcohol use in the ADHD group compared with the control group were reported in the Milwaukee study (Barkley et al., 2008). The Pittsburgh study (Molina et al., 2014) reported increased alcohol use disorder in the ADHD group, which also demonstrated antisocial personality disorder in addition to ADHD.

However, the New York study (Klein et al., 2012), the Berkeley Girls study (Hinshaw et al., 2012) and the MTA (Hechtman et al., submitted) all found no increased levels of alcohol use disorder in the ADHD group compared with the control group.

Non-alcoholic Substance Use

In the Montreal study (Hechtman & Weiss, 1986), more subjects in the ADHD group had stopped using drugs in the last three years. Similarly, the Massachusetts study (Biederman et al., 2012) reported higher rates of substance use disorder in the ADHD group versus the control group.

In the New York study (Klein et al., 2012), substance use disorder was three times more common in the ADHD versus the control group, particularly if the ADHD symptoms persisted. These researchers hypothesized a pattern in which the persistence of ADHD symptoms increased the prevalence of antisocial personality disorder, which, in turn, increased the rate of substance use disorder in the ADHD group.

The persistence of ADHD also was implicated in the MTA study (Hechtman et al., submitted) with regard to substance use disorder, with the ADHD symptom-persistent subgroup exhibiting increased marijuana and other substance use compared with the symptom-desistent and control groups, which were very similar in this regard.

Lifetime use of substances (marijuana), however, did not differ significantly between the ADHD versus the non-ADHD groups in the Pittsburgh study (Harty, Pedersen, Gnagy, Pelham, & Molina, 2015). In adolescence, however, 20% of the ADHD group had used other illicit substances (hallucinogens, inhalants) compared with 7% of the control group (Molina & Pelham, 2003).

The Berkeley Girls study (Hinshaw et al., 2012) also reported no differences between the ADHD and control groups with regard to any substance use disorder.

Even though the Milwaukee study reported increased misuse of prescription drugs (Barkley et al., 2008), no differences in the use of marijuana, cocaine, or speed were noted between the ADHD and control groups.

Increased cigarette smoking was noted in the ADHD versus the control group in a number of studies: Milwaukee (Barkley et al., 2008), Pittsburgh (Molina & Pelham, 2014) with an increase in conduct disorder, and in the Massachusetts study (Biederman et al., 2012).

It has been hypothesized by Biederman, Petty, Hammerness, Batchelder, and Faraone (2012) that cigarette smoking may constitute a gateway drug because it increases the rate of alcohol use, which, in turn, can lead to other substance use disorders.

The picture of alcohol and other substance use disorder in adults with ADHD varies; some studies show increases compared with controls and others report no differences. Again, studies vary in their location, nature of subjects (e.g., age, gender, comorbidity, persistence of ADHD), how the sample was recruited, and when they were evaluated. It is evident that persistence of ADHD, along with comorbidity with antisocial personality disorder or conduct disorder, exerts a strong influence on continued alcohol and substance use disorder in adulthood.

Risky Sexual Behavior

There is general consensus among the studies that have explored risky sexual behavior, such as Milwaukee (Barkley et al., 2008), Pittsburgh (Flory, Molina, Pelham, Gnagy, & Smith, 2006), and the MTA (Hechtman et al., submitted), that the ADHD group had earlier sexual intercourse, more sexual partners, used less contraception, had more teenage pregnancies and offspring, and more sexually transmitted diseases. In adulthood, the increase in sexually transmitted diseases in the combined ADHD group (15% vs. 7%) compared with the control group is possibly related to the increased number of sexual partners (Klein et al., 2012) particularly in the persistent ADHD group, and the larger number of offspring may be an outcome of the larger number of teenage pregnancies.

Risky Driving

The Montreal study reported an increased number of driving accidents in the ADHD group compared with the control group (Weiss & Hechtman, 1993).

The Milwaukee study (Barkley et al., 2008; Fischer, Barkley, Smallish, & Fletcher, 2007) also reported more car crashes, as well as more driving licenses suspended and revoked in the ADHD versus the control group. In addition, increased reckless driving and more driving infractions were documented in the ADHD group where symptoms persisted in adulthood.

The New York study (Ramos Olazagasti et al., 2013) and the Pittsburgh study (Thompson, Molina, Pelham, & Gnagy, 2007) linked risky driving (increased driving infractions) and at-fault driving accidents to coexisting conduct disorder and antisocial personality disorder, suggesting these disorders and not ADHD accounted for these difficulties.

By contrast, the Berkeley Girls study did not document any increases in risky driving behavior in the ADHD versus the control groups (Hinshaw et al., 2012).

Social Functioning

Problems in social relationships in adults with ADHD have been documented in a number of studies. The Montreal study (Weiss & Hechtman, 1993) showed that the ADHD group had more social problems at work and in their personal lives. The New York study (Klein et al., 2012) also showed social problems in adulthood with 31.1% of the ADHD group versus 11.8% of the control group having been divorced. The Pittsburgh study also documented social problems, such as few friends, negative friends influencing SUD and delinquency, and intimate partner impairment, with physical and verbal aggression (Wymbs et al., 2012).

If ADHD symptoms improve, some of the social difficulties appear to diminish. However, work, financial, alcohol and substance abuse problems, and risky sexual and driving behavior can all have a significantly negative impact on social functioning.

Finances and Money Management

Only the Milwaukee study (Barkley et al., 2008) explored money management in the ADHD versus control groups in detail. The study found that the ADHD group with persistent ADHD symptoms (ADHD+H) had the most financial difficulties compared with the control group, with the ADHD symptom-desistent group between the two. The ADHD+H group was more likely to buy on impulse, miss required rent or car payments, have no savings, have poor credit rating, and were more likely to have to declare bankruptcy. Increased gambling also was documented in this group, but this was thought to be related to antisocial personality disorder versus ADHD.

Physical Health

Only two studies, New York (Klein et al., 2012) and Milwaukee (Barkley et al., 2008), explored physical health in detail. Interestingly, both found obesity to be a greater problem in the ADHD group than in the control group. The figures were very comparable. In the New York study (Cortese, Ramos Olazagasti et al., 2013), 41% of the ADHD group and 21% of the control group were judged to be obese via body mass index scores. In the Milwaukee study (Barkley et al., 2008), 40% of the ADHD group and 20% of the control group were judged to be obese.

The New York study (Klein et al., 2012) also showed that the ADHD group had more emergency room visits (31% vs. 21%) and more head injuries (9% vs. 3%) compared with the control group (Ramos Olazagasti et al., 2013).

The Milwaukee study (Barkley et al., 2008) showed that the ADHD group was more likely to be hospitalized for serious injury (60%–69%) and accidental poisoning (11%–14%) compared with the control group (42% and 3%, respectively). The physical health of family members was also worse, particularly in the ADHD group with persistent ADHD compared with the ADHD desistent and control groups.

Given the increased unemployment, poorer financial circumstances, increased alcohol and substance abuse, increased risky sexual and driving behavior, and increased rates of divorce, it is not surprising that subjects with ADHD would have more physical health problems, as evidenced by more emergency room visits and hospitalizations, than subjects without ADHD.

All these problems undoubtedly contribute to a larger number of suicide attempts and deaths in the ADHD group. The New York study (Klein et al., 2012) documented a 7% death rate in the ADHD group compared with a 3% rate in the control group. The MTA (Hechtman et al., submitted) likewise found that the ADHD group had ten deaths compared with one in the control group.

CONTROVERSIES AND DISCREPANCIES IN OUTCOME FINDINGS

Bipolar Disorder

A remaining discrepancy and controversy concerns the high rate of Bipolar I disorder in the Massachusetts study (Biederman, Petty et al., 2009) compared with the other studies. This may be a function of subject recruitment at that particular site or a problem with DSM-IV diagnostic criteria for Bipolar disorder in children and adolescents. The introduction of the Severe Mood Dysregulation disorder diagnosis in DSM-5 may clarify this issue, however, because some of the patients previously diagnosed with Bipolar I disorder in the Massachusetts study may well receive the Severe Mood Dysregulation disorder diagnosis instead.

Similarities versus Differences in Outcomes between Girls and Boys with Attention Deficit Hyperactivity Disorder

The Massachusetts study (Biederman et al., 2012), which initially consisted of 140 boys and 140 girls with ADHD, and 120 boys and 122 girls without ADHD, was in a position to explore potential differences between girls and boys in adult outcomes. The Massachusetts study revealed no such gender differences in outcome.

One repeatedly saw, however, that the Berkeley Girls study (Hinshaw et al., 2012) differed from the other prospective follow-up studies with mainly male populations on types of comorbidities, increased suicidality, and increased self-injurious behavior, with no increases in delinquency, alcohol or substance use disorder, or driving risks. Thus, the outcomes in adulthood seen in the Berkeley Girls study were different, both from the Massachusetts study and the other prospective follow-up studies.

One possible reason is that a portion of the Berkeley Girls sample consisted of girls with the inattentive subtype and this may have influenced results. Many of these differences, however, also were noted for girls with the ADHD combined subtype.

The reasons for the differences in the outcomes of girls in the two studies remain unclear and need further exploration.

PREDICTORS OF OUTCOME

Persistence of Attention Deficit Hyperactivity Disorder Symptoms

The persistence of ADHD symptoms into adulthood is one of the most important predictors of adult outcome. In almost all of the studies, persistence of ADHD symptoms was associated with negative educational, occupational, emotional, psychiatric, social, alcohol use, and substance use disorder outcomes as well as increased risky driving, sexual, and criminal behavior.

The Massachusetts study (Biederman, Petty, Evans, Small, & Faraone, 2010) tried to identify factors that may predict persistence of ADHD. These factors included:

(a) Comorbidities such as Disruptive Behavior Disorder, Oppositional Defiant Disorder, Conduct Disorder, Mood and Anxiety Disorder
(b) Familial ADHD, particularly parental ADHD

(c) Psychosocial adversity, such as poverty, abuse, neglect
(d) Neuroimaging abnormalities in the default network, posterior cingulate cortex, and medial prefrontal cortex (Mattfeld et al., 2014).

Neuroimaging abnormalities also were found in the New York study (Cortese, Imperati et al., 2013; Proal et al., 2011). Cortese et al. (2013) explored structural brain connectivity via fractional anisotropy (FA), an index related to white matter structural properties. The ADHD group showed decreased FA compared with controls in tracts involving high-level as well as sensorimotor functions. There were no differences between ADHD persisters and remitters. With regard to gray matter, Proal et al. (2011) found that the cortex was thinner in the ADHD group than in the comparison group in the dorsal attentional network, limbic area, right caudate, right thalamus, and bilateral cerebellar hemispheres. Thus, areas implicated in the top-down control of attention, emotion regulation, and motivation appeared most affected. There was some suggestion that individuals with remitted ADHD had thicker cortex compared with those with persistent ADHD in the medial occipital cortex, insula, and parahippocampal, and prefrontal regions. This suggests compensatory maturation of prefrontal, cerebellar, and thalamic circuits.

Comorbidity—Oppositional Defiant Disorder, Conduct Disorder, and Antisocial Personality Disorder

Many children with Oppositional Defiant Disorder (ODD) do not progress to Conduct Disorder (CD) and many with CD do not develop Antisocial Personality Disorder (ASPD). However, the combination of ODD/CD in childhood and in the adolescence of children with ADHD has a negative impact on adolescent and adult outcome. It increases the likelihood of developing antisocial personality disorder and negatively affects educational, occupational, and social outcomes, increasing risk for alcohol use and SUD, as well as delinquency and risky sexual and driving behavior. It also appears to increase suicidal attempts and self-injurious behavior in girls with ADHD.

IQ and Cognitive Functioning

It appears that IQ and cognitive executive functioning predict academic/educational achievement and work performance. They also influence social and overall global functioning. Problems with response inhibition also have been associated with increased suicidal ideation, suicidal attempts, and nonsuicidal self-injuries in the Berkeley Girls study (Rinsky & Hinshaw, 2011).

Parents and Parenting Practices

Parental mental health (Roy et al., submitted), in particular parental ADHD, may have an impact on persistence of ADHD in offspring (Biederman et al., 2010) and on academic performance in children (Langberg et al., 2011). Poorer parental education also has been associated with decreased high school performance in the ADHD child (Kent et al., 2011). Parenting practices, particularly lack of appropriate supervision and limit setting, have been linked to increased levels of CD and SUD in children with ADHD (Walther et al., 2012) and the persistence of ADHD symptoms (Roy et al., submitted).

Stimulant Treatment

As outlined in the treatment chapter, most studies do not document either positive or negative effects of childhood stimulant treatment on adult outcome. The Montreal study (Hechtman, Weiss, & Perlman, 1984) suggested that stimulant treatment in childhood may improve self-esteem and social skills in adulthood.

The Milwaukee study (Barkley, Fischer, Smallish, & Fletcher, 2003) found that subjects with ADHD who received no stimulant treatment had higher rates of speed and prescription drug use, so some protection may be experienced from that treatment.

Only the Massachusetts study (Biederman, Monuteaux, Spencer, Wilens, & Faraone, 2009; Biederman et al., 2008) suggested that treatment with stimulants in childhood resulted in better adolescent and adult outcome with fewer repeated grades; less mood, anxiety, and disruptive behavior disorders; reduced SUD; and decreased risk of smoking.

Social Functioning

Social impairment in childhood and adolescence predicts adult social impairment. Furthermore, the Pittsburgh study (Molina et al., 2014) has clearly shown that social impairment often leads to association with peers who use and approve of drug use, resulting in increased drug and alcohol use.

Extreme social impairment, however, results in very few social contacts and less access to substances and, consequently, less use. Poor peer relationships in childhood and adolescence also may increase anxiety and depression (Bagwell et al., 2006). Childhood peer rejection also may result in adolescent academic problems, low achievement, school suspensions, and adolescent peer rejection (Hinshaw et al., 2006).

Stressful Life Events

The Pittsburgh study (Marshal, Molina, Pelham, & Cheong, 2007) documented that subjects with ADHD experience more controllable and uncontrollable stressful life events. These can include increased family stress (via parental alcoholism) and increased school stresses. Coupled with fewer coping skills, these result in increased alcohol or substance use in the patient with ADHD.

In the Berkeley Girls study (Guendelman, Owens, Galan, Gard, & Hinshaw, 2016) childhood maltreatment produced increased suicide attempts, internalizing disorders, eating disorders, and decreased sense of self-worth.

Psychosocial adversity, which can include stressful life events, was also a factor identified in the Massachusetts study (Biederman et al., 2010), which predicted the persistence of ADHD and the multiple negative outcomes associated with such persistence.

Socioeconomic Status and Race

Generally speaking, socioeconomic status (SES) and race did not appear to predict long-term outcome. Most studies did not have an equally distributed range of SES participants or significant racial diversity. With few exceptions, most participants were White and middle class. This was true for the Montreal, New York, Milwaukee, and Massachusetts studies. The MTA was perhaps the most socioeconomically and ethnically diverse, but these factors did not significantly impact adult outcome.

SUMMARY

Outcomes in adults with ADHD are not uniform. They vary and generally can be described as falling into three groups. Those who have fairly normal outcome, which does not differ from matched normal controls (about 30%) (Weiss & Hechtman, 1993). Those who continue to have significant symptoms of the syndrome with impaired functioning in academic, occupational, social, and emotional domains (50% of the group). Finally, a small subgroup, about 10% to 20%, who have significant negative outcome with poor educational attainment, poor work history, marked unemployment, significant alcohol/substance use disorder, and important psychiatric antisocial symptoms.

Persistence of ADHD, along with comorbid ODD/CD/ASPD, influences the negative outcome in this last group. Underlying problems in brain development also may influence this negative outcome (Cortese, Imperati et al., 2013; Mattfeld et al., 2014; Proal et al., 2011).

Given that ADHD is a chronic condition that continues into adulthood, treatment (involving both medication and psychosocial treatments) needs to address both ADHD and comorbid conditions and needs to continue ongoingly with varying intensity and careful follow-up. Only with such an approach can we hope to provide better adult outcomes for our patients with ADHD.

REFERENCES

Bagwell, C. L., Molina, B. S. G., Kashdan, T. B., Pelham, W. E., & Hoza, B. (2006). Anxiety and mood disorders in adolescents with childhood attention-deficit/hyperactivity disorder. *Journal of Emotional and Behavioral Disorders, 14*(3), 178–187. doi:10.1177/10634266060140030501

Barkley, R. A., Fischer, M., Smallish, L., & Fletcher, K. (2003). Does the treatment of attention-deficit/hyperactivity disorder with stimulants contribute to drug use/abuse? A 13-year prospective study. *Pediatrics, 111*(1), 97–109.

Barkley, R. A., Fischer, M., Smallish, L., & Fletcher, K. (2006). Young adult outcome of hyperactive children: adaptive functioning in major life activities. *Journal of the American Academy of Child and Adolescent Psychiatry, 45*(2), 192–202. doi:10.1097/01.chi.0000189134.97436.e2

Barkley, R. A., Murphy, K. R., & Fischer, M. (2008). *ADHD in Adults: What the Science Says*. New York: Guilford Press.

Biederman, J., Faraone, S. V., Keenan, K., & Tsuang, M. T. (1991). Evidence of familial association between attention deficit disorder and major affective disorders. *Archives of General Psychiatry, 48*(7), 633–642.

Biederman, J., Monuteaux, M. C., Mick, E., Spencer, T., Wilens, T. E., Silva, J. M., . . . Faraone, S. V. (2006). Young adult outcome of attention deficit hyperactivity disorder: a controlled 10-year follow-up study. *Psychological Medicine, 36*(2), 167–179. doi:10.1017/S0033291705006410

Biederman, J., Monuteaux, M. C., Spencer, T., Wilens, T. E., & Faraone, S. V. (2009). Do stimulants protect against psychiatric disorders in youth with ADHD? A 10-year follow-up study. *Pediatrics, 124*(1), 71–78. doi:10.1542/peds.2008-3347

Biederman, J., Monuteaux, M. C., Spencer, T., Wilens, T. E., Macpherson, H. A., & Faraone, S. V. (2008). Stimulant therapy and risk for subsequent substance use disorders in male adults with ADHD: a naturalistic controlled 10-year follow-up study. *American Journal of Psychiatry, 165*(5), 597–603. doi:10.1176/appi.ajp.2007.07091486

Biederman, J., Petty, C. R., Byrne, D., Wong, P., Wozniak, J., & Faraone, S. V. (2009). Risk for switch from unipolar to bipolar disorder in youth with ADHD: a long term prospective controlled study. *Journal of Affective Disorders, 119*(1-3), 16–21. doi:10.1016/j.jad.2009.02.024

Biederman, J., Petty, C. R., Evans, M., Small, J., & Faraone, S. V. (2010). How persistent is ADHD? A controlled 10-year follow-up study of boys with ADHD. *Psychiatry Research, 177*(3), 299–304. doi:10.1016/j.psychres.2009.12.010

Biederman, J., Petty, C. R., Woodworth, K. Y., Lomedico, A., Hyder, L. L., & Faraone, S. V. (2012). Adult outcome of attention-deficit/hyperactivity disorder: a controlled 16-year follow-up study. *Journal of Clinical Psychiatry, 73*(7), 941–950. doi:10.4088/JCP.11m07529

Cortese, S., Imperati, D., Zhou, J., Proal, E., Klein, R. G., Mannuzza, S., . . . Castellanos, F. X. (2013). White matter alterations at 33-year follow-up in adults with childhood attention-deficit/hyperactivity disorder. *Biological Psychiatry, 74*(8), 591–598. doi:10.1016/j.biopsych.2013.02.025

Cortese, S., Ramos Olazagasti, M. A., Klein, R. G., Castellanos, F. X., Proal, E., & Mannuzza, S. (2013). Obesity in men with childhood ADHD: a 33-year controlled, prospective, follow-up study. *Pediatrics, 131*(6), e1731–e1738. doi:10.1542/peds.2012-0540

Fischer, M., Barkley, R. A., Smallish, L., & Fletcher, K. (2007). Hyperactive children as young adults: driving abilities, safe driving behavior, and adverse driving outcomes. *Accident; Analysis and Prevention, 39*(1), 94–105. doi:10.1016/j.aap.2006.06.008

Flory, K., Molina, B. S., Pelham, W. E., Jr., Gnagy, E., & Smith, B. (2006). Childhood ADHD predicts risky sexual behavior in young adulthood. *Journal of Clinical Child and Adolescent Psychology, 35*(4), 571–577. doi:10.1207/s15374424jccp3504_8

Guendelman, M. D., Owens, E. B., Galan, C., Gard, A., & Hinshaw, S. P. (2016). Early-adult correlates of maltreatment in girls with attention-deficit/hyperactivity disorder: Increased risk for internalizing symptoms and suicidality. *Development and Psychopathology, 28*(1), 1–14. doi:10.1017/S0954579414001485

Harty, S. C., Pedersen, S. L., Gnagy, E. M., Pelham, W. E., & Molina, B. S. G. (2015). ADHD and marijuana-use expectancies in young adulthood. *Substance Use & Misuse, 50*(11), 1470–1478. doi:10.3109/10826084.2015.1018545

Hechtman, L., Swanson, J. M., Sibley, M. H., Stehli, A., Owens, E. B., Mitchell, J. T., . . . Nichols, J. Q. Functional adult outcomes 16 years after childhood diagnosis of attention-deficit/hyperactivity disorder: MTA results. Manuscript submitted for publication.

Hechtman, L., & Weiss, G. (1986). Controlled prospective fifteen year follow-up of hyperactives as adults: non-medical drug and alcohol use and anti-social behaviour. *Canadian Journal of Psychiatry, 31*(6), 557–567.

Hechtman, L., Weiss, G., & Perlman, T. (1984). Young adult outcome of hyperactive children who received long-term stimulant treatment. *Journal of the American Academy of Child Psychiatry, 23*(3), 261–269.

Hinshaw, S. P., Owens, E. B., Sami, N., & Fargeon, S. (2006). Prospective follow-up of girls with attention-deficit/hyperactivity disorder into adolescence: Evidence for continuing cross-domain impairment. *Journal of Consulting and Clinical Psychology, 74*(3), 489–499. doi:10.1037/0022-006X.74.3.489

Hinshaw, S. P., Owens, E. B., Zalecki, C., Huggins, S. P., Montenegro-Nevado, A. J., Schrodek, E., & Swanson, E. N. (2012). Prospective follow-up of girls with attention-deficit/hyperactivity disorder into early adulthood: continuing impairment includes elevated risk for suicide attempts and self-injury. *Journal of Consulting and Clinical Psychology, 80*(6), 1041–1051. doi:10.1037/a0029451

Kent, K. M., Pelham, W. E., Jr., Molina, B. S., Sibley, M. H., Waschbusch, D. A., Yu, J., . . . Karch, K. M. (2011). The academic experience of male high school students with ADHD. *Journal of Abnormal Child Psychology, 39*(3), 451–462. doi:10.1007/s10802-010-9472-4

Klein, R. G., Mannuzza, S., Olazagasti, M. A. R., Roizen, E., Hutchison, J. A., Lashua, E. C., & Castellanos, F. X. (2012). Clinical and functional outcome of childhood attention-deficit/hyperactivity disorder 33 years later. *Archives of General Psychiatry, 69*(12), 1295–1303. doi:10.1001/archgenpsychiatry.2012.271

Kuriyan, A. B., Pelham, W. E., Jr., Molina, B. S., Waschbusch, D. A., Gnagy, E. M., Sibley, M. H., . . . Kent, K. M. (2013). Young adult educational and vocational outcomes of children diagnosed with ADHD. *Journal of Abnormal Child Psychology, 41*(1), 27–41. doi:10.1007/s10802-012-9658-z

Langberg, J. M., Molina, B. S., Arnold, L. E., Epstein, J. N., Altaye, M., Hinshaw, S. P., . . . Hechtman, L. (2011). Patterns and predictors of adolescent academic achievement and performance in a sample of children with attention-deficit/hyperactivity disorder. *Journal of Clinical Child and Adolescent Psychology, 40*(4), 519–531. doi:10.1080/15374416.2011.581620

Mannuzza, S., Klein, R. G., & Moulton, J. L. (2008). Lifetime criminality among boys with attention deficit hyperactivity disorder: a prospective follow-up study into adulthood using official arrest records. *Psychiatry Research, 160*(3), 237–246. doi:10.1016/j.psychres.2007.11.003

Marshal, M. P., Molina, B. S., Pelham, W. E., & Cheong, J. (2007). Attention-deficit hyperactivity disorder moderates the life stress pathway to alcohol problems in children of alcoholics. *Alcoholism, Clinical and Experimental Research, 31*(4), 564–574. doi:10.1111/j.1530-0277.2007.00340.x

Mattfeld, A. T., Gabrieli, J. D., Biederman, J., Spencer, T., Brown, A., Kotte, A., . . . Whitfield-Gabrieli, S. (2014). Brain differences between persistent and remitted attention deficit hyperactivity disorder. *Brain, 137*(Pt 9), 24232428. doi:10.1093/brain/awu137

Molina, B. S., & Pelham, W. E., Jr. (2003). Childhood predictors of adolescent substance use in a longitudinal study of children with ADHD. *Journal of Abnormal Psychology, 112*(3), 497–507.

Molina, B. S., & Pelham, W. E., Jr. (2014). Attention-deficit/hyperactivity disorder and risk of substance use disorder: developmental considerations, potential pathways, and opportunities for research. *Annual Review of Clinical Psychology, 10*, 607–639. doi:10.1146/annurev-clinpsy-032813-153722

Molina, B. S., Walther, C. A., Cheong, J., Pedersen, S. L., Gnagy, E. M., & Pelham, W. E. (2014). Heavy alcohol use in early adulthood as a function of childhood ADHD: developmentally specific mediation by social impairment and delinquency. *Experimental and Clinical Psychopharmacology*, *22*(2), 110–121. doi:10.1037/a0035656

Proal, E., Reiss, P. T., Klein, R. G., Mannuzza, S., Gotimer, K., Ramos-Olazagasti, M. A., . . . Castellanos, F. X. (2011). Brain gray matter deficits at 33-year follow-up in adults with attention-deficit/hyperactivity disorder established in childhood. *Archives of General Psychiatry*, *68*(11), 1122–1134. doi:10.1001/archgenpsychiatry.2011.117

Ramos Olazagasti, M. A., Klein, R. G., Mannuzza, S., Belsky, E. R., Hutchison, J. A., Lashua-Shriftman, E. C., & Castellanos, F. X. (2013). Does childhood attention-deficit/hyperactivity disorder predict risk-taking and medical illnesses in adulthood? *Journal of the American Academy of Child and Adolescent Psychiatry*, *52*(2), 153–162. e154. doi:10.1016/j.jaac.2012.11.012

Rinsky, J. R., & Hinshaw, S. P. (2011). Linkages between childhood executive functioning and adolescent social functioning and psychopathology in girls with ADHD. *Child Neuropsychology*, *17*(4), 368–390. doi:10.1080/09297049.2010.544649

Robb, J. A., Sibley, M. H., Pelham, W. E., Jr., Foster, E. M., Molina, B. S., Gnagy, E. M., & Kuriyan, A. B. (2011). The estimated annual cost of ADHD to the U.S. education system. *School Mental Health*, *3*(3), 169–177. doi:10.1007/s12310-011-9057-6

Roy, A., Hechtman, L., Arnold, L. E., Swanson, J. M., Sibley, M. H., Molina, B. S. G., & Howard, A. (Submitted). Childhood factors affecting persistence and desistence of ADHD in adulthood: results from the MTA. Manuscript submitted for publication.

Thompson, A. L., Molina, B. S., Pelham, W., Jr., & Gnagy, E. M. (2007). Risky driving in adolescents and young adults with childhood ADHD. *Journal of Pediatric Psychology*, *32*(7), 745–759. doi:10.1093/jpepsy/jsm002

Walther, C. A., Cheong, J., Molina, B. S., Pelham, W. E., Jr., Wymbs, B. T., Belendiuk, K. A., & Pedersen, S. L. (2012). Substance use and delinquency among adolescents with childhood ADHD: the protective role of parenting. *Psychology of Addictive Behaviors*, *26*(3), 585–598. doi:10.1037/a0026818

Weiss, G., & Hechtman, L. (1993). *Hyperactive Children Grown Up: ADHD in Children, Adolescents, and Adults* (2nd ed.). New York: Guilford Press.

Weiss, G., Hechtman, L., Milroy, T., & Perlman, T. (1985). Psychiatric status of hyperactives as adults: a controlled prospective 15-year follow-up of 63 hyperactive children. *Journal of the American Academy of Child Psychiatry*, *24*(2), 211–220.

Wymbs, B., Molina, B., Pelham, W., Cheong, J., Gnagy, E., Belendiuk, K., . . . Waschbusch, D. (2012). Risk of intimate partner violence among young adult males with childhood ADHD. *Journal of Attention Disorders*, *16*(5), 373–383. doi:10.1177/1087054710389987

INDEX